Herpes Zoster and Postherpetic Neuralgia,
2nd Revised and Enlarged Edition

Pain Research and Clinical Management

Pain Research and Clinical Management

Volume 11

Herpes Zoster and Postherpetic Neuralgia, 2nd Revised and Enlarged Edition

Edited by

C. Peter N. Watson
Department of Medicine, University of Toronto and 1 Sir Williams Lane, Toronto, ON M9A 1T8, Canada

Anne A. Gershon
Division of Pediatric Infectious Diseases, Columbia University College of Physicians and Surgeons, 650 West 168th Street (BB 4-427), New York, NY 10032, USA

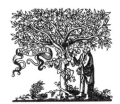

2001
ELSEVIER
AMSTERDAM • LAUSANNE • NEW YORK • OXFORD • SHANNON • SINGAPORE • TOKYO

First edition 1993
Second revised and enlarged edition 2001

Library of Congress Cataloging in Publications Data
A catalog record from the Library of Congress has been applied for.

ISBN: 0-444-50679-9 (hardbound)
ISBN: 0-444-50681-0 (paperback)
ISBN: 0921-3287 (series)

∞ Printed on acid free paper.

Printed in the United States of America.
10 9 8 7 6 5 4 3

Dedication

to Edgar Hope-Simpson

" If [we] have seen further, it is by standing
on the shoulders of giants"

Sir Isaac Newton, 1675

Shingles,

by Susan Telling (patient–poet)

Oh skin
so pale and thin –
who would guess what's hidden in –
So nicely healed
you conceal
a multitude of spikes and nails.
How you have failed
what you cover up so well.

Oh sly skin –
you fox, you sin.
Wretched liar –
scars and fire
grabbing me from sleep at night
lightning bolts, stabbing strikes,
and always more to come –
you're never done.
Unnerving snake, cleaving thing
unending fate, seething sting –

Oh fallen skin
you betrayed –
sores are gone
flames stayed.

Oh skin –
Oh Judas organ,
nerves within.
Your domain
my shingled body –
All my pain.

Acknowledgements

This book would not have been possible without Judy, Emily, Simon, Dorothy Barnes, Verna and Robert Watt. Angela Baird was indispensible in not only typing my manuscripts but advising and editing as well.

Preface to the Second Edition

A new edition of this book is surely welcome since so much new information has appeared since the first edition in 1993. And yet, the challenge remains urgent and acute since we remain largely unable to prevent or treat the disease in spite of the promise of the new knowledge. The challenge is tempting because of the two long latent periods between the first signal that trouble is on its way and the appearance of the disease. I will be reading this book with great anticipation to learn how the subject progresses.

The first latent period may last over seventy years between the original attack of chickenpox and the onset of zoster. It has been known since 1983 that particles of the varicella virus hibernate in dorsal root and trigeminal ganglia (Gilden et al., 1983; Hyman et al., 1983). We still need to know which type of nerve cell is the host and to be quite sure that non-neuronal cells are not alternative sites. The latent period ends with the massive reactivation of the latent virus. Even if the new attenuated virus vaccine for children were to eliminate the virus completely, our successors would still be treating herpes zoster in the 22nd century unless reactivation can be prevented. The present best hope for the prevention of reactivation lies in an understanding of the immune system. The evidence for that lies in the striking increase of herpes zoster with age coupled with its appearance in patients with immune suppression or with immune deficiency. The problem is by no means simple because these patients develop the localised condition of herpes zoster and do not have a recurrence of widespread chickenpox showing that they must retain a generalised immunity to varicella. In spite of this, trials of a vaccine to boost immunity in middle age are already under way (Levin et al., 1998). Trials of this type will require very long range planning and the patience of Job and will be a statistical nightmare.

The second latent period begins with the explosive reactivation of the virus and proceeds until sufficient damage has been done to produce the permanent state of postherpetic neuralgia. I will be discussing in my own chapter on pain what those changes might be. Since we do not know for certain the stage at which the changes become irreversible, we do not know which stage is essential for the development of the chronic state. Obviously the acute pain usually starts long before the herpes zoster presumably due to direct irritation of the sensory cells before the virus particles have been transported from the dorsal root ganglion cell to the periphery and into the skin where the shingles appears. Herpes zoster is an epidermal disease without an equivalent in muscle or viscera which may point to the cutaneous nerve cells as the crucial vector. It is not known if the pain only period is sufficient to produce enough damage to prolong into postherpetic neuralgia. The recognition of zoster sine herpete obviously presents a great diagnostic challenge but has become convincing where the virus is identified (Goon et al., 2000). The acute viral infection clearly spreads within the ganglion and even this route is not obvious. For example herpes zoster of the first division of the trigeminal nerve is common and yet a histological examination of the Gasserian ganglion does not reveal any obvious barrier to localise spread in only one division of the ganglion. Chapters in this book will discuss the undoubted occasional serious penetration of the acute infection into central structures but it is not clear if this plays a role in the eventual chronic state (Gilden et al., 2000). Zoster can be associated with motor signs but it is not clear if this represents a direct extension of viral infection or is secondary to inflammatory and vascular involvement.

The most contentious question covered by several chapters is whether the vigorous treatment of the acute phase of herpes zoster influences the later development of postherpetic neuralgia. A clear answer to this question is crucial in the understanding of mechanisms. Treatment to relieve or shorten the patients' period of acute discomfort may be fully justified but I look forward to reading statistically convincing evidence that early treatment has a pre-emptive effect on the postherpetic state.

Knowledge of the details of this second latent period has obviously been hindered by the lack of an animal model of the condition. This may be at an end with the publication of a short report (Fleetwood-Walker et al., 1999). They followed the methods in a previous report (Sadzot-Delvaux et al., 1995) and tissue cultured a latent varicella zoster virus which was known to infect dorsal root ganglian cells. They injected a massive dose (4×10^6 infected cells) into the foot pad of rats. Within 4–5 days the animals exhibited a marked allodynia and hyperalgesia which persisted for the next 30 days of observation. The exploration of these animals should provide much new knowledge.

The final chapters of this book analyse the most important practical clinical consequence of the disease which is the crippling pain. My own chapter will be a brief comment on the considered opinions of the real experts such as Rowbotham and colleagues and Watson and colleagues. There is no doubt that the pain is of multiple origin incorporating the consequences of both nerve cell destruction and of inflammation. To unravel such a pain, it is necessary to identify the factors which are necessary in its production from the factors which incidentally coincide with its production but are not necessary. Only then could a rationale therapy evolve. The fact that most people recover from herpes zoster is good for them but confusing for those who believe that there is a single simple therapy. In the first edition of this book, Watson identifies over forty therapies which is the same as saying that none work reliably. Hopefully with the publication of this edition, we all move a little towards understanding prevention and cure.

References

Fleetwood-Walker, S.M., Quinn, J.P., Wallace, C., Blackburn-Muro, G. et al. (1999) Behavioural changes in the rat following infection with varicella-zoster virus. J. Gen. Virol., 80: 2433–2436.

Gilden, D.H., Vafai, A., Shtram, Y., Becker, Y., Devlin, M. and Wellish, M. (1983) Varicella-zoster virus DNA in human sensory ganglia. Nature, 306: 478–480.

Gilden, D.H., Kleinsmidt-De Masters, B.K., La Guardia, J.J., Mahalingham, R. and Cohrs, R.J. (2000) Neurologic complications of the reactivation of varicella-zoster virus. New Eng. J. Med., 324: 635–645.

Goon, P., Wright, M. and Fink, C. (2000) Ophthalmic zoster sine herpete. J. R. Soc. Med., 93: 191–192.

Hyman, R.W., Ecker, J.R. and Tenser, B.B. (1983) Varicella-zoster virus RNA in human trigeminal ganglia. Lancet, 2: 814–816.

Levin, M.J., Barker, D., Goldblatt, E. et al. (1998) Use of live attenuated varicella-zoster virus in zeropositive people 55 years of age and older. J. Infect. Dis., 178: S109–112.

Sadzot-Delvaux, C., Debrus, S., Nickels, A., Piette, J. and Rentier, B. (1995) Varicella-zoster virus latency in the adult rat is a useful model for human latent infection. Neurology, 45: 18–20.

Patrick D. Wall
Center for Neuroscience Research,
Hodgkin Building, King's College London,
London SE1 1UK, UK

Preface to the Second Edition

The terrible pain of herpes zoster and postherpetic neuralgia is a challenge to all of us who try to understand persistent pain and attempt to relieve it. The severe pain in the acute stage makes the patient miserable, but there is the hopeful expectation that it will eventually vanish. When the pain persists in the chronic stage for months or years after the initial attack, the patient is devastated. Because these pains are relatively common, especially as the proportion of older people increases in our Western societies, it is gratifying that Dr. Peter Watson and Dr. Anne Gershon have edited this book which provides, in a single volume, up-to-date knowledge about every aspect of the syndrome.

The first edition of this book, published in 1993, received wide acclaim. In this new edition, Dr. Watson and Dr. Gershon are joined by outstanding authorities on the multiple facets of herpes zoster and postherpetic neuralgia. An impressive amount of knowledge has accumulated in recent years, and this book enriches our knowledge not only about this particular syndrome but about chronic pain in general. It is a valuable contribution to the literature on pain which deals with all the basic scientific information on the acute and chronic stages of herpes zoster as well as the recent exciting developments in the treatment of this awful affliction.

Postherpetic neuralgia has a special place in the history of theories of pain. William Noordenbos made this syndrome the foundation for his theory of pain in which he proposed that the selective destruction of large fibers by the herpes virus produces uninhibited transmission of small-fiber inputs through the dorsal horns. Noordenbos' brilliant little book was an inspiration to me and Patrick Wall, and led to our discussions that eventually resulted in the gate control theory of pain. Important progress has been made in recent years in controlling the pain of postherpetic neuralgia. Several effective treatment modalities are described in this book and more people are now obtaining relief than was thought possible a decade ago. Regrettably, there are people who are still not helped. This book is certain to influence its readers to carry out basic and clinical research. It will, hopefully, lead to a more thorough understanding of the problems and to pain relief for those who continue to suffer.

Ronald Melzack
E.P. Taylor Professor of Psychology,
McGill University,
1205 Dr. Penfield Avenue,
Montreal, PQ H3A 1B1, Canada

Introduction

The purpose of the second edition of this book has not changed, that is, to provide a source for current data regarding the varicella zoster virus and its complications for caregivers, clinical and basic scientists and our patients, the ultimate focus of all our labours. This edition is most fortunate in having as co-editor Anne Gershon who, as an eminent authority on this virus, has been indispensable.

Postherpetic neuralgia (PHN) has proven itself to be a major clinical model for the study of the more general problem of neuropathic pain. Most of what we know about nerve injury pain in humans, particularly regarding treatment, arises from this condition and painful diabetic neuropathy and the research results are quite similar.

This book is meant to be a useful stepping stone to further developments although the reader will certainly encounter information that is well established. Much of our understanding requires corroboration and stimulating ideas are presented in this volume about which our contributors do not always agree.

Some information remains much the same, such as the use of nerve blocks and surgery for PHN. Gerhard Fromm is now deceased, but his chapter from the first edition (with a commentary by Barry Sessle) remains as a tribute to him and because it continues to be very relevant. New chapters include Edgar Hope-Simpson's fascinating account of his ground-breaking epidemiological research, recent data on latency, the neurological and ocular complications of zoster, and new and stimulating concepts about the pathophysiology of this pain.

Recent studies provide new data about epidemiology and virology and further evidence against the utility of steroids to prevent PHN. The therapeutic advances include further data on the effectiveness of antidepressants and new information about gabapentin, opioids and the lidocaine skin patch. The exciting prospect of preventing PHN by vaccination and early, aggressive, multimodal therapy of herpes zoster are exciting future possibilities.

Finally, I want to thank my co-editor, Anne Gershon, and our many and authoritative contributors for taking the time to collaborate on this volume. This book would also not have been possible without Judy, Emily, Simon, Dorothy Barnes, Verna and Robert Watt, and Angela Baird.

C. Peter N. Watson, MD, FRCP(C)
Toronto, Canada

Introduction

It has been a great pleasure to be involved in the development and production of a second edition of this important volume on herpes zoster. Due to the advances in molecular biology, much new information has recently come to light on VZV, which is extremely difficult to propagate in vitro. Molecular biology has given researchers an alternative to standard virological approaches which require culture of a virus. Readers will therefore find exciting and up-to-date information on the basic biology of VZV and latent infection in this second edition. Many of these advances in our knowledge may be utilized in the future in the development of vaccines to prevent zoster. Readers will also find up-to-date information on the use and misuse of antiviral drugs and information helpful in the management of immunocompromised patients with zoster. This has become possible as more experience has been gained on the use of antivirals to treat and/or prevent zoster. Finally, a timely assessment of how vaccination can potentially be used to prevent zoster in high risk patients is included in this volume. This possibility is truly hopeful, and by the time a third edition of this volume appears, definitive information may have become available and might even have become "standard of care". That is certainly our hope.

Anne A. Gershon
New York, NY, USA

List of Contributors

Neena Abraham
MS Unit, Dalhousie University Medical School, Sir Charles Tupper Medical Building, Room 2L-A2 (2nd Floor-Link), Halifax, NS B3H 4H7, Canada.

Ann M. Arvin
Department of Pediatrics, Microbiology and Immunology, Stanford University School of Medicine, Stanford, CA 94305, USA.

Ralf Baron
Klinik für Neurophysiologie, Christian-Albrechts-Universität, D-24098 Kiel, Germany.

David Bowsher
Pain Research Institute, Clinical Sciences Building, University Hospital Aintree, Liverpool L9 7AL, UK; and Honorary Consultant Neurologist, Mersey Regional Centre for Pain Relief, Walton Hospital, Liverpool, UK.

Mary Chipman
Department of Public Health Sciences, University of Toronto, Toronto, ON M9A 1T8, Canada.

Randall J. Cohrs
Department of Neurology, University of Colorado Health Sciences Center, 4200 East 9th Avenue, Mail Stop B182, Denver, CO 80262, USA.

John H. Deck
Department of Pathology, University of Toronto, Toronto, ON M9A 1T8, Canada.

Robert Dworkin
Department of Anesthesiology, University of Rochester School of Medicine and Dentistry, 601 Elmwood Avenue, Box 604, Rochester, NY 14642, USA.

Howard L. Fields
UCSF Pain Clinical Research Center, and Departments of Neurology and Physiology, University of California, San Francisco, San Francisco, CA 94115, USA.

Perry G. Fine
Department of Anesthesiology, and Pain Management Center, University of Utah Health Sciences Center, Salt Lake City, UT 84108, USA.

Gerhard H. Fromm (deceased)

Department of Neurology, University of Pittsburgh School of Medicine, Pittsburgh, PA 15261, USA.

Anne A. Gershon

Department of Pediatrics, Division of Pediatric Infectious Diseases, Columbia University College of Physicians and Surgeons, 650 W. 168th Street, New York, NY 10032, USA.

Donald H. Gilden

Department of Neurology, University of Colorado Health Sciences Center, 4200 East 9th Avenue, Mail Stop B182, Denver, CO 80262, USA.

Maija Haanpää

Peijas Hospital, Sairaalakatu 1, Fin-01400 Vantaa, Finland

Edgar Hope-Simpson

46 Chesterton Park, Cirencester, Gloucestershire GLY 1XT, UK.

James J. LaGuardia

Department of Neurology, University of Colorado Health Sciences Center, 4200 East 9th Avenue, Mail Stop B182, Denver, CO 80262, USA.

Myron J. Levin

University of Colorado School of Medicine, Pediatric Infectious Diseases, 4200 East Ninth Avenue, C-227, Denver, CO 80262, USA.

John D. Loeser

Departments of Neurological Surgery and Anesthesiology, University of Washington, Box 356470, Seattle, WA 98195-6470, USA.

Barry A.S. Lycka

920 10665 Jasper Avenue, Edmonton, AB T5J 3S9, Canada.

Ronald Melzack

E.P. Taylor Professor of Psychology, McGill University, 1205 Dr. Penfield Avenue, Montreal, PQ H3A 1B1, Canada.

T. Jock Murray

Dalhousie Multiple Sclerosis Research Unit, Dalhousie University Medical School, Sir Charles Tupper Medical Building, Room 2L-A2 (2nd Floor-Link), Halifax, NS B3H 4H7, Canada.

Anne Louise Oaklander
Departments of Anesthesiology, Neurology and Pathology, Massachusetts General Hospital, Harvard Medical School, Boston, MA, USA.

Deborah Pavan-Langston
Department of Ophthalmology, Harvard Medical School, and Massachusetts Eye and Ear Infirmary, Clinical Virology, 243 Charles Street, Boston, MA 02114, USA.

Richard T. Perkin
Varicella-Zoster Research Foundation, 40 East 72nd Street, New York, NY 10021, USA.

Karin L. Petersen
UCSF Pain Clinical Research Center, Department of Neurology, University of California, San Francisco, San Francisco, CA 94115, USA.

John T. Philbrick
Department of Medicine, University of Virginia School of Medicine, Box 494, Charlottesville, VA 22908, USA.

Barbara T. Post
Northridge Internal Medicine, University of Virginia School of Medicine, 2955 Ivy Road, Suite 305, Charlottesville, VA 22901, USA.

Michael C. Rowbotham
Departments of Neurology and Anesthesia, University of California, San Francisco, and UCSF Pain Clinical Research Center, 1701 Divisadero Street, Suite 480, San Francisco, CA 94115, USA.

Ken Schmader
Division of Geriatrics, Department of Medicine and the Center for the Study of Aging and Human Development, Duke University Medical Center, Durham VA Medical Center, Durham, NC 27710, USA.

Barry J. Sessle
Faculty of Dentistry, University of Toronto, 124 Edward Street, Toronto, ON M5G 1G6, Canada.

R. Gary Sibbald
Department of Medicine, University of Toronto, Room BW4-658, 585 University Ave., Toronto, ON M5G 2C4, Canada.

Patrick D. Wall

Center for Neuroscience Research, Hodgkin Building, King's College London, London SE1 1UK, UK.

C. Peter N. Watson

Department of Medicine, University of Toronto and 1 Sir Williams Lane, Toronto, ON M9A 1T8, Canada.

Richard Whitley

Department of Pediatrics, Microbiology and Medicine, University of Alabama at Birmingham, The Children's Hospital of Alabama, Suite 616, ACC, 1600 Seventh Avenue South, Alabama, AL 35233, USA.

Diane Williamson

Dermatology Day Care and Wound Healing Clinic, Sunnybrook and Women's College Health Sciences Centre, Toronto, ON M5G 2C4, Canada.

Contents

A Tribute

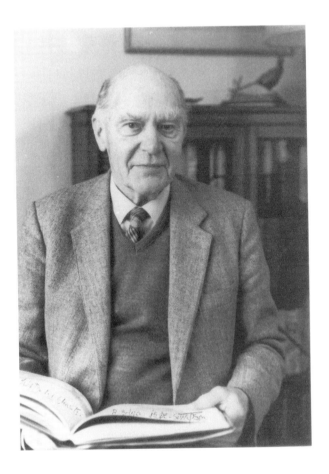

R. Edgar Hope-Simpson, O.B.E., F.R.C.G.P.

C. Peter N. Watson

"A man with powers of observation, well-trained in the wards and with strong natural propensities ... an absorbing desire to know the truth, an unswerving steadfastness in its pursuit and an open, honest heart ... may reach the higher levels of scholarship."
William Osler, 1849–1919, "A Student Life"

"The doctor is first and foremost a student of nature observing, recording, classifying and analysing"
John Ryle, 1931

The work of Edgar Hope-Simpson became known to me in the early 1980s. I became interested in the treatment of postherpetic neuralgia and read his 1975 publication on this condition in his general practice population. It was not until later that I realized his extraordinary accomplishment, as described in his 1965 paper, that established a firm foundation for the common origin of herpes zoster and varicella and the concept of viral latency and natural immunity. I also became cognizant of his earlier 1954 paper which compared varicella in the Shetland Island of Yell with varicella caught from cases of shingles both on the same island and from his own general practice population in Cirencester. His conclusion was that there was no difference in the characteristics of the disorders and that the virus must be the same. Perhaps only an epidemiologist would truly fully appreciate his perseverance and the meticulous observation and record keeping necessary in following his general practice population over 16 years. The 1965 paper described the first 16 years of what subsequently became an even more prolonged 26 years of study. As well, he has made significant contributions related specifically to influenza, pellagra, rubella, staphylococcal infections, Sendai virus, the common cold, and herpes simplex. More generally, his published research reveals an overall interest in the epidemiology of diseases in general practice.

Dr. Hope-Simpson is an original, one of those singularly brilliant individuals driven by intellectual curiosity about life. He would flourish in any situation in any time.

We can add to this an insight from an interview with Dr. David Carrington in which Dr. Hope-Simpson responds to a question about what to do with the very difficult cases of postherpetic neuralgia. Dr. Hope-Simpson states that, "A kindly understanding doctor, who will keep in touch with his patients even with postherpetic neuralgia for a very long time, is extremely valuable therapeutically." What follows is a fascinating account of his life's investigations written especially for this book.

References

Hope-Simpson, R.E. (1954) Studies on shingles. Is the virus ordinary chickenpox virus? Lancet, 25: 1299–1302.

Hope-Simpson, R.E. (1965) The nature of herpes zoster: a long-term study and a new hypothesis. Proc. Roy. Soc. Med., 58: 9–20.

Roland, C.G., Sir William Osler 1849–1919 (1982) The Hannah Institute for the History of Medicine.

Ryle, J.A. (1931) The physician as naturalist. Address to the Cambridge University Medical Society, April 29, 1931. Guy's Hosp. Rep., xxxi: 278.

Herpes Zoster and Postherpetic Neuralgia, 2nd Revised and Enlarged Edition
Pain Research and Clinical Management, Vol. 11
Edited by C.P.N. Watson and A.A. Gershon

Some early investigations into the nature of herpes zoster and postherpetic neuralgia

R. Edgar Hope-Simpson, O.B.E., F.R.C.G.P. [*]

General Practioner and Director (1946–1992), Epidemiological Research Unit, Cirencester, Gloucestershire, UK

1. Introduction

Medical history can often be instructive, especially the mistakes that inevitably come to light. Shingles (herpes zoster), is exceptionally interesting because of the difficult questions that it is still posing, despite being one of the easiest human ailments to identify.

In the United Kingdom, general practitioners had an almost unique opportunity for pursuing observational research because many of them were serving a fairly stable population of several thousand persons of all ages and both sexes for 30 years or more. They could characterise all the patients on their National Health Service list by age, sex, location and occupation.

The general practitioner is consulted about every case of zoster in his practice population because it is such a striking malady. Few others have had this opportunity to study its natural presentation in a characterised community. Sadly the opportunity was fleeting because GPs are now amalgamating into large groups lacking the personal list. Furthermore, the population is becoming increasingly nomadic.

This chapter, after a brief recapitulation of the history of research into the pathology of zoster, describes studies of its natural history, chiefly by a small epidemiological research unit established by the Medical Research Council and the Public Health Laboratory Service in a general practice in Cirencester, Gloucestershire, England.

2. The pathology of zoster

The characteristic distribution of zoster on one side of a single body segment has been recognised for centuries. Some ancient physician encountering the very rare condition of bilateral zosters girdling the trunk at the same level must have christened the disease 'cingulum', a girdle, anglicised as 'shingles'.

As long ago as 1831, Richard Bright recognised that the segmental distribution of the zoster eruption reflected the sensory innervation of the skin of the involved somite (Bright, 1831). A generation later Von Bärensprung (1862) demonstrated by autopsy the morbid changes in the relevant sensory nerve and ganglion, and so confirmed Bright's inference.

But to Head and Campbell (1900), we owe the first detailed demonstration of the morbid anatomy of zoster in an astonishing paper in the Journal *Brain*. Their method is worthy of record. Henry Head, consultant physician at University College Hospital, London, became interested in a large number of elderly patients with zoster, seen in his outpatient sessions and in his private practice. He asked his friend Dr. A.W. Campbell, Director of a large

* Correspondence to: Dr. R.E. Hope-Simpson, 46 Chesterton Park, Cirencester, Gloucestershire, UK. Phone: +44 (1285) 654530.

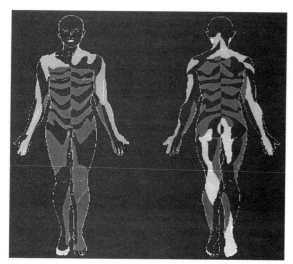

Fig. 1. Neurosegmental anatomy of the human body illustrated by the surface distributions of zoster eruptions. The affected sensory nerves and ganglia were identified by autopsy. Reproduced with permission from *Brain* (adapted from Head and Campbell, 1900).

infirmary in the Midlands, to notify him when any elderly inmate developed zoster.

As soon as Head received notice of a case he despatched his medical artist to make an accurate drawing showing the distribution of the zoster on the body surface. He then waited for the demise of such patients, a long wait at times because even in elderly persons, zoster is not lethal. When notified of the death, Head himself travelled to the infirmary to perform a meticulous autopsy. Twenty of these are recorded in their paper, enabling them to demonstrate how each zoster eruption is linked to a sensory ganglion by its afferent nerve, illustrating the damage to the nerve and ganglion, and, in some cases, to the relevant spinal tract, even as far as the brain. The results provided for the first time an accurate diagram of the neurosegmental anatomy of the human body (Fig. 1).

3. The relationship between zoster and varicella

Long before 1892, when Von Bokáy noticed the phenomenon, parents, grandparents and family doctors must also have been aware that children in con-

tact with a zoster sufferer often developed varicella (Von Bokáy, 1909). It must also have been common knowledge that only children unprotected by a previous attack of varicella developed the disease from contact with a zoster, so it is difficult to understand the prolonged argument as to the nature of the zoster-induced illness — was ordinary (O-varicella) a different disease from zoster-induced (Z-varicella)? Yet for many years thereafter the nature of Z-varicella was strongly debated.

The experiments of Kundratitz (1925) showed that children developing 'varicella' from inoculation with zoster vesicle fluid could also transmit the agent to cause 'varicella' in companions. Those findings were confirmed by Bruusgaard (1932), but they only proved that Z-varicella is naturally infectious and made no contribution to understanding the relationship between Z- and O-varicella.

Abrahamson (1944), faced with an outbreak of varicella among children in hospital, successfully protected those in contact with cases by inoculating them with stored plasma of blood taken from a patient convalescent from an attack of herpes zoster. The findings suggested that O- and Z-varicella are identical, caused by the same as yet unidentified pathogen. Unfortunately, one could not be sure that the hospital outbreak was not one of Z-varicella. Seiler (1949) conducted an epidemiological study in Edinburgh from which he concluded that, though clinically similar, they were different diseases caused by different agents.

4. Z-varicella

4.1. A new approach to the Z-varicella problem

This was the situation when in 1952 the small epidemiological research unit in Cirencester considered that it had developed an appropriate technique for tackling the problem anew (Hope-Simpson, 1952). A solution was essential for an understanding of the nature of zoster itself.

Nearly a century earlier Panum (1846), studying a measles epidemic in the Faröe Islands, had

TABLE I

Bionomic features of host–parasite cycles of three human epidemic pathogens

	Pathogen		
	Measles	Varicella	Mumps
Mean serial interval (days)	10	14	17
Infectiousness (%)	75.6	61.0	31.1
Mean age of host (years)	5.6	6.7	11.5
Age that 90% have been attacked (years)	8.3	10.7	29.0

drawn attention to the distinction between the incubation period – from infection to illness – and the serial interval – between illnesses in donor and recipient. The Cirencester team had found that precise measurements of these bionomic features gave much information about the host–parasite reproductive cycles of the pathogens causing measles, mumps and varicella, although none of their infective agents had yet been identified (Hope-Simpson, 1948). This encouraged them to find a method, the household exposure attack rate on susceptible contacts, to measure the infectiousness of each agent. Each disease was found to possess its own highly individual and consistent pattern of these bionomic characters (Table I).

The average age of those attacked in any community was also determined by these characteristics, though the actual averages differed according to the composition of the study population.

It seemed reasonable to suppose that this simple observational method could settle the Z-varicella problem. Should the Z-varicella pathogen differ from that causing O-varicella it would possess a different set of bionomics and no cross-protection would be expected, unless the pathogens happened to be related, in which case there might be limited cross-protection. Similar bionomics and complete cross-protection would be strong evidence of identity, proving that zoster is a second manifestation of the varicella pathogen.

The bionomics of O-varicella having already been recorded from epidemics in the Cirencester population, all that was now needed was to obtain compara-

ble data from Z-varicella outbreaks stemming from contact with persons suffering from zoster.

4.2. The investigation into Z-varicella

The investigation proved to be unworkable in the Cirencester population, surrounded as it was by large towns. Information about the origins of alleged Z-varicella cases was untrustworthy, and subsequent experience has emphasised the wisdom of extreme care in confirming the validity of data.

A search of the literature found a letter in the 1946 British Medical Journal (BMJ) from Peterson and Black describing how an attack of zoster in the teacher had initiated an outbreak of varicella in her little school on the Shetland island of Yell (Peterson and Black, 1946). Here seemed to be ideal material for the epidemiology of Z-varicella. A letter to the authors elicited the name and address of the teacher but added: "It is happening again. A crofter in the hamlet of Herra has zoster, and his five school-aged children seem to be developing varicella." A later letter confirmed the varicella, and a third announced the spread of varicella in other schoolchildren.

The opportunity was too good to be missed. Yell was a small remote island of scattered crofts, hamlets and a few little villages. Access to the Shetland capital Lerwick on the adjoining island called Mainland was limited. The whole research unit – field-worker, secretary and GP — went to Yell for 3 weeks in August 1954.

The varicella epidemic, which had begun in mid-March, was just ending and it seemed to have followed the expected sequence from the family of the Herra crofter with zoster (Fig. 2A). His children had provided the first epidemic-generations during the Easter school holiday, except for the youngest child who provided the first of the three cases in Herra Junior School.

In the Senior School at mid-Yell, the first generation of the epidemic consisted of a single case in a girl who initiated the long epidemic there, numbering 80 more cases. It seemed natural that she had done so because the date of her illness indicated that she must have become infected during the Easter

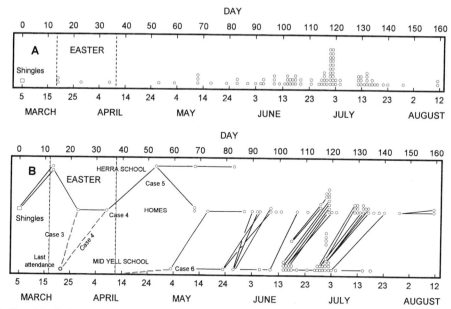

Fig. 2. (A) Varicella epidemic in 1954 in Shetland island of Yell. (B) The Yell epidemic analysed by schools and home cases. Lines indicate transmissions. Note origin of main epidemic from case 6.

holiday when the Herra crofter's family were infectious, and as their cousin, she would probably have visited them then.

Every case had been carefully studied and checked except this sixth case. The girl lived in a rather inaccessible croft. Nevertheless, considering her as the originator of the main epidemic, the team felt it wise to confirm that she had at Easter visited her Herra cousins. They walked from mid-Yell to the sea-loch, rowed themselves across to the north shore and walked several miles through the heather.

It was a sad but salutary lesson. She ought to have been visited first, not last. She had not seen her Herra cousins having spent the Easter holiday with other cousins living in Lerwick who had themselves been ill with varicella. She had been infected by them and had transmitted their strain to cause the epidemic in mid-Yell school.

The dejected team retraced their steps to mid-Yell pondering the catastrophe. One ray of hope seemed able to redeem the waste of time, money and labour, namely that the Lerwick cousins might themselves have caught varicella directly or indirectly from a zoster sufferer. The team accordingly travelled to

Lerwick, but, although they succeeded in tracing that strain from person to person far back into the previous year, they encountered no transmission from zoster. The conclusion was bitter, that only the five Herra children and four others had suffered Z-varicella. The main Yell epidemic was one of O-varicella (Fig. 2B).

4.3. An unexpected reprieve

Just when the unit team had reluctantly decided to abandon hope of solving the problem of the nature of Z-varicella a fortunate coincidence transformed the situation. Most Shetlanders are of Norse derivation and possess 'Saga' memories. They then had no newspaper on Yell and seemed to need none. The mid-Yell shopkeeper said: "Doctor, I hear you're working on shingles and chickenpox. Doubtless you've heard of Mr. O... of Sandwick Bay? No? Well he had shingles 12th August 1945 and his wee granddaughter had chickenpox 29th August, I think, but you'd better ask him." At Sandwick Bay, the team found the information correct, and Mr. O... directed them to other zoster households, and so they were shuttled back and forth across the island. They amassed in this way, and from the teacher whose school outbreak was reported in the BMJ letter, enough material to establish the bionomics of Z-varicella on reliable data. The host–parasite relationship of Z-varicella proved to be identical to that of O-varicella in Yell and in Cirencester.

But nature had also provided clinching evidence of their identity because data about persons with a history of O-varicella at household risk of infection with Z-varicella and vice versa showed that they were completely cross-protected. Had there been no cross-protection, some 60% should have developed varicella (Hope-Simpson, 1954). Zoster is clearly caused by the O-varicella pathogen (Table II).

Unknown to the Cirencester team, Weller and Stoddard (1952) in Enders' laboratory, Boston, MA had at last isolated varicella virus, and Weller and Coons (1954) had shown that it was identical with virus isolated from zoster lesions, hence its present name VZ virus.

5. VZ virus

5.1. The pathogenesis of zoster

The finding that VZ virus causes both varicella and zoster raises questions about the natural history of this human parasite. In order to obtain a comprehensive view, the Cirencester team studied all the 192 cases of zoster that had occurred in the general practice population, circa 3600 persons during the 16 years 1947–1962 (Hope-Simpson, 1965).

Henry Head, from hospital outpatient experience of many years, had considered that zoster was yet another acute exanthem *sui generis* coming in epidemics, like measles and rubella, zoster also being caught directly from other persons with zoster (personal communication). Barnett (1950), aware of a link between zoster and varicella, considered that zoster occurs when persons, in whom immunity from varicella is waning, again encounter VZ virus, a hypothesis that would help to explain the higher incidence in elderly persons.

TABLE II

Serial intervals and infectiousness and cross-protection between O- and Z-varicella

Bionomic features	O-varicella		Z-varicella
	Cirencester	Yell	Yell
Serial interval (no. of transmissions)	178	32	14
Average cycle (days)	14.0	14.0	15.1
Infectiousness (no. exposed)	282	77	30
Transmissions	172	45	19
Rate (%)	61.0	58.4	63.3
Cross-protection (no. of challenges)	–	28	13
Transmissions	–	0	0

The Cirencester team's findings fail to support either hypothesis. Both Head and Barnett suffered the disadvantage that neither had any knowledge of the composition of the community from which their zoster experience arose, nor could they know the overall picture of the disease. The team was fortunate in caring for a fully characterised general practice population continuously for many years, so it was simple to calculate the age specific incidence of zoster, the household contacts and the movement of varicella through the community because they dealt with every case of zoster in that community.

Zoster did not come in epidemics. It came continuously throughout the 16 years with random increases that showed no geographical association. Four years saw epidemics of varicella with high incidence, three of which were accompanied by the lowest incidences of zoster. Contrary to Barnett's supposition from which, as from Head's, zoster should have been most abundant in varicella years, it was almost as if varicella is inimical to production of zoster.

Moreover, of 318 persons in domiciliary contact with a person with zoster none developed zoster nor did any of 1287 similarly in contact with varicella. Neither hypothesis could be correct.

A third hypothesis that had been gaining acceptance suggested that latency of the VZ virus must somehow be involved. Before discussing it in more detail, one needs to examine the overall picture of zoster in the community.

5.2. The natural presentation of herpes zoster

Zoster was found by us to be coming at an average rate of 3.4 cases/1000/annum. McGregor (1957), recorded a higher rate of 4.8 in a more rural area. There was a persistent increased prevalence during the warmer half of the year, a feature that continued during the subsequent decennium.

The age-specific incidence (Fig. 3 and Table III) shows a rapid increase during infancy and adolescence from 0.79/1000/annum to reach about 2.2 and remain around that rate from 20 to 50 years of age.

Thereafter, the incidence rate increases as steeply as in the first 20 years of life, to reach 12.2/1000 in octogenarians, 15-fold that in those under 10 years old and 5.5 times that of persons between 20 and 50 years old. We shall see that this age-related behaviour is a host–parasite feature of importance in understanding the epidemiology of zoster.

The effect of gender also is of great interest. Males were popularly supposed to be preferentially attacked, but the situation is more complex. In the

TABLE III

Annual rate of zoster per 1000 of population per annum by decennia [1]

Age range (years)	Rate/1000
0–9	0.79
10–19	1.63
20–29	2.15
30–39	2.03
40–49	2.37
50–59	6.55
60–69	6.68
70–79	7.31
80+	12.19

[1] Unpublished data from the 26-year study.

26-year study, there was little difference between the experience of the sexes before the age of 50 years, but in the next decade of age, twice as many women developed shingles and they maintained their lead into old age. We shall look again at the important age-related gender difference.

The anatomical location of the segments attacked is also important in understanding the nature of zoster. Most cases attack a single sensory ganglion. An eruption that overflows onto adjacent somites does not necessarily indicate that more than one ganglion is involved, because abundant anastomotic twigs link each sensory nerve with adjacent areas (Weddell and Miller, 1962). Rare simultaneous zosters usually affect widely separate segments of the body often on opposite sides.

Fig. 4a illustrating the distribution of 185 zosters shows that the somite incidence is not random. Some ganglia are much more subject to attack than others. The distribution is nearly symmetrical, 91 on the left, 94 on the right, a finding that corroborates the accuracy of the picture.

The research team was struck by the similarity of the accumulated zoster distributions to that of the rash of varicella — centripetal. Stern (1937) had assembled 46 zoster distributions onto a single body diagram back and front, and he had also noted its resemblance to the exanthem of varicella (Fig. 4b). The 394 cases seen by Head show a similar distribution of zosters (Head and Campbell, 1900).

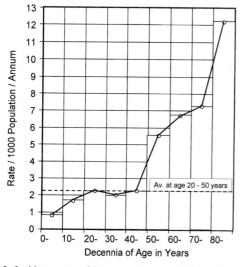

Fig. 3. Incidence rate of herpes zoster per 1000 of Cirencester general practice population annually by 10-year age groups. Twenty-six-year Cirencester study.

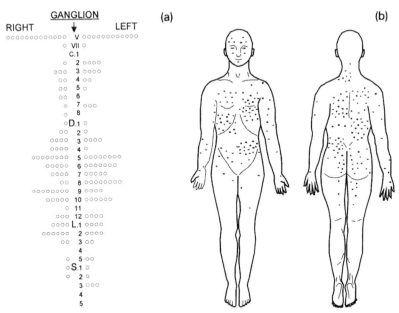

Fig. 4. (a) Segmental distribution of 185 consecutive cases of zoster in 16-year Cirencester study. Reproduced with permission of *Proc. R. Soc. Med.* (Hope-Simpson, 1965). (b) Forty-six zosters assembled onto single body diagram back and front. From Stern, 1937 with permission of *Br. J. Dermatol.*

Herpes zoster used to be thought to confer permanent immunity against subsequent attacks, but this is not so. Head recorded only three second attacks among 400 cases of zoster, whereas in the 192 Cirencester cases, eight were second attacks and one a third (Head and Campbell, 1900). Second attacks among persons who have already suffered a zoster are at least as common as first attacks in the general population. Four of the eight second attacks involved the same sensory ganglion as the first attack, an unexpected finding suggesting that ganglia in which reactivation from latency occurs are more liable to develop zoster than others, the reason perhaps being a greater load of latent 'provirus'.

6. Hypotheses

6.1. The hypothesis of varicella-zoster virus latency

It was not enough to disprove two hypotheses and accept latency by default. The virus had been found to belong to the herpes viruses, a group of micro-organisms that is notable for latent potential — but what was the evidence for latency in the natural behaviour of VZ virus?

Firstly, if zoster is caused by reactivation of latent varicella virus, one cannot develop zoster unless one has already had an attack of varicella — but is this always true? What about the six children under 10 years old among the 192 zoster cases in the Cirencester series? It was found that each had already had varicella, even a 2-year-old boy with zoster who had had his varicella when 6 months old.

In the general practice in Cirencester, zoster was once encountered in all three children in one family (Hope-Simpson, 1974). The oldest, a girl of 10 years, and her younger sisters all had zoster at different times, and all three had had varicella during the same epidemic previously. This observation suggests a genetic involvement in susceptibility to zoster, perhaps caused by deficient immune defences.

Winkelmann and Perry (1959) recorded zosters in seven children under 6 years old. All of them, even three 2-year-olds had already had varicella except for one, a baby aged 7 months.

Lomer (1889) records zoster in a 4-day-old boy, and Feldman (1952) reports his own patient with neonatal zoster and nine others from the literature. Such cases present an obstacle to the hypothesis of VZ virus latency after varicella in explaining zoster. Fortunately, a clue to the problem of neonatal zoster was found in some of these accounts. For example, during the third month of her pregnancy with the infant reported by Lomer, the mother spent a whole day with a friend who was suffering from zoster. Lomer had no inkling of the importance of this history, having regarded the encounter as a psychological precipitant. The mother of Feldman's infant had herself had zoster either just before or in the early stage of that pregnancy. Three siblings of Poulsen's (Poulsen, 1955) 15-month-old infant with ophthalmic zoster had had varicella 3 months before his birth.

It seems that zoster over 2 years of age is usually preceded by varicella, whereas in younger children, the encounter with VZ virus has occurred in the womb, though records of the latter have depended on good fortune.

6.2. Detailed hypotheses

The Research Unit team was now faced with so many questions about details of the host—parasite relationship of the VZ virus that they framed a series of suppositions that seemed to explain their findings and that might be verifiable.

(1) The primary infection of a susceptible human with VZ virus is like that of ectromelia in mice as described by Fenner (1948). It gains a foothold in the nasopharynx, where it produces a little lesion for perhaps 7 days while it multiplies. Next comes the primary viraemia in which a small batch of virus invades the circulation, the virus promptly being removed from the blood stream by the reticuloendothelial system, where it continues to multiply. Then comes a second much larger viraemia a fortnight or more after the infection, causing illness in the host as the virus is carried all over the body, lodging in skin and mucous membranes, where it causes the varicella exanthem, erythematous spots that become vesicles and later pustules and crusts. Virus shed from the spots infects susceptible human companions and accomplishes the parasite's reproductive cycle.

(2) This parasitic cycle does not complete the viral behaviour. Numerous varicella spots involve sensory nerve endings in the skin and in the mucous membranes, and all these nerve terminals receive an aliquot of virus particles that have already become defective, so that they cause no injury to the sensory nerves up which they travel to become latent in the first nucleated cells they encounter, namely the neurones and supporting cells of the sensory ganglia. Here they dwell for the remainder of the host's life, for most of the time causing no perceptible damage.

(3) The neural route to the sensory ganglia seems more plausible than the haematogenous because the accumulated zoster pattern on a diagram of the human body (in Fig. 4a,b) reproduces the distribution of the varicella rash. Three separate investigations in different localities and at different dates showed the same result. The more intense the area of varicella rash, the greater the quantity of VZ particles reaching the related neural ganglia. The more heavily parasitised ganglia will probably be the more liable to suffer reactivating virus successfully causing zoster. It is difficult to imagine how a haematogenous distribution could consistently produce this pattern of zosters. The picture is remarkable, almost everyone carrying lifelong a latent infective virus colony in most of the sensory ganglia. Presumably all these symbiotic colonies are liable to be reactivated to pathogenicity (Fig. 5).

(4) It is proposed that in all infected ganglia reactivation is recurring sporadically without ill-effect because the immunity conferred by the initial attack of varicella smothers the pathogenic explosion. The recurrences themselves ensure that the specific immune defences of the human host are usually kept continuously

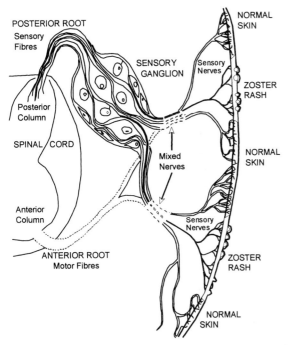

Fig. 5. Diagram of zoster pathology. Affected neurones and sensory nerves in white. Reproduced with permission of *Proc. R. Soc. Med.* (Hope-Simpson, 1965).

at a level that prevents ill effects. Contact with extraneous VZ virus also contributes to alert the defences. Specific antibody content of the blood has been shown to increase in immune parents whose children have varicella.

(5) Sooner or later, a reactivation may occur in a sensory ganglion when the specific immunity has declined below a critical value. There follows a race between reactivating virus and the rising immune reaction to it. Most virions gaining access to the circulation are rapidly neutralised, though Lewis (1958) found a few ectopic varicelliform vesicles on careful body search of all his zoster patients. Inside the sheath of the sensory nerve the virus, partially protected from the body defences, finds its route of escape into the skin and mucous membranes around the nerve endings served by the affected ganglion. Now fully pathogenic, it damages not only the ganglion, nerve and body surface tissues, but also the sensory tracts in spinal cord and brain.

(6) Evidence in favour of this strange picture — a lifelong competition going on in all of us between our immune defences and the enormous number of little colonies of reactivating VZ virus — may be found in the age distribution of zoster (Fig. 6). In children, successful reactivations causing zoster are not only rare, but usually very mild. Pain is negligible, the surface eruption is small and the spots discrete. The frequency of zosters increases with age, until at age 20 years, virtually everyone has received the dose of VZ virus as varicella that makes it possible to develop zoster. From young adulthood to middle age, say aged 20—50 years, the incidence remains static around 2.2/1000/annum. Thereafter it increases rapidly, presumably *pari passu* with diminution of immune potential caused by ageing.

(7) It is not only the incidence that increases with ageing, but the severity of the disease. Declining immunity permits such enormous multiplication of the pathogen that a mild complaint is transformed into a formidable illness.

(8) Diseases, medication and other substances that impair human immunity, provide evidence of the competition between immune defence and VZ virus. Lead, arsenic, drugs used in order to prevent transplant rejection, steroids, X-radiation, leukaemia, etc. render VZ virus highly dangerous. Varicella and zoster become potentially lethal, and the zosters may be complicated by a varicelliform rash — zoster generalisatus.

7. Postherpetic neuralgia (PHN)

In young persons, zoster seldom causes much pain, but with increasing age, it causes more and increasingly protracted pain. Postherpetic pain differs from that occurring before and during the eruption and is not much eased by analgesics. It seems to be imprinted in the brain and may persist for years. PHN commonly succeeds the severe zosters of elderly persons, and if they have not been forewarned of such a

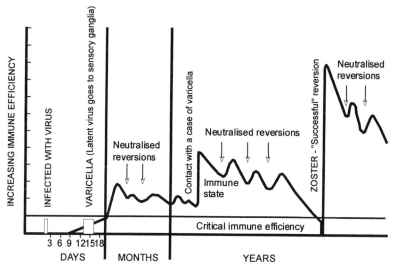

Fig. 6. Suggested biology of VZ virus: latency in neural ganglia and reactivations in continual competition with immune defences of the human body. Reproduced with permission of *Proc. R. Soc. Med.* (Hope-Simpson, 1965).

sequel and assured of continued help from the doctor, the continual pain may mislead the patient into fearing that cancer has been missed, or it may cause depression that has led to suicide.

Even the severest PHN gradually eases over months and years. Antidepressants, anticonvulsants and opioids have been found to be of help (Hope-Simpson, 1967), see Chapter 22.

Removal of the affected sensory ganglion does not cure the PHN. It seems likely that PHN arises when neurological damage occurs during the acute stage of the zoster. Again it seems that the multiplicity of reactivated VZ virus and effectiveness of the immune-systems of the host is determining the result. Treatment of this very serious malady of the elderly is being sought along the lines of prevention of varicella by vaccine, diminution of VZ virus during varicella and zoster by virucides, and enhancing the immune systems of the body.

The age and gender relationship of VZ virus infection are puzzling. Severity of varicella and zoster lesions, incidence of zoster in the community, incidence of PHN in zoster cases, and severity and chronicity of the pain are all age-related and differ between male and female sufferers (see Fig. 7a,b).

Fig. 7a shows that in the Cirencester general practice population in the 26-year study, the experience of zoster had been much the same in males and females under 50 years old, but the percentage then jumped from 5 to 19% in females, whereas in males in their 50s, the increase was much less, from 7 to 11%, and the percentage in older women continued to exceed that of the older men.

Fig. 7b shows that males with zoster began to have PHN in their 30s, but women with zoster did not suffer PHN until they were 50 years old, and the proportion after zoster in octogenarians was females 40%, males only 25%. It would be valuable to know what difference in the make up of the sexes is responsible for such a striking disparity in age-related incidence of zoster and PHN.

Severity and duration of PHN also increase with age, but no attempt has been made to see if these features also differed with the gender of the zoster patient.

8. The biological significance of herpes zoster

If varicella is the evolutionary adaptation whereby VZ virus becomes transmitted from host to host and achieves survival as a species, what biological purpose is served by zoster, a second evolutionary adaptation of the virus in the same host species

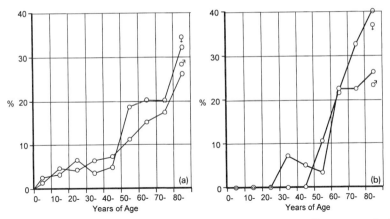

Fig. 7. (a) Percentage of GP population suffering zoster, by gender and age. Twenty-six-year Cirencester study. (b) Percentage of zoster patients developing postherpetic neuralgia by gender and age. Twenty-six-year Cirencester study.

which is only occurring after the varicella — usually many years after? What benefit can zoster confer on the virus?

VZ virus possesses the attributes of a very ancient parasite of mankind. The virus has become closely cell-adapted and, whatever the pristine severity of the disease, it is now usually mild, seldom killing human hosts on whom it depends. It seems to have come to terms with the human host species, and it has few near-relative viruses that are parasitic on other species of host. How did it survive in prehistoric times?

Mankind has been aggregated into great cities for only a brief period of evolutionary time, and varicella virus requires communities of around 250,000 to survive solely by continuous transmission from cases of varicella (Bartlett, 1957). Among prehistoric humans living in groups of 100 or less, with little inter-communication between groups, the virus would inevitably have become extinct had it depended solely on varicella for survival. It must, therefore, have developed some additional evolutionary adaptation, and in herpes zoster, we find the ideal solution to its problem.

All the members of the small communities of susceptible neoliths having caught varicella would become immune carriers of latent virions in their sensory ganglia for the remainder of their lives. Years later, when most infected neoliths had died and the community again consisted largely of susceptible

persons born after the varicella epidemic, a surviving elder would develop zoster. VZ virus would again cause an epidemic of varicella in the new generation of neoliths and the VZ virus species would continue to survive as a human parasite.

If, as suggested by the findings of the Cirencester Unit, zoster is postponed by extraneous contact with VZ virus, it would postpone zoster in the neolithic groups until varicella had long been absent and the group again consisted largely of susceptibles — an elegant refinement of the evolutionary adaptation (Hope-Simpson, 1968). In remote communities, such as that in Yell in the 1950s, VZ virus seemed still to have been surviving by these means.

References

Abrahamson, A.W. (1944) Varicella and herpes zoster: an experiment. Br. Med. J., i: 812–813.

Barnett, C.H. (1950) The relationship between herpes zoster and varicella. Med. Pr., 223: 126–128.

Bartlett, M. (1957) J. Roy. Statist. Soc., 120: 48.

Bright, R. (1831) Rep. Med. Cases, London, 2. i: 383.

Bruusgaard, E. (1932) Mutual relationship between zoster and varicella. Br. J. Dermatol., 44: 1.

Feldman, G.V. (1952) Herpes zoster neonatorum. Arch. Dis. Childh., 27: 126–127.

Fenner, F. (1948) Pathogenesis of the acute exanthemata — an interpretation based on experimental investigation with mousepox (infection ectromelia of mice). Lancet, ii: 915–920.

Head, H. and Campbell, A.W. (1900) The pathology of herpes

zoster and its bearing on sensory localisation. Brain, 23: 353–523.

Hope-Simpson, R.E. (1948) The period of transmission in certain epidemic diseases. Lancet, ii: 755–769.

Hope-Simpson, R.E. (1952) Infectiousness of communicable diseases in the household, (Measles, Chickenpox and Mumps). Lancet, ii: 549–564.

Hope-Simpson, R.E. (1954) Studies on shingles. Is the virus ordinary Chickenpox virus? Lancet, ii: 1299–1302.

Hope-Simpson, R.E. (1965) The nature of herpes hoster: a long-term study and a new hypothesis. (First Albert Wander Lecture). Proc. R. Soc. Med., 58: 1: 9–20.

Hope-Simpson, R.E. (1967) Herpes zoster in the elderly. Geriatrics, 22: 151–159.

Hope-Simpson, R.E. (1968) The epidemiology of viruses: antigenicity and evolution. Proc. Roy. Soc. Med., 62: 1138.

Hope-Simpson, R.E. (1974) Zoster in three children in a family. Br. Med. J., iii: 626 (letter).

Kundratitz, K. (1925) Wien. Klin. Wschr., 38: 502.

Lewis, G.W. (1958) Zoster sine herpete. Br. Med. J., ii: 418–419.

Lomer (1889) Zbl. Gynäk. 13: 778.

McGregor, R.M. (1957) Herpes zoster, Chickenpox and cancer in general practice. Br. Med. J., i: 84–87.

Panum, P.L. (1846) Observations made during the epidemic of measles on the Faroe Islands in the year 1846. New York (reprinted 1940).

Peterson, P.H. and Black, S.A.B. (1946) Varicella herpetiformis. Br. Med. J., i: 762.

Poulsen, P.A. (1955) Zoster ophthalmicus. Report of a case in a child of sixteen months. Acta Med. Scand., 151: 131–134.

Seiler, H.E. (1949) The mechanism of herpes zoster and its relationship to chickenpox. J. Hyg. Camb., 47: 253–262.

Stern, E. (1937) The mechanism of herpes zoster and its relationship to chickenpox. Br. J. Dermatol., 49: 263–271.

Von Bärensprung, F.G.F. (1862) Beitrage zur kentniss des zoster. Ann. Charité-Krankenh. Berlin, 10: 96–104.

Von Bokáy, J. (1909) Uber den Atiologischen zusammenhang der varicellen mit gewissen fallen von herpes zoster. Wien. Klin. Wschr. (Suppl.), 39: 1323.

Weddell, G. and Miller, S. (1962) Cutaneous sensibility. Annu. Rev. Physiol., 24: 199–222.

Weller, T.H. and Coons, A.H. (1954) Fluorescent antibody study with agents of varicella and herpes zoster propagated in vitro. Proc. Soc. Exp. Biol., 86: 789–794.

Weller, T.H. and Stoddard, M.B. (1952) Intranuclear inclusion bodies in cultures of human tissue inoculated with varicella vesicle fluid. J. Immunol., 68: 311–319.

Winkelmann, R.K. and Perry, H.O. (1959) Herpes zoster in children. J. Am. Med. Assoc., 171: 876–880.

Herpes Zoster and Postherpetic Neuralgia, 2nd Revised and Enlarged Edition
Pain Research and Clinical Management, Vol. 11
Edited by C.P.N. Watson and A.A. Gershon

CHAPTER 2

Making a difference: the VZV Research Foundation

Richard T. Perkin [*]

President, VZV Research Foundation, 40 East 72nd Street, New York, NY 10021, USA

1. Life at a crossroads

In 1989, as I was nearing my 59th birthday, I seriously contemplated the next phase of my professional and civic life. My career had long centered on public media, including television documentary syndication, and the charitable boards on which I served related to the arts, education, science and wildlife conservation.

My interest in the sciences had been spurred by my father, the late Richard S. Perkin, co-founder of The Perkin-Elmer Corporation, which has made many pioneering contributions to the fields of science, instrumentation and astronomy.

In sum, I had a wonderful life, largely due to my wife, Leslie, and my three children.

Life had been good to me and I wanted to give something back.

As I pondered my next move, little did I realize that the inspiration for a new and dramatically different stage of my life would not originate within myself, but, rather, from my then 82-year old mother. Deeply moved by the excruciating pain she was experiencing as a shingles and, later, a post-herpetic neuralgia (PHN) sufferer, I resolved to answer her plea for "someone to do something about this terrible disease" by doing something myself. And within two years, I established the Varicella-Zoster Virus (VZV) Research Foundation.

As the Foundation celebrates its tenth anniversary, it remains the world's only nonprofit organization solely fostering research and education on the varicella-zoster virus and VZV infections.

2. A powerless witness to pain

My mother was a classic stoic. She came from a generation of men and women who simply did not complain, especially about pain. But, for my mother, that all changed in September 1989. She had been experiencing severe headaches following cataract surgery, which both she and I dismissed as simply post-operative discomfort. However, over the next few days, these headaches became totally unbearable for her and she began complaining of unrelenting pain, a sign that something was terribly wrong.

My mother pleaded with me to find a way to relieve her suffering, but the nature of her illness eluded me, as it did her doctor. In fact, it took a second visit to his office, and the appearance of the tell-tale blisters, to secure a diagnosis of ophthalmic shingles.

* Correspondence to: R.T. Perkin, President, VZV Research Foundation, 40 East 72nd Street, New York, NY 10021, USA. Phone: +1 (212) 472-3181; Fax: +1 (212) 861-7033; E-mail: rtp@vzvfoundation.org

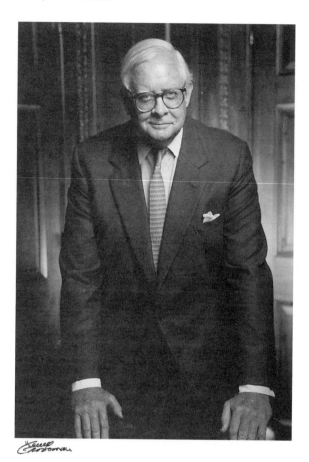

Richard T. Perkin. (Photo by Henry Grossman.)

Antiviral therapy helped ease the pain, but shortly thereafter it returned, only this time there was no rash and the pain was much more intense. I learned that the shingles had progressed to PHN, which, I now know, is more common in ophthalmic shingles sufferers.

I also learned that my mother's stoicism had not served her well in this instance since, according to her doctor, shingles must be treated within 24 to 72 hours of the appearance of the rash. Prompt medical attention could have potentially reduced the severity and duration of shingles and the likelihood of PHN.

My mother repeatedly asked me to help her, but, not being a doctor and lacking a firm understanding of VZV infections, I was, in essence, a powerless witness to her pain.

This was about to change.

3. The search for knowledge

In 1990, my mother's condition worsened and, in desperation, I began a full-time search for any and all information about shingles and PHN. It was a challenging search, since VZV infections are multidisciplinary.

Shingles' origins lie in chicken pox, which is pediatric. Shingles manifests itself on the skin, so it is dermatologic. It involves the nervous system, so it is neurological. It afflicts primarily older individuals, so it is geriatric. It can affect the eye, so it is ophthalmic. It is an infectious disease, so it has public health implications. The pain of shingles and PHN involves the fields of pain medicine and management, and anesthesiology. And even psychology and psychiatry become relevant when one considers the mental and emotional anguish VZV disease often inflicts.

The number of VZV-related fields seemed endless. So I set out to consult with many of the best minds in the field of VZV. Without exception, they all sympathized with my mother's plight, but it soon became apparent that, with shingles, there unfortunately were no black and white answers.

4. The roots of the foundation

My search for knowledge on VZV did not yield what I had hoped would be the means to end my mother's suffering, but, rather, the means to begin an organized effort to focus worldwide attention — and, hopefully, some resources — on VZV.

Organization and focus was precisely what was needed in this field, as I soon discovered. In fact, I was astonished to learn that, despite significant strides made by scientists worldwide, they were not unified in their efforts. Moreover, there was relatively little research being conducted, largely due to a lack of funding. And shingles and PHN were not top-of-mind among health professionals and the general public, with little awareness of their widespread incidence and potential severity.

Motivated by these troubling realities, and the fact that there was no single organization dedicated to VZV infections — a necessity if research and education on the virus was going to proliferate — I set about trying to remedy this. I sought the counsel of many experts in the field of VZV, chief among them Dr. Anne A. Gershon, professor of pediatrics at Columbia University, who is renowned for her work on the chicken pox vaccine. I also consulted with Louis R. Gary, chairman of the Manhattan Institute for Cancer Research in New York City. Nearly ten years later, they continue as my mentors in their respective areas of expertise — science and medicine, and the non-profit arena.

The VZV Research Foundation was established in the spring of 1991. Our key objectives remain constant: to foster scientific research on VZV and to educate the public and health-care professionals about VZV infections.

5. Leading the fight against VZV infections

The VZV Research Foundation is guided by a Board of Directors and has a Scientific Advisory Board (SAB) chaired by Dr. Gershon and consisting of more than thirty scientists from around the world who are expert in VZV. Many leading universities and institutions are represented on the SAB, including the Centers for Disease Control and Prevention (CDC) and the National Institutes of Health (NIH). Members include two pioneers in VZV research: Dr. Michiaki Takahashi, professor emeritus at Osaka University, who developed the chicken pox vaccine; and Dr. Thomas Weller, professor emeritus at Harvard School of Public Health and a Nobel Laureate, who first isolated the varicella-zoster virus.

Since its inception, the VZV Research Foundation has served as an information resource for VZV sufferers and their families, and to scientific and medical professionals who study or treat the virus. Its primary activities to date include:

- Sponsorship of five international scientific conferences, in addition to scientific symposia, workshops and roundtables at scientific meetings around the world.
- Provision of ten, two-year research fellowships

totaling more than $1 million to (1) investigate the reasons for the virus' reemergence, (2) develop new vaccines to prevent chicken pox and shingles in the immunocompromised, and (3) seek out new treatments for PHN.

- Development of educational materials for scientists and physicians, including continuing medical education (CME) courses, and publication of the proceedings of our scientific conferences in leading journals.
- Creation of educational materials and programs for the general public, including: (1) informational booklets; (2) a website (www.vzvfoundation.org); (3) a toll-free, VZV Information Line; (4) a television and radio public service campaign; and (5) public health forums attended by hundreds of shingles and PHN sufferers.
- Establishment of the VZVRF Scientific Achievement Award honoring those who have made significant contributions to the study of VZV, including Dr. Takahashi and Dr. Weller. The other recipients of this award are: Dr. R. Edgar Hope-Simpson, a former general practitioner from Cirencester, United Kingdom, who refined the theory that shingles is caused by a reactivation of dormant varicella virus; the late Dr. Gertrude B. Elion, scientist emeritus at Glaxo Wellcome Inc. and a Nobel Laureate, whose research led to the creation of the first antiviral therapy for shingles; and Dr. Gershon, for not only her achievements in VZV research, but also her mentorship of a generation of scientists and clinicians.

6. FastForward: VZVRF's evolving role in VZV

The 21st century holds much promise of continuing innovations that will mark our lives as no previous century. Nowhere does this hold more significance than in the area of medical science. Dramatic proof of this was evidenced in June 2000 with the announcement of the completion of the first assembly of the human genome by Celera Genomics — a corporation which evolved from Perkin-Elmer — and the National Institutes of Health.

In the field of VZV, alone, we have witnessed some significant advances since our inception in 1991, including:

- the development of new antivirals to combat shingles;
- the U.S. approval of a chicken pox vaccine;
- the launch of a major study to explore shingles prevention through vaccination; and,
- the growing focus on new PHN pain therapies.

Against this backdrop, and with the sustained support of individuals, corporations and philanthropies, the VZV Research Foundation has embarked on several new initiatives.

In the area of scientific exchange, the VZV Research Foundation has recently launched an effort to explore the desirability and feasibility of universal vaccination against chicken pox throughout Europe. Issues under discussion include whether the American experience with the vaccine is a transposable model due to the many cultural differences and health-care delivery systems throughout Europe, which are largely driven by national policies. Other barriers to universal vaccination include the perception that chicken pox is a mild childhood illness, in addition to questions concerning whether sufficient coverage can be achieved and whether immunity will wane over time. The existence of breakthrough cases and the cost of vaccination are additional areas of concern. The VZVRF/European Working Group on Varicella Vaccination (EuroVar) is headquartered at the University of Liège in Belgium and is chaired by the head of our International Committee, Dr. Bernard Rentier. The work of the EuroVar is made possible by an unrestricted, educational grant from GlaxoSmithKline/Belgium.

In the area of research, the Foundation is launching a major effort to assist scientists in their efforts to learn more about the causes of PHN so that more effective treatments for PHN can be developed. This initiative involves the establishment of The VZVRF Ganglia Bank at Columbia University, which will work to secure human ganglia for study by researchers. The seed money for the Ganglia Bank, which will be directed by Dr. Gershon, was provided by The F.M. Kirby Foundation, Inc.

Organizationally, we are formalizing our presence in the United Kingdom through the establishment of a subcommittee of our Scientific Advisory Board. This prestigious scientific body will advise the Foundation on research and education initiatives in the UK.

In addition to continuing our current research and education programs, we will also (1) broaden the scope of reference materials for both the public and health professionals, (2) expand distribution of television public service announcements featuring celebrity spokespersons promoting shingles awareness, (3) enhance the interactive capabilities of our website and explore the possibility of online CME courses for physicians, and (4) increase direct public outreach through the sponsorship of free, informational health forums.

7. Closing thoughts from a *former* powerless witness

Great progress has been made in the field of VZV, but two serious hurdles remain.

(1) Insufficient funding for research. VZV researchers continue to find it difficult to compete for funding with 'headliner' diseases such as AIDS, heart disease and cancer. These and other diseases merit as many research dollars as are available, but so, too, do VZV infections. Only through greater funding, and a focused, interdisciplinary research effort, can science hope to unravel the reasons for the virus' reemergence and develop more effective therapeutic and preventive measures for VZV infections.

(2) Insufficient awareness of the potential severity of VZV infections among the public and health professionals. Patients and physicians equally must be educated about the signs and symptoms of shingles and the need for prompt medical attention as a means of potentially lessening the severity of the disease. Government must also be educated about the ever growing incidence of shingles and PHN, as our aged and immunocompromised populations increase.

By all accounts — and largely due to the support and encouragement of our foundation and corporate supporters, the general public and the scientific/medical community — the VZV Research Foundation has evolved over the past decade into a true leader in the fight against VZV infections. We look forward to continuing this fight in the 21st century.

We also look to the day when science and education ultimately triumphs over VZV infections. Such a victory will spare future generations of the pain and suffering currently experienced by millions of men and women around the world, including my late mother.

Gladys Perkin eventually lost the sight in her left eye from ophthalmic shingles. And until her death on November 28, 2000, she suffered terribly from the lingering pain of PHN.

It was her plea to me ten years ago to "do something" which left an indelible mark that never failed to inspire me.

To learn more about the work of the Foundation, please contact: Richard T. Perkin, President, VZV Research Foundation, 40 East 72nd Street, New York, NY 10021 USA.
E-mail: rtp@vzvfoundation.org
Tel.: +1 (212) 472-3181; Fax: +1 (212) 861-7033
Website: www.vzvfoundation.org

Herpes Zoster and Postherpetic Neuralgia, 2nd Revised and Enlarged Edition
Pain Research and Clinical Management, Vol. 11
Edited by C.P.N. Watson and A.A. Gershon

The belt of roses from hell [1]: historical aspects of herpes zoster and postherpetic neuralgia

Neena Abraham and T. Jock Murray [*]

MS Unit, Dalhousie University Medical School, Sir Charles Tupper Medical Building, Room 2L-A2 (2nd Floor-Link), Halifax, NS B3H 4H7, Canada

The chief of Queensland demons makes himself visible at great assemblies, and as he is not only the author of disease, but also of mischief and wisdom, he fitly makes his appearance as a serpent. To the present day there are people in Great Britain who have seen the disease serpent when exhibiting himself in the annoying illness called Shingles. One physician suffered so extremely as in moments of excessive pain to touch the rough scales of the imagined serpent with his hand.

Black (1967), p. 10

The deep, boring, stabbing or lancing pain of herpes zoster has been recognized since the days of the early Greeks. It caused physicians to devise forms of relief which varied as the practices of medicine changed as the dominant world view and the theories of the cause of the diseases evolved (Grossman, 1985).

Little is said of herpes zoster in the Hippocratic collection, perhaps because the ancient physician considered skin lesions as deformities and not disease. However, the significance of the Greek term 'herpes', which means something that creeps, is commonly employed in the earliest epoch of Greek medicine to designate chronic cutaneous diseases. The Roman Pliny used the word zona for the rash. According to Galen, herpes implied "a process that extended from one part to another in a serpiginous way" (Cumston, 1926). Today the Greek term herpes is linked with zoster, a Greek term for the belt a warrior used to secure his armour. Thus, together the term herpes zoster aptly describes the erythematous rash that creeps around one side of its victim. It is also appropriate that the common word 'shingles' has been used to describe this painful condition. Shingles is also an ancient term derived from the Latin word *cingere*, 'to grind'. This disease is certainly one which creeps round the girdle of one side of the body.

The Anglo-Saxon leechbooks of the Middle Ages provide ample evidence of the occurrence of herpes zoster. The Leechbook of Bald is the most important document to have survived from the Anglo-Saxon period. This book was the second leechbook belonging to a physician, or leech, known as Bald (Rubin, 1974, p. 55). The leechbooks were probably compiled as instructional texts and are rich in

* Correspondence to: Dr. T.J. Murray, MS Unit, Dalhousie University Medical School, Sir Charles Tupper Medical Building, Room 2L-A2 (2nd Floor-Link), Halifax, NS B3H 4H7, Canada. Fax: +1 (902) 494-2074; E-mail: jock.murray@dal.ca

[1] Anonymous (1979). Shingles: A belt of roses from hell.

a variety of surgical techniques based more upon traditional ideas than on any knowledge of pathological process. In many cases, alternative remedies are cited and hence the leech gives the illusion of considerable choice in his day to day practice. In reality, many of the necessary ingredients for those folk cures were too exotic for the local leech. In these leechbooks reference is made to the "Circular adle (disease)" which can be identified with certainty as herpes zoster (Rubin, 1974, p. 57). Treatment of this condition, or any kind of wound "whether internally or externally" consisted of a prescribed salve of "waybroad beaten and mixed with old lard, the fresh is of no use. Take waybroad seed, crush it small, shed it on the wound and soon it will be better" (Rubin, 1974, p. 60). This type of folk therapy for zoster recurs over the centuries in history. Barbers, bathkeepers, magicians, alchemists, surgeons, Indians, settlers, Victorian physicians — all who pursued the art of healing, prescribed herbal remedies. Herbs were considered invaluable on account of their healing and curative powers. Culpeper, in his book (1653) on herbal remedies, recommends cinquefoil, nightshade and cow parsnip, and advises that "the juice of the herb and berries, with oil of roses and a little vinegar, beaten in a mortar, is good to anoint all hot inflammations in the eyes. It is good for the shingles, and painful sores with heat and putrefaction" (Culpeper, 1985). In old England women applied the blood of a black cat's tail to the affected area. Whereas among New England wisemen, the blood of a perfectly black hen "will cure rheumatism, shingles, or, in fact, anything if applied externally" (Black, 1967, p. 117).

It was not until 1831 that the neurological basis of herpes zoster was suspected. It was then that Richard Bright suggested that the characteristic distribution of the rash was due to segmental nerve involvement (Bright, 1831). Romberg noted its relationship to neuralgia in 1855 (Romberg, 1855). Ten years later, Von Barensprung completed studies which identified the dorsal root ganglion corresponding to the level of the skin rash (Von Barensprung, 1861, 1862) shown to be similar in the trigeminal ganglion by Hutchinson (1864).

When epidemics of herpes zoster were reported (Weiss, 1890) the idea that it was an infection became prominent. Nielsen believed arsenic could cause herpes zoster and thought this did not rule out the possibility that it was an underlying infection (Nielsen, 1893).

Sir William Gowers discussed neuralgic pain from herpes and noted that Sir William Jenner in his lectures, used to illustrate the "obstinate persistence" of this pain in the elderly by the instance of a man who endured the excision of his skin in the area of pain, without anaesthetic, in the unsuccessful hope that it would give him relief. Finding none, he shot himself (Gowers, 1888). Osler also referred to a patient whose intractable neuralgia drove him to suicide (Osler, 1892).

Although herpes zoster is a disease quite distinct from herpes simplex, it is very closely allied to chicken pox. In 1892, Von Bokay established that zoster and varicella were different manifestations of the same etiological process (Von Bokay, 1909). Following this initial discovery, Sir Henry Head and A.V. Campbell (1900) undertook the most comprehensive pathological study of herpes zoster published as a 170 page article in Brain. [2] They discovered that the pathological changes of herpes zoster were usually limited to one dorsal root ganglion or to the sensory ganglion of a cranial nerve and the closest corresponding nerve root. They noted that certain spinal root ganglia were more often affected than others. These were the second, third and fourth cervical, the thoracic from the second downwards, and the first lumbar ganglia.

Of the cranial ganglia the gasserian (trigeminal) was noted to be most commonly attacked, usually its internal part which is related to the ophthalmic division (Head and Campbell, 1900). Sir Henry Head also found that a number of patients presented symptoms and signs highly suggestive of zoster but without its characteristic rash. This complication of herpes zoster was coined 'zona fruste' by Widal (1907)

---

[2] An offprint of this classical article, signed by Head, was for sale for $1850 U.S.

and 'zoster sine herpete' by Weber (1916). Head (1910) described a series of 416 cases of herpes zoster, noting that in a few cases vesicles were found across the mid-line. He described one case with involvement of T8 on the left and T10 on the right. Twenty-two of his cases were trigeminal, 18 in the first division, 2 in the second and 2 in the third. This selective choice "amid ganglion-cells adds another to zona's unsolved problems", commented Kinnier Wilson (Wilson, 1940, p. 676). Head's (1910) research also revealed that the ratio was almost 2:1 for males:females. This is quite opposed to most subsequent studies which have shown an equal sex incidence. He noted the increased occurrence in various months, particularly in the spring, and suggested occasional epidemics. This has been proven not to be true. It is difficult to know how to interpret Head's patient material. He cites 75% of his cases as being under age 25, which is entirely opposed to other studies (Bruusgaard, 1932) and current experience, which indicates that it is rare in children and most common in the elderly.

Ludwig Nielsen of Copenhagen wrote of the observation that herpes zoster occurred in patients treated with arsenic (Nielsen, 1893). Others had noted that herpes zoster was seen in cases of psoriasis, chorea, 'nervous debility' and carbon monoxide poisoning treated with arsenic. He noted that Kaposi and others thought it was coincidental, even though it occurred in 1.8% of the cases of psoriasis, as both conditions were common. Nielsen noted, however, that no cases were seen in 200 cases of psoriasis treated with potassium iodide. Nielsen describes details of 10 cases of arsenic induced zoster.

An unusual observation was made in 1901 with epidemic zona described as a feature of arsenic poisoning from adulterated beer (Reynolds, 1901). Yet, to Kinnier Wilson: "How a metal like arsenic can activate the virus or aid its entry can hardly even be guessed" (Wilson, 1940, p. 683). He goes on to state that "most cases recover without a hitch". In the acute state he recommended rest and 'febrifuge', and if pre-herpetic neuralgia developed it was treated by anodynes (Wilson, 1940, p. 683).

F. Parkes Weber described two cases of herpes zoster associated with a varicella-like eruption. He added it was doubtless a mere coincidence that a four-year-old boy who was on the ward with one of the patients developed varicella ten days later when he was discharged home (Weber, 1916b). At the turn of the century there were twenty such reports of the association of herpes zoster with a simultaneous varicella, including a French report of 26 cases. Weber reviewed the literature on this topic (Weber, 1916a).

It was not until 1919 that the zoster virus was positively identified. Using only a light microscope, Paschen was able to successfully identify the zoster virus (Parry, 1973) thereby setting the stage for the work of Netter and Urbain (1926). These two scientists completed the earliest serological studies on Paschen's isolated virus in an attempt to test for its antibody. In 1926, Netter and Urbain convincingly showed the similarity of antigens in the vesicle fluids from zoster and varicella eruptions. Finally, Blank and Rake (1955) were able to successfully prove the relationship between varicella and zoster, first suggested by Von Bokay in 1892. They suggested that it was analogous to a primary and recurrent manifestation of the same herpetic process.

Traditionally there have been two main platforms in the debate regarding the mode of transmission of herpes zoster. One school of thought believes that the virus is transmitted by exposure (Palmer et al., 1985), while others subscribe to the theory that it is caused by reactivation of the latent virus (Miller and Brunell, 1970). Glynn et al. (1990) conducted a retrospective study of 1019 patients with acute zoster infection. Their research failed to demonstrate a relationship between the two infections and concluded it was unlikely that the varicella-zoster virus is infective or that re-exposure to the virus caused reactivation of the latent virus. Another major contribution to our current knowledge about zoster is the extensive work done by Hope-Simpson (1965) (see Chapter 1). The Hope-Simpson hypothesis that zoster is due to reactivation of a latent VZ virus found in sensory ganglia during a time of declining immunity, is widely accepted today (Huff, 1988).

Since these early discoveries, research into herpes zoster has focused on methods of treatment.

As modern therapeutics unveil new drugs and treatments, these have been put to the test in the therapy of this "belt of roses from hell" (Anonymous, BMJ, 1979). As the area of the acquired immunodeficiency syndrome (AIDS) dawned, researchers found new challenges in the search for a better treatment for herpes zoster and its accompanying neuralgia. The immunosuppressed population with AIDS and cancer, as well as the elderly are especially susceptible to herpes zoster.

The plight of the sufferer was recently described by Thomas C. Thomsen, an advertising writer who wrote an advice book for other patients, as he felt there was a dearth of information to guide sufferers. He had been suffering with postherpetic neuralgia since 1986 (Thomsen, 1994).

Prevention of herpes zoster may be available in the near future in the form of vaccination against varicella. Until recently, all the physician had to offer patients afflicted with this ailment were analgesics, sympathy, and a liberal dose of hope. New understanding of the underlying infection, new drugs for relief, and inroads to effective prevention will characterize the future.

References

Anonymous (1979) Quoted in: Shingles: A belt of roses from hell. BMJ, 1: 5.

Black, W.G. (1967) Folk Medicine: A Chapter in the History of Culture. Kraus Reprint, Nendeln-Lichtenstein.

Bruusgaard, E. (1932) Mutual relation between zoster and varicella. Br. J. Dermatol. Syph., 44: 1.

Blank, H., and Rake, G. (1955) Viral and Rickettsial Diseases of the Skin, Eye, and Mucous Membranes of Man. Little, Brown and Co., Boston, MA, p. 71.

Bright, R. (1831) Reports of Medical Cases. London, Vol. 2, Part 1, p. 383.

Culpeper, N. (1985), Complete Herbal. Omega Books, St. Paul, MN, p. 206. (Originally published in 1653.)

Cumston, C.G. (1926) The history of herpes from the earliest times to the nineteenth century. Ann. Med. Hist., 8: 284.

Glynn, C. et al. (1990) Epidemiology of shingles. J. R. Soc. Med., 83: 617–619.

Gowers W.R. (1888) A Manual of Disease of the Nervous System. T.P. Blakston, Son and Co, Philadelphia, PA, p. 22.

Grossman, R. (1985) The Other Medicines: An invitation to Understanding and Using them for Health and Healing. Doubleday and Company, New York, p. 123.

Head, H. (1910) Herpes zoster. In: C. Allbutt and H.D. Rolleston (Eds.), A System of Medicine, Vol. 7. MacMillan and Company, London, 2nd ed., pp. 470–492.

Head, H. and Campbell, A.W. (1900) The pathology of herpes zoster and its bearing on sensory location. Brain, 22: 353–523. (This elegant 170 page paper was recently reprinted in an abridged 12 page summary in Med. Virol., 1997; 7: 131–143.)

Hope-Simpson, R.E. (1965) The nature of herpes zoster: a long-term study and a new hypothesis. Proc. R. Soc. Med., 58: 9–20.

Huff, J.C. (1988) Current Problems in Dermatology: Herpes Zoster (monograph). Yearbook Medical Publishers, p. 14.

Hutchinson, J. (1864) Clinical report on herpes zoster frontalis ophthalmicus. Ophtha Hosp. Rep., 1864; 3: 72; 5: 191. 1867-9; 6: 181.

Miller, L.A. and Brunell, P.A. (1970) Zoster, reinfection or activation of latent virus. Am. J. Med., 49: 480–483.

Nielsen, L. (1893) On the Appearance of Herpes Zoster during the Administration of Arsenic. New Sydenham Society, London, p. 167, p. 174, p. 578.

Netter, A. and Urbain, A. (1926) Relations between herpes zoster and chickenpox: serologic study of 100 cases of herpes zoster. C. R. Soc. Biol., 94 (Jan.): 98–100.

Osler, W. (1892) The Principles and Practice of Medicine. Appleton and Co., New York, p. 961.

Palmer, S.R. et al. (1985) An outbreak of shingles. Lancet, 2: 1108–1111.

Parry, W.H. (1973) Communicable Diseases: An Epidemiological approach. The English Universities Press Ltd., London, p. 52.

Reynolds, E.S. (1901) An account of the epidemic outbreak of arsenical poisoning occurring in beer drinkers in North of England and the Midland counties in 1900. Med.-Chir. Trans. London, 84: 409–452.

Romberg, M.H. (1955) A Manual of the Nervous Diseases of Man. The Sydenham Society, London.

Rubin, S. (1974) Medieval English Medicine. David and Charles, Newton Abbey, UK and Barnes and Noble, New York, USA.

Thomsen, T.C. (1994) Shingles and postherpetic neuralgia. Cross River Press, Cross River, New York.

Von Barensprung, F.G.F. (1861) Die Gurtelkrankheit, Ann. Char.-Krankenh. Berlin, 9: 40–238.

Von Barensprung, F.G.F. (1862) Beiträge zur Kenntnis des Zoster. Ann. Char.-Krankenh. Berlin, 10: 96–104.

Von Bokay, I. (1909) Über den ätiologischen Zusammenhang der varicellen mit gewissen fallen von Herpes Zoster. Wein Klin. Wochenschr. (suppl.), 39: 1323.

Weber, F.P. (1916a) Herpes zoster; its occasional association with a generalized eruption and its occasional connection with muscular paralysis; also an analysis of the literature of the subject. Int. Clin. Philadelphia, 3: 185.

Weber, F.P. (1916b) Two cases of Herpes Zoster associated with a generalized eruption of varicella spots: one of the cases followed by oculomotor paresis, mydriasis and frontal anesthesia. Br. J. Dermatol., Jan–Mar, p. 1–14.

Weiss, E. (1890) Epidemic zoster. Arch. Dermatol. Syph., p. 629.

Widal, G.F.I. (1907) Le Zona fruste. J. Med. Chir. Prat., 78: 12.

Wilson, S.A.K. (1940) Neurology, Vol. 1, A.N. Bruce (Ed.). Edward Arnold and Co., London, p. 676, p. 683.

Herpes Zoster and Postherpetic Neuralgia, 2nd Revised and Enlarged Edition
Pain Research and Clinical Management, Vol. 11
Edited by C.P.N. Watson and A.A. Gershon

CHAPTER 4

The varicella-zoster virus

Ann M. Arvin [*]

*Department of Pediatrics and Microbiology and Immunology, Stanford University School of Medicine,
Stanford, CA 94305, USA*

1. Introduction

Varicella-zoster virus (VZV) is a human alphaherpesvirus that causes varicella (chicken pox) during primary infection and establishes latency in dorsal root ganglia; reactivation of latent VZV results in herpes zoster. VZV is one of the eight herpesviruses responsible for human disease; among these viruses, it is related most closely to herpes simplex virus 1 (HSV-1), which is the prototype of the alphaherpesviruses (Arvin, 1995; Cohen and Straus, 1995). VZV also shares many genetic similarities with simian varicella virus (SVV) (Gray et al., 1993). Contemporary investigations of VZV as an infectious agent began with the detection of multinucleated cells in cultures of human skin cells on allantoic membranes following inoculation with zoster vesicle fluid (Goodpasture and Anderson, 1944) and the isolation of the virus in cell culture (Weller, 1953). Confirmation of the virologic relationship between varicella and zoster was proved by restriction endonuclease analysis of VZV DNA from varicella lesions and a subsequent episode of zoster in the same individual (Straus et al., 1984). Further evidence that zoster is due to reactivation of the original infecting strain of VZV is provided by the analysis of isolates from episodes of zoster in recipients of the live attenuated varicella vaccine, which have been shown to be caused by the vaccine Oka strain (Hayakawa et al., 1984; Williams et al., 1985).

2. The viral genome, replication and the virion structure

2.1. Organization of the genome

VZV is the smallest of the alphaherpesviruses, with a genome consisting of approximately 125 kilobase pairs (kb). The genome is organized as unique long (UL) and short (US) sequences, each of which is flanked by repeated sequences, referred to as internal (IR) and terminal repeats (TR) (Fig. 1). The complete sequence of the VZV Dumas genome was reported in 1986 (Davison and Scott, 1986); the parent Oka and the vaccine Oka strains have also now been sequenced, and genetic differences have been described (Gomi et al., 2000; Argaw et al., 2000). The VZV genome has at least 69 unique open reading frames (ORFs) and three genes that are duplicated in the repeats (ORFs 62/71, 63/70; ORFs 64/69) (reviews: Ruyechan and Hay, 2000; Cohen and Straus, 1995). Although VZV has the smallest genome, the TRL/IRL is larger in VZV than the

* Correspondence to: Dr. A.M. Arvin, Department of Pediatrics and Microbiology and Immunology, Stanford University School of Medicine, Stanford, CA 94305, USA.

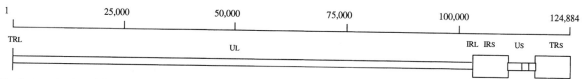

Fig. 1. Organization of the VZV genome. The VZV genome is a linear double-stranded DNA molecule. It consists of long unique and short unique sections, each of which is flanked by repeats. Genes duplicated in the repeat regions are ORF62/71, 63/70 and 64/69; origins of replication are located in each of the repeats of the short unique segment.

other alphaherpesviruses. Because of the repeat regions, VZV DNA can be synthesized as molecules that vary in the orientation of UL and US, although in VZV, few virion DNA molecules have UL in the inverse orientation. The VZV genome also has five regions in which a series of nucleotides is repeated, which are designated R1 (ORF11), R2 (ORF14), R3 (ORF22), R4 (US repeat regions, two copies) and R5 (within an intragenic region of UL). Most VZV genes are expressed from unique promoters, although some genes located on the same strand have a downstream polyadenylation site in common, as illustrated by VZV ORF46–49. The linear order of genes in the VZV genome resembles HSV-1, but recombination at sites between the US and the IRs or TRs seems to have resulted in transfer of genes into the VZV repeat regions. For example, VZV ORF64 is the homologue of HSV US10, but ORF64 is located in the IR-S and is duplicated as ORF69 in the TR-S, whereas HSV US10 is present as a single copy in the US region. VZV differs from other alphaherpesviruses in having only two glycoprotein genes in the US region; of note, VZV lacks the gene for gD, which is essential in HSV, as well as any gG homolog. Conversely, VZV has five ORFs not found in HSV, including ORFs 1, 2, 13, 32 and 57.

2.2. Events in replication

The kinetics of VZV transcription and replication have not been defined because cell-free virions cannot be recovered in sufficient titers to allow synchronous infection of tissue culture cells at a high multiplicity. VZV genes are probably expressed as α (immediate-early, IE), β (early, E) and γ (late) genes, as is characteristic of other herpesviruses. No direct evidence is available for VZV, but the linear DNA

molecule is presumed to circularize by ligation of the termini, by analogy with HSV; after replication, VZV DNA must be cleaved into genome full length genome segments, and packaged into capsids.

2.3. Virion formation

The physical structure of the VZV virion consists of an icosahedral capsid within which the full length viral DNA genome is packaged. The capsid is surrounded by the tegument, made up of several viral proteins that act to initiate DNA replication when the virus enters the host cell. Of these tegument proteins, the IE62 transactivating protein is predominant. The virion envelope is the outermost component of the complete virus particle; this lipid membrane contains glycoproteins that are presumed to mediate cell entry.

2.4. Genetic stability

The VZV genome exhibits relative genetic stability during in vitro propagation, to the degree that changes can be detected by restriction digest analysis of viral DNA using multiple enzymes (Cohen and Straus, 1995). Although VZV isolates of diverse origins have variable restriction enzyme profiles, altered patterns of viral replication in cell culture have not been associated with spontaneously occurring genetic variations. The exception is a newly identified VZV strain with a mutation in gE, which exhibits accelerated cell–cell spread, increased numbers of cell surface virions and increased infectivity in the SCIDhu skin model (Santos et al., 1998, 2000). This change in VZV phenotype is due to a single amino acid substitution at residue 150 in the ectodomain of gE, and represents a gE antibody 'escape mutant'. Inhibition of thymidine kinase expression can be induced by passage of VZV in the presence of acyclovir or related antiviral agents and mutants with downregulation of gC synthesis can be recovered by plaque purification from VZV strains passed in fibroblasts (Kinchington et al., 1990). The availability of new sequencing technologies is beginning to reveal genetic differences between VZV strains; comparing the sequences of the vaccine strain of VZV Oka and its parent strain has received particular attention (Gomi et al., 2000; Argaw et al., 2000). Current evidence suggests that prominent differences that are associated with changes in amino acid residues occur in ORF62. Mutations are also relatively common in ORF14, which encodes gC, but the other VZV glycoproteins of vaccine Oka show few changes.

3. The viral proteins

The functions of some VZV proteins have been defined but the contributions of others are presumed from the sequence homologies with HSV proteins of known function (Kinchington and Cohen, 2000) (Table I). Many of the other VZV genes have sequence relationships to HSV ORFs but functions are not identified for the prototype. Two genes that encode glycoproteins, ORF5 which encodes gK, and ORF68 which encodes gE, are required for VZV replication (Mo et al., 1999; Mo and Arvin, unpublished data). Several VZV genes are dispensable in tissue culture (Table I). However, it is important to note that some of these ORFs, including ORFs 14, 47, and 66 are required infectivity or for optimal replication in differentiated human cells in vivo (Moffat et al., 1998a,b).

The major nucleocapsid protein of VZV is encoded by ORF40, with ORF33.5 being a putative assembly protein. Seven VZV ORFs resemble gene products required for origin-dependent DNA synthesis in HSV. These genes and their known or putative functions are ORF28: polymerase catalytic subunit; ORF16: polymerase processivity, accessory to ORF28 protein; ORF29: major single strand DNA

binding protein; ORFs 6, 52, 55: heterotrimeric helicase/primase complex; and ORF51: origin binding protein.

Several VZV gene products that are incorporated into the virion tegument during assembly of mature virions have transactivating functions for other viral genes. These proteins are encoded by ORFs 4, 10, 61, and the duplicated genes, 62/71 and 63/70; ORF61 also has transrepressor activity (Ruyechan and Hay, 2000; Spengler, 2000; Kinchington et al., 1992). A number of VZV genes encode proteins that have enzyme functions. Of these, ORF47 and ORF66 gene products are serine/threonine protein kinases. The ORF8 gene product is a dUTPase, ORF13 encodes thymidylate synthetase and ORFs 18 and 19 gene products are the small and large subunit ribonucleotide reductases, respectively. The genome also has genes for protease (ORF33), thymidine kinase (ORF36), deoxyribonuclease (ORF48) and uracil-DNA glycosylase (ORF59). Several of these genes have been shown to be dispensable for replication in tissue culture (Table I).

The seven VZV glycoproteins that have been characterized are gB, gC, gE, gH, gI, gK and gL; a putative ORF for gM is present by genome sequencing. The order of their location along the linear genome is: ORF5, gK; ORF14, gC; ORF31, gB; ORF37, gH; ORF50, gM; ORF60, gL; ORF67, gI; and ORF68, gE (Kinchington and Cohen, 2000; Kinchington et al., 1986). The glycoproteins of the VZV envelope are presumed to mediate cellular attachment and penetration, as well as fusion of infected cell membranes and cell to cell spread of the virus. VZV gB, like other herpesviral gB proteins, is highly conserved and probably acts during attachment and fusion of the virus to cell membranes. VZV gE is a multifunctional protein that forms heterodimers with gI, and gI has a chaperone function for gE intracellular trafficking. VZV gI is necessary for replication in Vero cells, and while VZV lacking gI replicated in fibroblasts and melanoma cells, virus yields are lower, normal syncytial formation is disrupted and gE trafficking is altered (Mallory et al., 1997; Cohen and Nguyen, 1997). VZV gH and gL form a complex likely to be involved in cell–cell fusion and virion

TABLE I

VZV genes with known or putative functions

VZV gene	Established or predicted function and location	Dispensable in tissue culture	HSV homolog
1	membrane protein	yes	
4	transactivator, tegument protein		ICP27
10	transactivator, tegument protein	yes	VP16
61	transactivator, transrepressor	yes	ICP0
72, 71	transactivator, tegument protein		ICP4
63, 70	tegument		ICP22
47	protein kinase	yes	VP18.8
66	protein kinase	yes	
6	presumed helicase-primase		
8	dUTPase	yes	
9A	syncytia formation	yes	
13	thymidylate synthetase	yes	
16	presumed polymerase processivity		UL42
17	presumed viral host shut off		UL41
18	ribonucleotide reductase, small subunit		
19	ribonucleotide reductase, large subunit	yes	
28	DNA polymerase		
29	ssDNA binding protein		ICP8
32	probable substrate for ORF47 kinase	yes	
33	protease		VP24
33.5	assembly protein		VP22
36	thymidine kinase	yes	
40	major nucleocapsid protein		VP5
48	deoxyribonuclease		
51	origin binding protein		
52	presumed helicase/primase		UL8
55	presumed helicase primase		UL5
57	?	yes	
59	uracil-DNA glycosylase	yes	

egress from infected cells. VZV gK is a structural glycoprotein and is required for replication (Mo et al., 1999).

Among the other VZV genes, ORF1 encodes a membrane protein of unknown function which is not essential for replication in tissue culture. ORF9A is not essential but its disruption alters syncytia formation. ORF17 is homologous to HSV UL41, which is the viral host shut off protein. Of the genes present in VZV and not HSV, ORF32 is a probable substrate for the ORF47 kinase; the function of ORF57 is not known but it is dispensable in tissue culture. A novel protein of unknown function has been identified recently as a product of an ORF S/L

gene; deletion of this gene disrupts attachment of infected cells (Annunziato et al., 2000).

4. Characteristics of VZV infection in vitro

4.1. Tissue culture cells

VZV can be isolated in cultures of primary, diploid or transformed human cells and can be propagated in nonhuman cells, including monkey kidney cells and guinea pig embryo fibroblasts (review: Gershon et al., 1998). VZV-infected cells are visible by immunohistochemical staining methods within 4 to 10 h after inoculation. Cytopathic effects (CPE) appear 2 to 7 days after inoculation of vesicle fluid. CPE is characterized by syncytial formation. Infectious foci consist of rounded, refractile cells that become mult-inucleated giant cells with enlarged nuclei, abnormal nucleoli, and marginated chromatin. VZV virions are enclosed in membrane-lined vacuoles within the cytoplasm (Grose and Ng, 1992). Complete and partial virions, lacking a nucleocapsid, are visible by EM and CPE is associated with the formation of 'viral highways' that have virions visible on their surfaces (Olson and Grose, 1998). The replication of VZV is highly cell associated; virus is not released into supernatant and propagation requires the transfer of intact infected cells or an infected cell inoculum disrupted by trypsin, sonication, or freeze–thawing. Low quantities of cell-free virus can be obtained by sonication and gradient purification but the ratios of PFU to uninfected cells achieved range from 1 : 5 to 1 : 10. VZV is most infectious when the virion envelope is preserved and replication is also relatively temperature-dependent, with optimal growth at 32–33°C. Exposure to high temperatures (56–60°C), or storage above −70°C reduces or destroys infectivity.

4.2. VZV proteins dispensable or essential in vitro

A number of VZV genes can be deleted without altering the kinetics of VZV replication in cell culture and without changing CPE; these genes include those encoding thymidine kinase, dUTPase, thymidylate synthetase, uracil DNA glycosylase, the ORF47 and ORF66 serine/threonine protein kinases, ORF10 virion associated transactivator, the gene products of ORF32 and ORF57, and the glycoprotein, gC (Kinchington and Cohen, 2000). Other genes are dispensable for replication but plaque morphology is altered; when gI (ORF67) is deleted, or its expression is blocked, VZV mutants exhibit a small plaque phenotype with distortion of polykaryocyte formation in melanoma cells and no growth is detected in Vero cells (Mallory et al., 1997; Cohen and Nguyen, 1997). Syncytial formation is also reduced if the products of both ORF8 and ORF9A are not expressed (Ross et al., 1997). Deletion of

the ORF S/L protein causes rapid detachment of infected cells and removal of both copies of the diploid gene, ORF64/69 results in formation of extensive syncytia and polykaryocytes that have many nuclei (M. Sommer and A.M. Arvin, unpubl. data). Deletion of ORF68, encoding gE, is not compatible with VZV replication and gK (ORF5) is also an essential gene. Deletion of both copies of the diploid gene, ORF63/70 also blocks infectivity (M. Sommer and A.M. Arvin, unpubl. data).

4.3. VZV infection in specialized cells in vitro

VZV replication has been studied in vitro using differentiated primary human cells or cell lines related to the cell types that are infected during pathogenesis in vivo. VZV can infect activated peripheral blood mononuclear cells (PBMC) from healthy adults but only 0.01% of T cells were positive by in situ hybridization (Koropchak et al., 1989); higher percentages of cord blood T cells (3–5%) were infected in vitro (Soong et al., 2000). Transformed T-cell lines can be used to investigate transient expression of VZV proteins but are not permissive for replication (Perera et al., 1992). The IE62 protein has the potential to transactivate all classes of VZV genes in vitro in a human T-cell line and abortive replication was observed in a CD4+ T-cell hybridoma line (II23 cells) (Zerboni et al., 2000). The nonpermissiveness of most PBMC, including resting T cells, for VZV replication in vitro parallels the low frequency of VZV-infected mononuclear cells that can be detected during acute varicella (Mainka et al., 1998). Some replication of VZV is also observed in EBV-transformed human B lymphocytes in vitro (Koropchak et al., 1989). Although keratinocytes can be infected, infectious virus yields were low (Sexton et al., 1992) and these cells, which release cell-free virus into cutaneous vesicle fluid in vivo, do not allow viral egress in vitro. Primary cells derived from nervous system tissue, including Schwann cells and astrocytes, can be infected with VZV (Gilden et al., 1983; Somekh and Levin, 1993). Experiments using fetal dorsal root ganglia showed that the supporting non-neuronal cells were more susceptible to CPE than neurons (Assouline et al., 1990). Infection of cultures containing both human fetal neurons and satellite cells in the presence of bromovinylarauracil (BVaraU) followed by withdrawal of the antiviral resulted in recovery of infectious VZV but the cells did not become persistently infected (Somekh and Levin, 1993). The neuroblastoma cell line (IMR-32), also supports VZV replication (Bourdon-Wouters et al., 1990).

4.4. Effects of VZV on cellular proteins and functions in vitro

Syncytial formation is the most characteristic effect of VZV on cells in culture but VZV also has more subtle effects. Examples of these effects include the downregulation of the usual constitutive expression of major histocompatibility (MHC) class I molecules on the surface of infected cells (Cohen, 1998; Abendroth et al., 2000a). This effect has the potential to interfere with clearance of VZV-infected cells by antigen-specific CD8 T cells. It is observed on T cells infected with VZV, which may facilitate viral transport to cutaneous sites (Abendroth et al., 2000b) as well as on fibroblasts, which may delay control of viral replication at cutaneous sites. MHC class I molecules transit the ER but are retained in the Golgi compartment of VZV-infected cells but the viral protein or proteins that mediate this effect have not been identified.

VZV also blocks the upregulation of MHC class II expression which is induced by IFN-γ, with inhibition occurring at the level cellular gene transcription through the Jak–Stat pathway (Abendroth et al., 2000a). Interference with MHC class II presentation of viral peptides may reduce the initial CD4 T-cell response and the lack of MHC class II expression on VZV-infected cells from varicella and zoster lesions in vivo indicates that these cells may be protected transiently from immune surveillance by CD4 T cells. VZV does not downregulate MHC class II expression on cells exposed to IFN-γ before infection; therefore, the transfer of virus to adjacent uninfected cells may be prevented, since local release of IFN-γ should make these secondarily infected cells subject to immune clearance. Among other examples of ef-

fects of VZV on cellular functions, the virus has the capacity to inhibit apoptosis mediated by Fas ligand (Hata et al., 2000). VZV gE and gE/gI expression in polarized epithelial cells in vitro may also enhance formation of cell–cell junctions (Mo et al., 2000).

5. Characteristics of VZV infection in vivo: animal models

Because VZV exhibits a highly restricted host range compared to other herpesviruses, especially HSV, animal models have not been used extensively to examine events in VZV replication in vivo. Non-human primates can be infected but usually remain asymptomatic, with the exception of gorillas and chimpanzees (Myers and Connelly, 1992; Cohen et al., 1996). When African green monkeys, *Erythrocebus patas*, and pygmy marmosets were infected with VZV, no infectious virus was recovered but VZV IgG antibodies were induced; VZV antiserum given before challenge blocked seroconversion in African green monkeys, suggesting that viral replication had occurred. Although VZV infection is limited in primates, the close genetic relationship between VZV and SVV suggests that studies of SVV infection in its natural host should provide new insights about VZV pathogenesis (Mahalingam et al., 1998). Although rodents, including suckling mice, do not have signs of disease, viral DNA can be detected in ganglia. Transfer of virus to dorsal root ganglia cells has been documented following subcutaneous inoculation of adult rats and intraperitoneal inoculation of suckling mice, and in mice after ocular infection (Annunziato et al., 1998). The guinea pig model reproduces some critical events in VZV pathogenesis, including viremia and ganglion infection, and can be used to evaluate the host response to viral antigens (Myers and Connelly, 1992; Lowry et al., 1992; Sabella et al., 1993). However, it is difficult to achieve infection reproducibly and many animals remain asymptomatic.

VZV tropism for certain human cell types can be examined in the SCIDhu mouse model (Moffat et al., 1995, 1998a,b). These animals have allografts of hu-

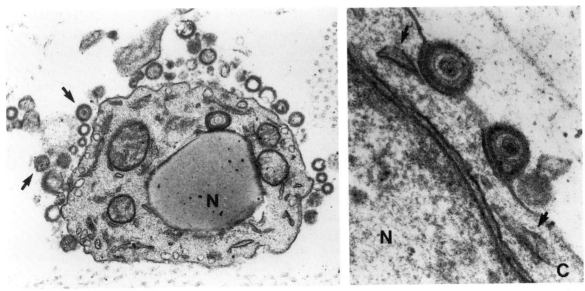

Fig. 2. VZV release from skin cells. Skin implants in SCIDhu mice were inoculated with a clinical isolate of VZV. This figure shows a transmission electron micrograph of skin cells 21 days after inoculation with a clinical isolate of VZV. Enveloped virions containing dense cores have dispersed from the cell. Residual vacuoles from which particles appeared to have exited the infected cell are visible adjacent to the cell membrane. Nucleocapsids are not visible in the nucleus (N) by this staining method. Magnification, ×24,000 (Moffat et al., 1998a).

man thymus/liver, containing CD4+, CD8+ and dual positive T cells, or human skin implants that can be inoculated with VZV. The model examines VZV pathogenesis in differentiated human cells without any immunomodulatory effect by the host response because the animals are immunodeficient. VZV infectivity for human T cells can be demonstrated by infectious focus assay and by flow cytometry; cell-free virus is released when T cells are infected with low passage VZV isolates. Infected skin implants develop epidermal vesicles with spread across the basement membrane to the dermis. Infected skin cells produce many virions by electron microscopy and infectious virus is released(Fig. 2; Moffat et al., 1998a).

6. Characteristics of VZV infection in vivo: pathogenesis in the human host

6.1. Entry

Primary VZV infection must begin with viral inoculation of mucous membranes, presumably of the respiratory tract. Nevertheless, infectious virus has not been recovered from this site in exposed individuals, in part because of the difficulty of ascertaining the occurrence of natural inoculation.

6.2. Site of primary replication and viral spread

As first suggested by Grose, VZV pathogenesis is thought to follow the Fenner model of mousepox (Grose, 1981). A number of the putative events in pathogenesis have not been documented, but infectious VZV is probably transferred first to regional lymph nodes; whether it replicates at this site is not known. Entry is presumed to be followed by a primary viremia with transport of the virus to the liver and other cells of the reticuloendothelial system. The occurrence of a secondary viremia in the last 4 or 5 days of the usual 10–21 day incubation period, or during the first 24 h of acute varicella has been proved by isolation of the virus from PBMC, by in situ hybridization and by PCR (Ozaki et al., 1986; Koropchak et al., 1991; Mainka et al., 1998). Secondary viremia is associated with VZV dissemination to cutaneous epithelial cells. The secondary viremia persists after the initial skin lesions appear, as shown by the recovery of VZV from 11% to 24% of PBMC samples taken within 24 h after the appearance of the varicella exanthem and its detection by in situ hybridization or PCR in 67% to 74% of cases (Koropchak et al., 1989; Sawyer et al., 1992). Cell-associated viremia is limited in the healthy host to only 0.01% to 0.001% of PBMC. The infected PBMC are cleared within 24 to 72 h after the rash appears. Which cell types are infected during natural infection has been difficult to determine but the permissiveness of human CD4+ as well as CD8+ T lymphocytes for VZV infection has been demonstrated in the SCIDhu model (Moffat et al., 1995).

VZV differs from the other human herpesviruses in that infectious virus is released into respiratory secretions, presumably from replication in epithelial cells of the mucous membranes, which allows airborne transmission of the virus (Grose, 1981; Asano et al., 1999). VZV is likely to be transported back to respiratory mucosal sites during the secondary viremia and must replicate there because transmission has been documented 24 to 48 h before the appearance of varicella rash. VZV is difficult to isolate from nasopharyngeal secretions during the preeruptive phase, but was found in 4.2% of cases and secretions are positive for VZV DNA by PCR when tested immediately before and after the onset of rash (Sawyer et al., 1992). Much of the transmissibility of VZV can be attributed to its skin tropism; high concentrations of cell-free virus are present in cutaneous vesicles, whether associated with varicella or zoster. The role of skin replication is illustrated by the observation that the vaccine strain has been transmitted only from individuals with vaccine-related rash (Tsolia et al., 1990).

6.3. Cellular and tissue tropism

The cell types that are involved in the pathogenesis of primary VZV infection include T cells, skin cells and neurons and satellite cells of the dorsal root ganglia. T-cell tropism appears to be essential but the site where these cells become infected and the

molecular mechanisms by which virus enters T cells have not been defined. Recent experiments indicate that VZV infects dendritic cells and that the virus can be transferred from these cells into T cells in vitro, events that could occur in regional lymph nodes or other reticuloendothelial tissues (A. Abendroth et al., pers. commun.). In skin, epidermal cells become the primary cells that support replication. How VZV reaches these cells is not certain; infected T cells may migrate from capillaries into skin tissue and release infectious virions (Moffat et al., 1995), or infectious virus may infect endothelial cells before spreading to adjacent epithelial cells. Viral inclusions and viral proteins have been observed in capillary endothelial cells and in adjacent fibroblasts, as well as in epithelial cells from VZV lesion biopsies (review: Arvin, 1998). In 1906, Tyzzer described the first changes in varicella skin lesions as consisting of vasculitis of the small blood vessels followed by appearance of enlarged, multinucleated epithelial cells with intranuclear eosinophilic inclusions (Tyzzer, 1906). Later events due to VZV replication include degeneration of epithelial cells, formation of multinucleated cells, and coalescence of fluid-filled vacuoles; larger lesions are associated with destruction of the germinal layer of the epithelium (Nikkels et al., 1995). Inflammatory cells increase as cutaneous lesions progress to ulceration, and dermal necrosis. VZV virions are present in the capillary endothelial cells and keratinocytes and cell-free virus is detected in vesicular fluid by electron microscopy. Macrophages contain virions in later stages of lesion progression. Immunohistochemical or in situ hybridization methods revealed expression of IE63 in keratinocytes initially, followed by gE, gB, and IE63 synthesis in keratinocytes, sebocytes, Langerhans cells, dermal dendrocytes, monocytes/macrophages, and endothelial cells; these VZV proteins were also detected in dermal nerves and in perineural type I dendrocytes (Annunziato et al., 2000). During replication in vivo, many VZV virions are released into vesicular fluid, accounting for the high rate of secondary spread among close contacts.

If VZV replication is not controlled by the host response, the virus exhibits a capacity to replicate extensively in other cell types (review: Arvin, 1998). Disseminated VZV is associated with lytic infection in differentiated cells that comprise the lungs, liver, central nervous system, and other organs (Myers, 1979). In the lungs, VZV infects the epithelial cells of the pulmonary alveoli and elicits a severe local inflammatory response; dense arrays of virions are visible in pulmonary epithelial cells. Transient replication in hepatic cells is probably a usual component of the pathogenesis of primary VZV infection but may progress to extensive cellular destruction. Some central nervous system infections with VZV represent direct viral invasion and infection of parenchymal cells (Takashima and Becker, 1979); VZV is also detected in brain cells in patients with multifocal leukoencephalitis and other neurologic manifestations are due either directly or indirectly to VZV (review: Gilden, 2000).

6.4. Persistence

Latent infection of cells in the dorsal root ganglia appears to be an invariable consequence of primary VZV infection (Gilden et al., 1983; Hyman et al., 1983; Straus et al., 1984; Furata et al., 1992). The viral determinants of virulence that are involved in this process are not known. The virus is presumed to be transported from mucocutaneous sites of replication by the neuronal cell axons to the dorsal root ganglia. Alternatively, the virus may reach sensory ganglia via infected PBMC independently of cutaneous replication. The dynamics of VZV interactions with neuronal and non-neuronal cells during latency have been perceived to differ significantly from the other human herpesviruses, for which episodes of asymptomatic reactivation can be demonstrated readily, as is the case for HSV, or the virus persists in circulating peripheral blood cells, as exemplified by HCMV and EBV. While VZV reactivation is difficult to document virologically unless skin lesions appear, subclinical VZV reactivation are likely to occur unless mechanisms for preserving latency are much more efficient in the case of VZV. Subclinical VZV viremia has been demonstrated (Devlin et al., 1992; Wilson et al., 1992; Schunemann et al.,

1998). Transcripts of VZV ORFs 21, 29, 62, and 63 have been detected and there is evidence that proteins of ORFs 4, 21, 29 and 62 are made in latently infected cells (Lungu et al., 1998). The molecular mechanisms of VZV latency are not understood, but the patterns of viral gene expression are quite different from the prototype, HSV-1, as described in subsequent chapters.

7. Virulence and attenuation

Although no systematic analyses have been done, the presumption from clinical experience is that naturally circulating strains of VZV do not differ significantly in their intrinsic virulence. The range of disease severity appears to be comparable in varicella epidemics that occur in different geographical locations and from year to year. Detailed information about the effects of genetic mutations on VZV virulence is quite limited. VZV gC-negative mutants have marked limitations in infectivity for human skin cells in the SCIDhu mouse model (Moffat et al., 1998a); VZV TK-negative viruses have been isolated from patients given prolonged acyclovir therapy, but no increases or decreases in pathogenicity have been described (Whitley, 1998). Investigations of VZV tropisms in the SCIDhu model indicate that the ORF47 gene product is a virulence determinant for T cells and skin (Moffat et al., 1998b). Eliminating the expression of ORF66, a second serine/threonine protein kinase unique to the alphaherpesviruses, was associated with decreased VZV infectivity for T cells but did not impair replication in skin (Moffat et al., 1998b).

The comparison of epidemiologically distinct VZV strains using polyclonal or monoclonal antibody reagents, suggests that there is very little antigenic diversity among VZV isolates. Japanese isolates have been shown to lack an epitope within the ORF10 gene product when compared with VZV strains from the United States and Europe, as assessed by reactivity to an antiserum generated to an ORF10 synthetic peptide (Kinchington and Turse, 1995). The ORF10 mutation and the gE ectodomain mutant identified in the United States (Santos et al., 1998) are the only examples of VZV antigenic variants that have been reported.

The live attenuated varicella vaccine is the first human herpesvirus vaccine licensed for clinical use in several countries (Takahashi, 1986; review: Arvin and Gershon, 1996; review: Krause and Klinman, 1995). The vaccine virus was derived from a clinical isolate of VZV, the Oka strain, and propagated in guinea pig embryo fibroblasts and WI38 cells. The vaccine strain of VZV Oka has been demonstrated to be attenuated for replication in healthy children and adults. In contrast to early experience in susceptible children who developed classic varicella after they were inoculated with VZV from vesicle fluid (von Bókay, 1909), administration of vaccine Oka virus by subcutaneous inoculation rarely produces any signs of infection. A comparative analysis of the vaccine virus in the SCID-hu mouse model demonstrated that vaccine Oka has a diminished capacity to replicate in human skin but remained infectious for T cells (Moffat et al., 1998a). The molecular mechanisms of attenuation of the Oka strain have not been identified, but can be pursued now that sequence comparisons are possible.

8. Host regulation of VZV replication

Virus–host interactions during primary VZV infection benefit the virus initially. Immune evasion during the incubation period, viremia and the first stages of cutaneous viral replication function to allow VZV transmission to susceptible contacts. The establishment of latency is also likely to occur in the early phase of infection. However, even during this interval, it is likely that uncontrolled VZV replication is prevented by mechanisms of innate immunity. Within a few days after the onset of the rash, or in some cases, just before lesions appear, adaptive humoral and cellular immune responses directed against VZV proteins develop. These responses evolve to a robust VZV-specific memory immunity that protects against illness upon subsequent exposures and preserves latency, or at least

blocks disease due to VZV reactivation until other factors, such as advanced age or immunosuppression impair memory immunity.

With respect to innate immune responses, interferon-alpha (IFN-α) is detected in serum when varicella lesions appear (Arvin et al., 1991; Wallace et al., 1994), and may limit early viral replication IFN-α. Natural killer (NK) cells can lyse VZV-infected fibroblasts and are enhanced by IFN-α and interleukin 2 (Bowden et al., 1985; Ito et al., 1986; review: Arvin, 1998). Granulysin is a novel cytolytic protein made by NK cells, as well as by antigen-specific CD8+ T lymphocytes. Granulysin promotes death of VZV-infected cells in vitro and inactivates intracellular virus (Hata et al., 2000).

The adaptive immune response to VZV includes the production of IgG, IgM, and IgA antibodies that bind many viral proteins (review: Gershon and LaRussa, 1998). Ant-VZV antibodies have neutralizing activity and function in antibody-mediated cellular cytotoxicity. Antibodies to gE and gI proteins neutralize VZV in the presence of complement (Litwin et al., 1992; Yao et al., 1993). Dominant antibody-binding epitopes of gE have been localized to residues 86–105, 116–135, and 56–75 (Fowler et al., 1995; Wu and Forghani, 1997). Antibodies to gB, gH and gC proteins have complement-independent neutralizing activity (Forghani et al., 1984). All of the major glycoproteins are also targets of VZV specific T cells (review: Arvin, 1998). VZV proteins other than the glycoproteins are also important targets of the host response. For example, antibodies to the viral thymidine kinase and regulatory proteins, such as IE62 and IE63 proteins are induced and regulatory/structural proteins as well as the viral glycoproteins, gB, gC, gE gH, gI, are recognized by VZV specific T-cells with helper and cytotoxic function.

Studies of VZV immune globulin prophylaxis show that passive antibodies present at or immediately after inoculation can restrict VZV replication. However, effective control of VZV infection requires the induction of active immunity mediated by VZV-specific T cells (review: Arvin, 1998). Intact cellular immunity appears to be important for terminating cell-associated viremia as well as limiting virus replication at localized cutaneous sites. T-cell responses to VZV proteins include production of cytokines of the TH1 type, including interleukin 2 (IL-2) and interferon gamma (IFN-γ). IFN-γ which potentiates the clonal expansion of virus-specific T cells, is detected in serum during acute varicella.

The balance between the virus and host is maintained for years after primary VZV infection by the persistence of adaptive immune responses. VZV memory T lymphocytes are maintained at frequencies of approximately 1 : 20,000–1 : 40,000 PBMC in immune adults (Levin and Hayward, 1996). Memory CD4+ and CD8+ CTL specific for VZV proteins are present at frequencies of about 1 : 150,000 PBMC. In immune adults, the mean percentage of VZV-specific CD4 T cells that produced IFN-γ was 0.12% by intracellular cytokine assay (Asanuma et al., 2000). Immune subjects also have persistent delayed hypersensitivity (DTH) responses to VZV skin test antigens (Kamiya et al., 1977). Cellular immunity is likely to be enhanced periodically in immune individuals by reexposure to cases of varicella or zoster. Although gene products of several VZV ORFs, including 21, 29, 62 and 63 may be expressed in neuronal cells during latency, it is presumed that immune surveillance is evaded because viral peptides can only be detected when complexed with MHC class I (Sadzot-Delvaux et al., 1997; Arvin et al., 1991). In contrast to other somatic cells, MHC class I expression by neurons requires IFN-γ induction. How latently infected satellite cells are protected from immune mechanisms is not certain, although co-stimulatory molecules necessary for T-cell recognition may not be expressed.

9. Summary

The current knowledge suggests that there is no definitive relationship between the infecting strain of wild-type VZV and virulence in the human host. The presumption is that host factors are more critical determinants of the outcome of the primary infection than the infecting strain, and that herpes zoster results when the host response is perturbed, rather than as a result of a differences in the propensity of VZV strains to reactivate from latency. However, these concepts may change as new methods to find and analyze VZV variants become available, as illustrated by the identification of the gE 'escape' mutant (Santos et al., 1998). Virologic mechanisms that might be associated with an enhanced or diminished risk of reactivation herpes zoster have not been described. Universal immunization with the attenuated Oka vaccine should provide an new insights about the relative contributions of viral and host factors to VZV-related disease. For example, the extent of initial viral replication could affect the propensity of VZV to cause herpes zoster. Triggering of viral reactivation certainly occurs even in the intact host; what factors allow viral gene expression to progress to lytic replication are not known. Nevertheless, the consequences of VZV reactivation can be modified by medical interventions, such as antiviral therapy or pain management, as described in this volume.

References

Abendroth, A., Slobedman, B., Lee, E., Mellins, E., Wallace, M. and Arvin, A.M. (2000a) Modulation of major histocompatibility class II expression by varicella zoster virus. J. Virol., 74: 1900–1907.

Abendroth, A., Lin, I., Ploegh, H. and Arvin, A.M. (2000b). Varicella zoster virus retains major histocompatibility complex class I molecules in the Golgi compartment of infected cells. J. Virology, in revision.

Annunziato, P., LaRussa, P., Lee, P., Steinberg, S., Lungo, O., Gershon, A.A. and Silverstein, S. (1998) Evidence of latent varicella-zoster virus in rat dorsal root ganglia. J. Infect. Dis., 178(Suppl. 1): 48–51.

Annunziato, P., Lungu, O., Gershon, A. and Silverstein, S. (2000) Varicella-zoster virus proteins in skin lesions: implications for a novel role of ORF29p in chicken pox. J. Virol., 74: 2005–2010.

Argaw, T., Cohen, J.I., Klutch, M. et al. (2000) Nucleotide sequences that distinguish Oka vaccine from parental Oka and other varicella-zoster virus isolates. J. Infect. Dis., 18: 1153–1157.

Arvin, A.M. (1995) Varicella-zoster virus. In: B. Fields, D. Knipe and P. Howley (Eds.), Virology. Lippincott-Raven Press, Philadelphia, PA, pp. 2547–2586.

Arvin, A. (1998) Varicella-zoster virus: Virologic and immunologic aspects of persistent infection. In: R. Ahmed and I. Chen (Eds.), Persistent Viral Infections. Wiley, New York, pp. 183–208.

Arvin, A.M. and Gershon, A.A. (1996) Live attenuated varicella vaccine. Annu. Rev. Microbiol., 50: 59–100.

Arvin, A.M., Sharp, M., Smith, S., Koropchak, C.M., Diaz, P.S., Kinchington, P., Ruyechan, W. and Hay, J. (1991) Equivalent recognition of a varicella-zoster virus immediate early protein (IE62) and glycoprotein I by cytotoxic T lymphocytes of either CD4+ or CD8+ phenotype. J. Immunol., 146: 257–264.

Asano, Y., Yoshikawa, T. et al. (1999) Spread of varicella-zoster virus DNA to family members and environments from siblings with varicella in a household. Pediatrics, 103: 61.

Asanuma, H., Sharp, M., Maecker, H.T., Maino, V.C. and Arvin, A.M. (2000) Frequencies of memory T cells specific for varicella-zoster virus, herpes simplex virus and cytomegalovirus determined by intracellular detection of cytokine expression. J. Infect. Dis., 181: 859–866.

Assouline, J.G., Levin, M.J., Major, E.O., Forghani, B., Straus, S.E. and Ostrove, J.M. (1990) Varicella-zoster virus infection of human astrocytes, Schwann cells, and neurons. Virology, 179: 834–844.

Bourdon-Wouters, C., Merville-Louis, M.P., Sadzot-Delvaux C. et al. (1990) Acute and persistent varicella-zoster virus infection of human and murine neuroblastoma cell lines. J. Neurosci. Res., 26: 90–97.

Bowden, R.A., Levin, M.J., Giller, R.H., Tubergen, D.G. and Hayward, A.R. (1985) Lysis of varicella-zoster virus infected cells by lymphocytes from normal humans and immunosuppressed pediatric leukemic patients. Clin. Exp. Immunol., 60: 387–395.

Cohen, J.I. (1998) Infection of cells with varicella-zoster virus down-regulates surface expression of class I major histocompatibility complex antigens. J. Infect. Dis., 177: 1390–1393.

Cohen, J.I. and Nguyen, H. (1997) Varicella-zoster virus glycoprotein I is essential for growth of virus in Vero cells. J. Virol., 71: 6913–6920.

Cohen, J. and Straus, S. (1995) Varicella-zoster virus and its replication. In: B. Fields, D. Knipe and P. Howley (Eds.), Virology. Lippincott-Raven Press, Philadelphia, PA, pp. 2547–2586.

Cohen, J.I., Moskal, T. et al. (1996) Varicella in chimpanzees. J. Med. Virol., 1996; 50: 289–292.

Davison, A.J. and Scott, J.E. (1986) The complete DNA sequence of varicella-zoster virus. J. Gen. Virol., 67: 1759–1816.

Devlin, M.E., Gilden, D.H., Mahalingam, R., Dueland, A.N. and Cohrs, R. (1992) Peripheral blood mononuclear cells of the elderly contain varicella-zoster virus DNA. J. Infect. Dis., 165: 619–622.

Forghani, B., Dupuis, K.W. and Schmidt, N. (1984) Varicella-zoster viral glycoproteins analyzed with monoclonal antibodies. J. Virol., 52: 55–62.

Fowler, W.J., Garcia, V.M. et al. (1995) Identification of im-munodominant regions and linear B cell epitopes of the gE envelope protein of varicella-zoster virus. Virology, 214: 531–540.

Furata, Y., Takasu, T., Fukuda, S. et al. (1992) Detection of varicella-zoster virus DNA in human geniculate ganglia by polymerase chain reaction. J. Infect. Dis., 166: 1157–1159.

Gershon, A.A. and LaRussa, P.S. (1998) Varicella vaccine. Pediatr. Infect. Dis. J., 146: 257–264.

Gershon, A.A., Steinberg, S.P. and Schmidt, N.J. (1998) Varicella-zoster virus. In: A. Balows, W.J. Hauseler, K.L. Herrman, H.D. Isenberg and H.J. Shadomy (Eds.), Manual of Clinical Microbiology. American Society for Microbiology, Washington, DC, pp. 900–911.

Gilden, D. (2000) Postherpetic neuralgia and other neurologic complications. In: A.M. Arvin and A.A. Gershon (Eds.), Varicella-zoster Virus: Virology and Clinical Management. Cambridge University Press, pp. 460–476.

Gilden, D.H., Vafai, A., Shtram, Y., Becker, Y., Devlin, M. and Wellish, M. (1983) Varicella-zoster virus DNA in human sensory ganglia. Nature, 306: 478–480.

Gomi, Y., Imagawa, T., Takahashi, M. and Yamanishi, K. (2000) Oka varicella vaccine is distinguishable from its parental virus in DNA sequence open reading frame 62 and its transactivation activity. J. Med. Virol., 61: 497–503.

Goodpasture, E.W. and Anderson, K. (1944) Infection of human skin, grafted on the chorioallantois of chick embryos with the virus of herpes zoster. Am. J. Pathol., 20: 447–455.

Gray, W.L., Gusick, N., Fletcher, T.M. and Pumphrey, C.Y. (1993) Characterization and mapping of simian varicella virus transcripts. J. Gen. Virol., 74: 1639–1643.

Grose, C. (1981) Variation on a theme by Fenner: the pathogenesis of chickenpox. Pediatrics, 68: 735–737.

Grose, C. and Ng, T.I. (1992) Intracellular synthesis of varicella-zoster virus. J. Infect. Dis., 166(Suppl. 1): S7–S12.

Hata, A., Kaspar, A., Krenksy, A., Zerboni, L., Krensky, A.M. and Arvin, A.M. (2000) Antiviral activity of granulysin against varicella-zoster virus. Viral Immunol., in press.

Hayakawa, Y., Torigoe, S., Shiraki, K., Yamanishi, K. and Takahashi, M. (1984) Biologic and biophysical markers of a live varicella vaccine strain (Oka): identification of clinical isolates from vaccine recipients. J. Infect. Dis., 149: 956–963.

Hyman, R.W., Ecker, J.R. and Tenser, R.B. (1983) Varicella-zoster virus RNA in human trigeminal ganglia. Lancet, 2: 814–816.

Ito, M., Bandyopadhyay, S., Matsumoto-Kobayashi, M., Clark, S.C., Miller, D. and Starr, S.E. (1986) Interleukin 2 enhances natural killing of varicella-zoster virus infected targets. Clin. Exp. Immunol., 65: 182–190.

Kamiya, H., Ihara, T., Hattori, A. et al. (1977) Diagnostic skin test reactions with varicella virus antigen and clinical application of the test. J. Infect. Dis., 136: 784–788.

Kinchington, P.R. and Cohen, J. (2000) Viral proteins. In: A.M. Arvin and A.A. Gershon (Eds.), Varicella-Zoster Virus: Virology and Clinical Management. Cambridge University Press, pp. 74–104.

Kinchington, P.R. and Turse, S.E. (1995) Molecular basis for a geographic variation of varicella-zoster virus recognized by a peptide antibody. Neurology, 45(Suppl. 8): S13–S14.

Kinchington, P.R., Remenich, J., Ostrove, J.M., Straus, S.E., Ruyechan, W.T. and Hay, J. (1986) Putative glycoprotein gene of varicella-zoster virus with variable copy numbers of a 42-base-pair repeat sequence has homology to herpes simplex virus glycoprotein C. J. Virol., 59: 660–668.

Kinchington, P.R., Ling, P., Pensiero, M., Moss, B., Ruyechan, W.T. and Hay, J. (1990) The glycoprotein products of varicella-zoster virus gene 14 and their defective accumulation in a vaccine strain (Oka). J. Virol., 64: 4540–4548.

Kinchington, P.R., Houghland, J.K., Arvin, A.M., Ruyechan, W.T. and Hay, J. (1992) Varicella zoster virus IE62 protein is a major virion component. J. Virol., 66: 359–366.

Koropchak, C.M., Solem, S.M., Diaz, P.S. and Arvin, A.M. (1989) Investigation of varicella-zoster virus infection of lymphocytes by in situ hybridization. J. Virol., 63: 2392–2395.

Koropchak, C.M., Graham, G., Palmer, J., Winsberg, M., Ting, S.F., Wallace, M., Prober, C.G. and Arvin, A.M. (1991) Investigation of varicella-zoster virus infection by polymerase chain reaction in the immunocompetent host with acute varicella. J. Infect. Dis., 163: 1016–1022.

Krause, P.R. and Klinman, D.M. (1995) Efficacy, immunogenicity, safety, and use of live attenuated chickenpox vaccine. J. Pediatr., 127: 518–525.

Levin, M.J. and Hayward, A.R. (1996). The varicella vaccine. Prevention of herpes zoster. Infect. Dis. Clin. North Am., 10: 657–675.

Litwin, V., Jackson, W. and Grose, C. (1992) Receptor properties of two varicella-zoster virus glycoproteins, gpI and gpIV, homologous to herpes simplex virus gE and gI. J. Virol., 66: 3643–3651.

Lowry, P.W., Solem, S., Watson, B.N., Koropchak, C.M., Kinchington, P.E., Ruyechan, W., Hay, J. and Arvin, A.M. (1992) Immunity in strain 2 guinea pigs inoculated with vaccinia recombinants expressing varicella-zoster virus glycoproteins I, IV, V or the immediate early gene 62. J. Gen. Virol., 73: 811–819.

Lungu, O., Panagiotidis, C., Annunziato, P., Gershon, A. and Silverstein, S. (1998) Aberrant intracellular localization of varicella-zoster virus regulatory proteins during latency. Proc. Natl. Acad. Sci. U.S.A., 95: 780–785.

Mahalingam, R., Wellish, M., White, T., Soike, K., Cohrs, R., Kleineschmidt-DeMasters, B.K. and Gilden, Dh. (1998) Infectious simian varicella virus expressing the green fluorescent protein. J. Neurovirol., 4: 438–444.

Mainka, C., Fuss, B., Geiger, H., Hofelmayr, H. and Wolff, M.H. (1998) Characterization of viremia at different stages of varicella-zoster virus infection. J. Med. Virol., 56: 91–98.

Mallory, S., Sommer, M. and Arvin, A.M. (1997) Mutational analysis of the role of glycoprotein I in varicella-zoster virus

replication and its effects on glycoprotein E conformation and trafficking. J. Virol., 71: 8279–8288.

Mo, C., Suen, J. et al. (1999) Characterization of varicella-zoster virus glycoprotein K (open reading frame 5) and its role in virus growth. J. Virol., 73: 4197–4207.

Mo, C., Schneeberger, E.E. and Arvin, A.M. (2000) The glycoprotein E of varicella-zoster virus facilitates translocation of tight junction proteins in polarized epithelial cells. J. Virol., 174: 11377–11387.

Moffat, J.F. and Arvin, A.M. (1998) Varicella-zoster virus infection of T-cells and skin in the SCID-hu mouse model. In: O. Zak and M. Sande (Eds.), Handbook of Animal Models of Infection. Academic Press, London.

Moffat, J.F., Stein, M., Kaneshima, H. and Arvin, A.M. (1995) Tropism of varicella-zoster virus for human CD4+ and CD8+ T lymphocytes and epidermal cells in SCID-hu mice. J. Virol., 69: 5236–5242.

Moffat, J.F., Zerboni, L. et al. (1998a) Attenuation of the vaccine Oka strain of varicella-zoster virus and role of glycoprotein C in alphaherpesvirus virulence demonstrated in the SCID-hu mouse. J. Virol., 72: 965–974.

Moffat, J.F., Zerboni, L., Sommer, M.H. et al. (1998b) The ORF47 and ORF66 putative protein kinases of varicella-zoster virus determine tropism for human T cells and skin in the SCID-hu mouse. Proc. Natl. Acad. Sci. U. S. A., 95: 11969–11974.

Myers, M. (1979) Viremia caused by varicella-zoster virus: association with malignant progressive varicella. J. Infect. Dis., 140: 229–232.

Myers, M.G. and Connelly, B.L. (1992) Animal models of varicella. J. Infect. Dis., 166(Suppl. 1): 48–50.

Nikkels, A.F., Debrus, S. et al. (1995) Localization of varicella-zoster virus nucleic acids and proteins in human skin. Neurology, 46: 47–49.

Olson, J.K. and Grose, C. (1998) Complex formation facilitates endocytosis of the varicella-zoster virus gE:gI Fc receptor. J. Virol., 72: 1542–1551.

Ozaki, T., Ichikawa, T., Matsui, Y. et al. (1986) Lymphocyte-associated viremia in varicella. J. Med. Virol., 19: 249–253.

Perera, L.P., Mosca, J.D., Ruyechan, W.T. and Hay, J. (1992) Regulation of varicella-zoster virus gene expression in human T lymphocytes. J. Virol., 66: 5298–5304.

Ross, J., Williams, M. and Cohen, J.I. (1997) Disruption of the varicella-zoster virus dUTPase and the adjacent ORF9A gene results in impaired growth and reduced syncytia formation in vitro. Virology, 234: 186–195.

Ruyechan, W. and Hay, J. (2000) DNA replication. In: A.M. Arvin and A.A. Gershon (Eds.), Varicella-zoster Virus: Virology and Clinical Management. Cambridge University Press, pp. 51–73.

Sabella, C., Lowry, P.W., Abbruzzi, G.M., Koropchak, C.M., Kinchington, P.R., Sadegh-Zadeh, M., Hay, J., Ruyechan, W.T. and Arvin, A.M. (1993) Immunization with the immediate-early tegument protein (Open Reading Frame 62) of varicella-zoster virus protects guinea pigs against virus challenge. J. Virol., 67: 7673–7676.

Sadzot-Delvaux, C., Kinchington, P., Rentier, B. and Arvin, A.M. (1997) Recognition of the latency-associated immediate early protein IE63 of varicella-zoster virus by human memory T lymphocytes. J. Immunol., 159: 2802–2806.

Santos, R.A., Padilla, J.A., Hatfield, C. and Grose, C. (1998) Antigenic variation of varicella zoster virus Fc receptor gE: loss of a major B cell epitope in the ectodomain. Virology, 249: 21–31.

Santos, R.A., Hatfield, C.C., Faga, B.P. et al. (2000) Varicella-zoster virus gE escape mutant VZV-MSP exhibits an accelerated cell-to-cell spread phenotype in both infected cell cultures and SCID-hu mice. Virology, 275: 306–317.

Sawyer, M.H., Wu, Y.N., Chamberlin, C.J. et al. (1992) Detection of varicella-zoster virus DNA in the oropharynx and blood of patients with varicella. J. Infect. Dis., 166: 885–888.

Schunemann, S., Mainka, C. and Wolff, M.H. (1998) Subclinical reactivation of varicella-zoster virus in immunocompromised and immunocompetent individuals. Intervirology, 41: 98–102.

Sexton, C.J., Navsaria, H.A., Leigh, I.M. and Powell, K. (1992) Replication of varicella zoster virus in primary human keratinocytes. J. Med. Virol., 38: 260–264.

Somekh, E. and Levin, M.J. (1993) Infection of human fetal dorsal root neurons with wild type varicella virus and the Oka strain varicella vaccine. J. Med. Virol., 40(3): 241–243.

Soong, W., Schultz, J.C., Patera, A.C., Sommer, M.H. and Cohen, J.I. (2000) Infection of human T lymphocytes with varicella-zoster virus: an analysis with viral mutants and clinical isolates. J. Virol., 74: 1864–1870.

Spengler, M., Fuyechan, W.T. and Hay, J. (2000) Physical interaction between two varicella-zoster virus gene regulatory proteins, IE4 and IE62. Virology, 272: 375–381.

Straus, S.E., Reinhold, W., Smith, H.A. et al. (1984) Endonuclease analysis of viral DNA from varicella and subsequent zoster infection in the same patient. N. Engl. J. Med., 311: 1362–1364.

Takahashi, M. (1986) Clinical overview of varicella vaccine: development and early studies. Pediatrics, 78: 736–741.

Takashima, S. and Becker, L.E. (1979) Neuropathology of fatal varicella. Arch. Pathol. Lab. Med., 103: 209–213.

Tsolia, M., Gershon, A., Steinberg, S. and Gelb, L. (1990) Live attenuated varicella vaccine: evidence that the virus is attenuated and the importance of skin lesions in transmission of varicella-zoster virus. J. Pediatr., 116: 184–189.

Tyzzer, E.E. (1906) The histology of skin lesions in varicella. J. Med. Res., 14: 361–392.

Von Bókay, J. (1909) Über den ätiologischen Zusammenhang der Varizellen mit gewissen Fällen von Herpes Zoster. Wien. Klin. Wochenschr., 22: 1323–1326.

Wallace, M.R., Woelfl, I., Bowler, W.A., Olson, P.E., Murray, N.B., Brodine, S.K., Oldfield, E.C. and Arvin, A.M. (1994) Tumor necrosis factor, interleukin-2 and interferon-gamma in adult varicella. J. Med. Virol., 43: 69–71.

Weller, T.H. (1953) The propagation in viro of agents producing inclusion bodies derived from varicella and herpes zoster. Proc. Soc. Exp. Biol. Med., 83: 340–346.

Whitley, R.J. (1998) Antiviral Therapy. Infectious Diseases. W.B. Saunders, Philadelphia, PA, 2nd ed., pp. 330–350.

Williams, D.L., Gershon, A., Gelb, L.D., Spraker, M.K., Steinberg, S. and Ragab, A.H. (1985) Herpes zoster following varicella vaccine in a child with acute lymphocytic leukemia. J. Pediatr., 106: 259–261.

Wilson, A., Sharp, M., Koropchak, C.M., Ting, S.F. and Arvin, A.M. (1992) Subclinical varicella-zoster virus viremia, herpes zoster and recovery of T-lymphocyte responses to varicella-zoster viral antigens after allogeneic and autologous bone marrow transplantation. J. Infect. Dis., 165: 119–126.

Wu, L. and Forghani, B. (1997) Characterization of neutralizing domains on varicella-zoster virus glycoprotein E defined by monoclonal antibodies. Arch. Virol., 142: 349–362.

Yao, Z., Jackson, W., Forghani, B. and Grose, C. (1993) Varicella-zoster virus glycoprotein gpI/gpIV receptor: expression, complex formation, and antigenicity within the vaccinia virus-T7 RNA polymerase transfection system. J. Virol., 67: 305–314.

Zerboni, L., Sommer, M., Ware, C.F. and Arvin, A.M. (2000) Varicella-zoster virus infection of a human CD4-positive T cell line. Virology, 19: 1207–1216.

Herpes Zoster and Postherpetic Neuralgia, 2nd Revised and Enlarged Edition
Pain Research and Clinical Management, Vol. 11
Edited by C.P.N. Watson and A.A. Gershon
© *2001 Elsevier Science B.V. All rights reserved*

CHAPTER 5

The epidemiology and natural history of herpes zoster and postherpetic neuralgia

Robert H. Dworkin [1,*] and Kenneth E. Schmader [2]

[1] *Department of Anesthesiology, University of Rochester School of Medicine and Dentistry, Rochester, NY 14642, USA and [2] Division of Geriatrics, Department of Medicine and the Center for the Study of Aging and Human Development, Duke University Medical Center, Geriatric Research, Education and Clinical Center, Durham VA Medical Center, Durham, NC 27710, USA*

1. Introduction

The objective of this chapter is to review the epidemiology and natural history of herpes zoster and postherpetic neuralgia. Epidemiology seeks to explain and comprehend diseases by studying the characteristics of diseases in populations. Those characteristics include morbidity, mortality, incidence and prevalence rates, and risk factors. The sources of epidemiological data on herpes zoster and postherpetic neuralgia include cohort studies, case-control studies, clinical trials, large case series, and case reports. We emphasize immunocompetent patients because data regarding the epidemiology and natural history of herpes zoster and postherpetic neuralgia in immunocompromised patients are discussed in detail elsewhere (Chapter 10; Schmader, 2000).

2. Herpes zoster

The varicella-zoster virus (VZV) establishes latency in sensory ganglia following primary varicella in-fection. Herpes zoster (shingles) is the reactivation of the virus and its spread from a single dorsal root or cranial nerve ganglion to the corresponding dermatome and neural tissue of the same segment (Hope-Simpson, 1954, 1965; Weller et al., 1958; Straus et al., 1984). Herpes zoster has the highest incidence of all neurological diseases, occurring annually in approximately 500,000 people in the United States and during the lifetimes of as much as 20% of the population (Kurtzke, 1984; Donahue et al., 1995).

The presentation of herpes zoster is variable. In approximately 75% of patients, a prodrome of dermatomal pain precedes the appearance of a characteristic unilateral rash (Rogers and Tindall, 1971; Cobo et al., 1986; Beutner et al., 1995; Dworkin et al., 1998; Haanpää et al., 1999). Although this prodrome begins several days before rash onset in almost all cases, a series of patients with prodromal pain preceding the appearance of the rash by 7 to more than 100 days has been reported (Gilden et al., 1991).

Thoracic dermatomes are the most commonly affected sites in herpes zoster and account for 50–

* Correspondence to: Dr. R.H. Dworkin, Department of Anesthesiology, University of Rochester School of Medicine and Dentistry, 601 Elmwood Avenue, Box 604, Rochester, NY 14642, USA. Phone: +1 (716) 275-3524; E-mail: robert_dworkin@urmc.rochester.edu

70% of all cases (Burgoon et al., 1957; McGregor, 1957; Hope-Simpson, 1965; Brown, 1976; Mazur and Dolin, 1978; Ragozzino et al., 1982a; Helgason et al., 1996). Cranial (especially the ophthalmic division of the trigeminal nerve), cervical, and lumbar dermatomes each account for 10–20% of cases, and sacral dermatomes are affected in 2–8% of cases (Burgoon et al., 1957; Mazur and Dolin, 1978; Ragozzino et al., 1982a; Helgason et al., 1996). The rash becomes pustular after several days, then forms a crust, and loss of all scabs usually occurs within 2–4 weeks (Burgoon et al., 1957).

Pain in the affected dermatome accompanies the rash in most patients. Those who did not have a painful prodrome typically begin to experience pain at rash onset or shortly afterwards. This acute herpes zoster pain gradually resolves before or shortly after rash healing in the majority of cases. Dermatomal pain without a rash, referred to as zoster sine herpete, has also been described (Lewis, 1958; Gilden et al., 1992). The recent finding of VZV DNA in the cerebrospinal fluid of two patients with prolonged radicular pain and no rash provides evidence of the this syndrome (Gilden et al., 1994).

Acute herpes zoster pain is often accompanied by decreased quality of life; severe acute pain interferes with patients' abilities to carry out normal activities of daily living and is, not surprisingly, associated with greater use of analgesic medications (Mauskopf et al., 1994; Lydick et al., 1995a,b). Although quality of life is adversely affected by herpes zoster, it returns to normal levels in most patients after recovery from the acute infection (Lydick et al., 1995b).

It has been hypothesized that older patients have more severe herpes zoster infections (Higa et al., 1988, 1992, 1997), but the results of several studies have not provided uniform support for this prediction. The results of these studies suggest that older age is not consistently associated with either greater acute pain severity or longer acute pain duration (Bamford and Boundy, 1968; Wildenhoff et al., 1979, 1981; Harding et al., 1987; Higa et al., 1988, 1992, 1997; Bean et al., 1993; Boon and Griffin, 1996; Dworkin et al., 1997b; Haanpää et al., 1999). Moreover, older age is not consistently associated

with either greater rash severity or longer rash duration (Burgoon et al., 1957; Wildenhoff et al., 1979, 1981; Harding et al., 1987; Higa et al., 1988, 1992, 1997; Bean et al., 1993; Decroix et al., 2000).

Significant associations between greater acute pain severity and presence of a prodrome (Haanpää et al., 1999) and greater rash severity and duration (Molin, 1969; Mauskopf et al., 1994; Lydick et al., 1995a; Harrison et al., 1999) have been reported. In other recent studies, however, no association was found between acute pain severity or allodynia and rash severity (Cioni et al., 1994; Haanpää et al., 1999, 2000). Acute pain severity was not significantly associated with presence of sensory deficits in the affected dermatome (Haanpää et al., 1999), electromyogram (EMG) motor abnormalities (Haanpää et al., 1997), or magnetic resonance imaging (MRI) abnormalities in the brainstem and cervical cord (Haanpää et al., 1998) during herpes zoster.

The relationships between the severity of acute pain in herpes zoster and several demographic and clinical variables were recently examined in two large samples of patients enrolled in clinical trials of an antiviral agent (Dworkin et al., 2000a). In these analyses, greater acute pain severity assessed within 72 h of rash onset was weakly but significantly associated with greater age, greater rash severity, and presence of prodromal pain or dysesthesias. Weak relationships among age, acute pain and other aspects of herpes zoster could account for the inconsistent results of previous studies.

2.1. Incidence of herpes zoster

The strongest research designs for providing epidemiological data about herpes zoster are large cohort studies. Large, multi-year cohort studies of zoster in the general population are summarized in Table I. The incidence of herpes zoster in these mostly immunocompetent community dwelling populations ranged from 1.2 to 3.4 per 1000 person-years. In the elderly (above 65 years old), investigators have reported an incidence of zoster that ranges from 3.9 to 11.8 per 1000 person-years. These studies differed in their methods of case ascertainment,

TABLE I

Cohort studies of herpes zoster

Author and time of study	Setting	Population		No. cases	Zoster incidence per 1000 person-years		
		Person-years	Age		All ages	Elderly (age)	Children (age)
Hope-Simpson, 1947–1962	Cirencester, UK	53,010	0– 99	192	3.4	7.8 (60–99)	0.74 (0–9)
Ragozzino et al., 1945–1959	Rochester, MN, USA	473,170	0– 75+	590	1.25	3.9 (65–75+)	0.4 (<14)
Guess et al., 1960–1981	Rochester, MN, USA	410,244	0– 19	173	–	–	0.42 (0–19)
Donahue et al., 1990–1992	Boston, MA, USA	500,408	0– 75+	1075	2.15	11.8 (65–75+)	0.47 (<14)
Schmader et al., 1987–1990	Durham, NC, USA	9,618	65–104	69	–	7.1 (65–104)	–
Helgason et al. and Petursson et al., 1990–1995	Iceland	229,547	0– 80+	457	2.0	4.6 (60–80+)	1.6 (0–19)

which may explain, in part, the nearly three-fold difference in the incidence of zoster among studies. The incidence of zoster in populations limited to immunosuppressed patients is substantially higher (Schmader, 2000). The likelihood of recurrent zoster was 4.1, 5.2, and 1.7% in the studies of Hope-Simpson (1965), Ragozzino et al. (1982a) and Donahue et al. (1995), respectively.

2.2. Morbidity and mortality of herpes zoster

The morbidity of zoster includes acute pain and chronic pain (discussed below), other neurological disorders, and ophthalmological, cutaneous, and visceral complications. In cohort studies (Ragozzino et al., 1982a; Galil et al., 1997), the types and estimated frequencies of neurological complications included motor neuropathy (1%), cranial polyneuritis (less than 1%), transverse myelitis (less than 1%), meningoencephalitis (less than 1%), and cerebral angiitis and stroke after ophthalmic zoster (less than 1%). Ophthalmological complications have been described in 2–6% of zoster cases, including keratitis, uveitis, iridocyclitis, panophthalmitis, and glaucoma (Burgoon et al., 1957; Ragozzino et al., 1982a; Galil et al., 1997). Bacterial infection of the rash and herpes gangrenosum occurred in zero to 2% in these series. Visceral involvement was not noted in these studies. Elderly and immunosuppressed patients with zoster are at greater risk for these complications. Reliable data on zoster mortality rates are unavailable because it is an unusual event and because

zoster-related deaths are not systematically reported in most countries. Nonetheless, over 100 zoster-related deaths are estimated to occur each year in England and Wales (Miller et al., 1993) and 1064 zoster-related deaths were reported in 1982–1990 in the United States (Weller, 1997).

2.3. Geographic distribution of herpes zoster

The great majority of the world's adults are latently infected with VZV and at risk for developing zoster. However, population based studies of zoster have not been performed in many parts of the world so there are little data to describe how zoster is distributed geographically. Varicella occurs more often in adolescence and adulthood in some tropical climates compared to temperate zones (Weller, 1983). Whether variations in age of onset of varicella alters age of onset of zoster or the incidence of zoster is unknown. Another potential geographic difference is residence in an urban versus rural environment. McGregor (1957) reported the occurrence of zoster over a seven year period in 2400 patients who were two-thirds suburban and one-third rural. Of suburban patients, 3.4% developed zoster compared to 3.3% of rural residents. In the Duke Established Populations for Epidemiological Studies of the Elderly (EPESE), urban residence did not increase the lifetime risk of zoster compared to rural residence (Schmader et al., 1995).

2.4. Temporal distribution of herpes zoster

Zoster happens periodically throughout the year in contrast to the well-documented seasonal pattern of varicella in temperate zones (Ragozzino et al., 1982a; Weller, 1983; Cooper, 1987; Paul and Thiel, 1996). For instance, within the same population in the United Kingdom, Cooper (1987) reported that the weekly incidence of zoster stayed level at 5 cases per 1000 person-years throughout the year 1984–1985 whereas the weekly incidence of varicella had a well-defined springtime peak as high as 20 cases per 1000 person-years and an autumn trough of roughly 6 per 1000 person-years.

Some investigators have provided data on the incidence of zoster over time. In Rochester, MN from 1945 to 1959, the incidence of zoster increased from 1.12 to 1.31 per 1000 person-years (Ragozzino et al., 1982a). In Scotland from 1955 to 1985, the number of zoster cases increased each year between 1969 and 1982, but the number of cases declined after 1982 (Wilson, 1986). Conversely, the incidence of zoster showed no yearly increase from 1947 to 1962 in England and from 1967 to 1983 in the United Kingdom (Hope-Simpson, 1965; Cooper, 1987). The most recent cohort study, from Boston in 1990–1992, reported the highest incidence of zoster, even after excluding zoster cases associated with HIV infection and cancer, but it is difficult to directly compare rates across time in these studies because of differences in study methodology (Donahue et al., 1995).

2.5. Risk factors for herpes zoster

2.5.1. Age

A fundamental epidemiological feature of zoster is a marked increase in incidence with aging. Hope-Simpson (1965) documented an incidence of 0.74 per 1000 person-years in children under 10 years old, 2.5 per 1000 person-years in adults aged 20–50 years, and 7.8 per 1000 person-years in those older than 60 years. Ragozzino et al. (1982a) found a similar dramatic increase with aging in Minnesota, where the incidence of zoster was less than 1 per 1000 person-years under 44 years old, but peaked

at 4–4.5 per 1000 person-years in persons over 75 years old. Donahue et al. (1995) confirmed this relationship when they reported an incidence of 1.9, 2.3, 3.1, 5.7 and 11.8 per 1000 person-years for the age groups 25–34, 35–44, 45–54, 55–64 and 65–75+ years, respectively.

The age at which the sharpest increase in zoster occurs is 50–60 years. Furthermore, the slope continues a marked upward course in the decades above 60 years. In the Duke EPESE (Schmader et al., 1995), the lifetime risk of zoster increased significantly with age even among individuals age 65 years and older (odds ratio, 1.20 for every five years, 95% confidence interval [CI], 1.10–1.31). From these studies, it is estimated that the lifetime incidence of zoster is 10–20% in the general population (Ragozzino et al., 1982a; Straus, 1993; Donahue et al., 1995; Schmader et al., 1995) and as high as 50% of a cohort surviving to 85 years of age (Hope-Simpson, 1965).

In children and adolescents, the incidence of zoster ranges from 0.42 to 1.6 per 1000 person-years in ages 0–19 years (Hope-Simpson, 1965; Guess et al., 1985; Donahue et al., 1995; Petursson et al., 1998). In children aged 0–9 years, the incidence ranges from 0.25 to 1.1 per 1000 person-years (Hope-Simpson, 1965; Guess et al., 1985; Petursson et al., 1998). The incidence of zoster during childhood is increased when primary VZV infection of the mother occurs during pregnancy or primary VZV infection of the child occurs during the first year of life (Timothy and Williams, 1979; Dworsky et al., 1980; Latif and Shope, 1983; Guess et al., 1985; Baba et al., 1986; Terada et al., 1993; Kakourou et al., 1998). Guess et al. (1985) reported that children who experienced chickenpox during the first year of life were 2.8 (95% CI, 1.6–4.7) times more likely to develop zoster during childhood than children who experienced chickenpox after the first year of life. The association of malignancy with zoster appears to be uncommon in childhood. Of 173 childhood zoster cases reported by Guess et al. (1985), only 3% occurred in children with malignancy. Of 118 zoster cases reported by Petursson et al. (1998), no children had an associated malignancy and one 19-year-old had Hodgkin's disease. Finally, childhood zoster is a much milder disease in immunocompetent children than in adults, especially with respect to pain (Brunell et al., 1968; Rogers and Tindall, 1972; Guess et al., 1985; Smith and Glaser, 1996; Kakourou et al., 1998; Petursson et al., 1998). For example, Petursson et al. (1998) reported that none of 118 patients with zoster aged 0–19 years developed pain that persisted 30 days or more after rash onset.

2.5.2. Human immunodeficiency virus infection and acquired immunodeficiency syndrome

The frequency and complications of zoster are significantly increased in patients with suppressed cell-mediated immunity, including human immunodeficiency virus infection (HIV) and/or acquired immunodeficiency syndrome (AIDS), certain cancers, organ transplants, immune-mediated diseases, and immunosuppressive treatments, compared to immunocompetent individuals. We summarize these studies briefly because they have been reviewed in detail elsewhere (Schmader, 2000).

HIV infection is a very strong risk factor for zoster. Cohort studies of zoster in HIV-infected individuals have examined HIV-seropositive and/or AIDS patients from HIV clinics or community dwelling homosexual men (Buchbinder et al., 1992; Rogues et al., 1993; Glesby et al., 1995; Holmberg et al., 1995; Veenstra et al., 1995; Moore and Chaisson, 1996; McNulty et al., 1997; Engels et al., 1999). The incidence of zoster in HIV-infected individuals varied from 29 to 51 per 1000 person-years, some 15–25 times greater than the incidence rates of zoster in the general population and 3–7 times greater than the incidence rates of zoster in the elderly. HIV infection increases zoster risk even in HIV-infected children, 27% of whom developed zoster an average of 1.9 years after varicella (Gershon et al., 1997). As with immunocompetent individuals, greater age increases the risk for zoster among HIV-infected adults, with the incidence increasing from less than 40 per 1000 person-years in individuals 49 years of age or younger to 225 per 1000 person-years in those 50–59 years of age (Buchbinder et al., 1992). Irrespective of age, the cumulative incidence of

zoster in HIV-infected persons is estimated to be 30–40% over approximately 10 years of follow-up. Several studies have demonstrated that patients who presented with zoster in areas of high HIV prevalence often had underlying HIV infection. Therefore, zoster may be the first clue to underlying HIV infection when it occurs in groups at high risk for HIV infection (Friedman-Kien et al., 1986; Sandor et al., 1986; Melbye et al., 1987; Colebunders et al., 1988; Van de Perre et al., 1988; Dehne et al., 1992; Panda et al., 1994; Tyndall et al., 1995). Zoster can occur at any stage of HIV/AIDS (Friedman-Kien et al., 1986; Melbye et al., 1987; Buchbinder et al., 1992; Rogues et al., 1993; Holmberg et al., 1995; McNulty et al., 1997; Engels et al., 1999).

The morbidity of herpes zoster is also greater in HIV-infected patients, who have an increased frequency of atypical skin lesions (3–11%), severe neurological complications (6–8%), ocular complications (6–11%), and a prolonged course compared to the elderly or the general population (Glesby et al., 1995; Veenstra et al., 1996). Studies differ on whether zoster is a risk factor for progression to AIDS or death. Most studies have not controlled CD4 count and viral load (Schmader, 2000); one study which did control for CD4 count found that zoster was not a risk factor for progression to AIDS or death (Veenstra et al., 1995).

2.5.3. Cancer

Malignancy is another important risk factor for zoster. In community dwelling cohort studies, cancer preceded zoster in 6% of the population and a past history of cancer significantly increased the lifetime risk of zoster in the elderly (Ragozzino et al., 1982a; Donahue et al., 1995; Schmader et al., 1995). In retrospective case series, investigators have described the frequency and clinical characteristics of zoster in Hodgkin's diseases, non-Hodgkin's lymphoma, leukemia, and lung cancer (e.g. Dolin et al., 1978; Rusthoven et al., 1988a; Bower et al., 1997; Schmader, 2000).

In the largest and strongest study of zoster in a cancer population, Rusthoven et al. (1988a) reported on zoster in patients older than 15 years who attended a comprehensive cancer center in Ontario, Canada from 1972 to 1980. They identified 766 episodes of zoster among 740 adult cancer patients among the more than 7000 new cases of cancer each year. The median age of the cancer patients with zoster was 57 years (range 16–99 years). The cumulative incidence rate of zoster in this population 5 years after diagnosis was 62.5 per 1000 person-years. The cumulative incidence was highest in Hodgkin's disease (14%), leukemia (10%), and non-Hodgkin's lymphoma (5%). The risk of second episodes was highest among patients with hematologic malignancies. Among solid tumors, the cumulative incidence was highest in treated patients with breast (2%), lung (2%), and gynecologic malignancies (1%). Hodgkin's disease, non-Hodgkin's lymphoma, and head and neck cancer were independent risk factors for disseminated zoster infection (Rusthoven et al., 1988b). Consistent with these data, multiple other studies have found that the risk of herpes zoster is greater in patients with hematological malignancies than in those with solid tumors and is greatest for Hodgkin's disease compared to all malignancies (Rusthoven, 1994; Schmader, 2000).

2.5.4. Organ transplants

Zoster commonly occurs in bone marrow, kidney, and heart transplant recipients. The incidence and risk factors for zoster in these patients are difficult to report because published studies have multiple limitations, including small numbers of patients with variable underlying diseases and treatment regimens, variable length of follow-up, and lack of knowledge about whether donors or recipients were VZV seropositive.

Despite these limitations, it appears that bone marrow transplant (BMT) recipients are particularly susceptible to developing zoster (Rusthoven, 1994). The frequency of zoster in BMT recipients ranges from 13 to 55% and the majority of cases occur within 12 months of transplantation (Schmader, 2000). Several studies have examined issues pertinent to BMT and zoster risk, including type of transplant (allogeneic vs. autologous), graft-versus-host disease, underlying disease, and pre-BMT ir-

radiation. On all these issues, study results conflict as to whether they increase zoster risk (Schmader, 2000). However, all studies agree that cutaneous dissemination (18–23%) and visceral involvement (13–14%) are more common in BMT recipients than in immunocompetent patients.

The amount of published data on zoster after renal and cardiac transplantation is small. Of four studies of renal transplant recipients, the frequency of zoster in renal transplant recipients was approximately 7–14% within 2–5 years of transplantation (Rifkind, 1966; Luby et al., 1977; Naraqi et al., 1977; Lo and Cheng, 1996). Most cases were localized zoster without serious complications. In the largest study, 14% of renal transplant patients developed zoster after a mean of 5 years of follow-up (Lo and Cheng, 1996). The median time to zoster onset was 7.6 months after transplant and 63% of cases occurred within 1 year of transplantation. Of two studies of cardiac transplant recipients, the frequency of zoster was 13% within 6 months of transplantation and 22% after 6 years of follow-up (Rand et al., 1977; Preiksaitis et al., 1983).

2.5.5. Systemic lupus erythematosus (SLE)

Studies of zoster and SLE are limited by retrospective chart reviews, referral bias, variable treatment regimens and time of follow-up, and small samples. Despite these limitations, studies have reliably documented a significant association between zoster and SLE. Researchers have reported a frequency of zoster of 13–21% in SLE patients and an incidence of 16–22 cases per 1000 person-years (Moutsopoulos et al., 1978; Kahl, 1994; Manzi et al., 1995; Moga et al., 1995).

In the largest study of SLE and zoster, Manzi et al. (1995) reported that 15% of 321 SLE patients developed zoster a median of 6.2 years (range 1 month to 29 years) after the diagnosis of SLE for an estimated incidence of 22 cases per 1000 person-years. In univariate analyses, compared to SLE controls, risk factors for herpes zoster included azathioprine, cyclophosphamide, nephritis, and malignancy. Zoster was usually localized and uncomplicated even during immunosuppressive therapy in all SLE studies. In addition, the appearance of zoster was not related to SLE activity because cases occurred when SLE disease activity was severe, mild, or inactive. The impact of immunological effects of SLE versus immunosuppressive therapy on the risk of herpes zoster was impossible to disentangle. However, a high frequency of zoster in SLE was reported before the use of immunosuppressants, which suggests that SLE-induced immune deficits play a role in zoster susceptibility (Hamaguchi et al., 1970). Zoster has also been reported in rheumatoid arthritis, polymyositis, and dermatomyositis, but the studies are case reports or case series and complicated by the use of immunosuppressants (Nagaoka et al., 1990; Antonelli et al., 1991).

2.5.6. Immunosuppressive treatments

Immunosuppressive treatments may increase the risk of zoster, but little information is available on the degree of risk. Additionally, it is often difficult to disentangle the effects of the underlying disease and its treatment on the risk of zoster. Radiation therapy, cancer chemotherapeutic agents, corticosteroids, post-transplant immunosuppressants, and agents for immune-mediated diseases are the agents that have been linked to zoster.

Several authors have reported a high frequency of radiation treatments in cancer patients with zoster (Schmader, 2000). Most studies did not include control groups. In one study that did include a control group, 31% of Hodgkin's disease patients who received radiation therapy developed zoster compared to 11% of Hodgkin's disease patients who did not receive radiation therapy, suggesting that radiation therapy alone predisposed to zoster (Schimpff et al., 1972). In a study of BMT recipients (Han et al., 1994), radiation therapy in pre-transplant conditioning significantly increased the risk of VZV infection, including zoster, post BMT. However, radiation therapy was not a significant risk factor for zoster in three other BMT studies (Schuchter et al., 1989; Wacker et al., 1989; Tzeng et al., 1995).

The occurrence of zoster has been reported in patients receiving cancer chemotherapy, but the studies could not control for the effects of the underlying cancer nor could they determine the degree of risk for zoster among different chemotherapeutic agents (Schmader, 2000). In a study of multiple immunosuppressive treatments in cancer, the cumulative 3-year incidence of zoster in Hodgkin's disease was highest in patients receiving induction chemotherapy, radiation therapy, and maintenance chemotherapy (27.3% of 185 patients) compared to radiation therapy alone (11.5% of 193 patients), induction chemotherapy alone (13.2% of 91 patients), and induction chemotherapy followed by radiation therapy (19.8% of 134 patients). These results remained significant after multivariate analysis (Guinee et al., 1985).

Clinical experience and case reports suggest that corticosteroids increase zoster risk but there are no well-designed, controlled studies of this relationship. A case-control study of prednisone and herpesvirus infections in HIV infection found no difference in VZV infection between treated (0%) and untreated patients (0.3%) within 30 days of prednisone treatment (Keiser et al., 1996). In two studies of SLE, the risk of zoster was higher in patients who received cyclophosphamide and azathioprine compared to those who were not administered these drugs (Kahl, 1994; Manzi et al., 1995).

2.5.7. Race and ethnicity

White populations in the United States and Europe have been the focus of most studies of zoster epidemiology. The Duke EPESE achieved an equal mix of black and white participants by using a stratified, random sampling technique in community dwelling elderly. Of 3206 subjects in this population, 4.6% of blacks and 16.1% of whites had a past occurrence of zoster (Schmader et al., 1995). After controlling for age, cancer, and demographic factors, blacks remained one-fourth as likely as whites to have experienced zoster (adjusted odds ratio, 0.25, 95% CI, 0.18–0.35, $P = 0.0001$). In a study of the prospective occurrence of zoster in the Duke EPESE (Schmader et al., 1998), 4.3% of blacks and 10.9% of whites developed zoster over 6 years. After controlling for the above variables, blacks remained significantly less likely to develop zoster (adjusted risk ratio, 0.35, 95% CI, 0.24–0.51, $P < 0.001$). Zoster case ascertainment in these studies had a false positive rate of 3% and false negative rate of 0%, which was not enough to explain these striking racial differences (Schmader et al., 1994). Hypothesized reasons for the differences include racial differences in VZV immunity, age at onset of varicella, and exposure to varicella over the life course (Dworkin, 1996).

Ross et al. (1995) reported significantly lower rates of zoster among 5601 white Hutterites with life-long residence in Manitoba compared to 5476 non-Hutterite white Canadian controls also living in Manitoba. The Hutterites had had 39% less varicella by age 10 years than the controls and a signifi cantly greater number of Hutterites of all ages were seronegative for VZV antibodies (Ross et al., 1997).

2.5.8. Gender and other demographic factors

There were no differences found in the incidence of zoster by gender in large cohort studies. Hope-Simpson (1965), Ragozzino et al. (1982a), and Donahue et al. (1995) reported that the incidence of zoster among males versus females was 3.6 vs. 3.2, 1.34 vs. 1.26 and 2.19 vs. 2.11 per 1000 person-years, respectively. Among elderly persons in the Duke EPESE (Schmader et al., 1995, 1998), being female, being married, and years of education did not significantly affect lifetime zoster risk or zoster incidence.

2.5.9. Physical trauma

In case reports, physical trauma and surgery have been linked to the development of zoster. However, there are no controlled studies of this phenomenon. Ragozzino et al. (1982a) reported that 1.9% of zoster cases had prior trauma, but the temporal relationship of the trauma to zoster and the percentage of trauma in non-zoster controls were not reported. Hope-Simpson (1965) noted that only two cases of zoster in his sample had preceding physical trauma.

2.5.10. Psychosocial factors

Psychological stress is often thought to play a role in the development of zoster. Stress and zoster was studied in 101 community dwelling elders over age

50 years with zoster (cases) and 101 randomly sampled controls without zoster (Schmader et al., 1990). Stressful life events were identified in these participants with the Geriatric Scale of Recent Life Events. The results showed no significant differences between cases and controls for any single life event or total life events. However, cases experienced negative life events significantly more often than controls at two months (26 vs. 10, odds ratio 2.64, 95% CI 1.13, 6.27, $P = 0.012$), 3 months (29 vs. 11, odds ratio 2.64, 95% CI 1.20, 6.04, $P = 0.007$), and 6 months (35 vs. 16, odds ratio 2.00, 95% CI 1.04, 3.93, $P = 0.012$) prior to zoster onset. Thus, while patients with zoster experienced the same kinds of life events in the year preceding the illness as did controls, recent events perceived as stressful were significantly more common among patients with zoster. The effect of acute (negative life events) and chronic (lack of social support) psychological stress on the risk of zoster in the elderly was studied prospectively in the Duke EPESE. After controlling for multiple demographic, health, and social factors, negative life events increased the risk of zoster, but the result was borderline for statistical significance (adjusted RR = 1.38, 95% CI 0.96 – 1.97, $P = 0.078$). The temporal aspects of the study design biased against finding a positive association between stressful life events and zoster because stressful life events were measured over 1 year and zoster was measured over the subsequent 3 years. No measures of social support were significantly associated with zoster (Schmader et al., 1998).

2.6. Herpes zoster as a risk factor for other diseases

As opposed to risk factors for zoster, investigators have studied zoster as a risk factor for cancer, diabetes mellitus, rheumatoid arthritis, multiple sclerosis (MS), SLE, and glioma. Prospective studies of patients with zoster did not demonstrate an increased risk for malignancy (Ragozzino et al., 1982b; Fueyo and Lookingbill, 1984; Wurzel et al., 1986). In a study of 590 zoster cases with over 9389 person-years of observation for the development of cancer in Rochester, MN, the relative risk for detection of cancer after zoster was not significantly increased compared to age- and sex-specific cancer rates in the entire Rochester population (Ragozzino et al., 1982b). Studies in the same population showed that zoster was not associated with rheumatoid arthritis or diabetes mellitus (Ragozzino and Kurland, 1982; Ragozzino et al., 1983).

In a retrospective study of 50 MS patients and 50 age- and sex-matched controls with psoriasis (Lenman and Peters, 1969), 10 MS cases reported a history of shingles compared to two controls ($P < 0.05$). In a retrospective case-control study of Hutterites and non-Hutterites in Canada, investigators noted 40 cases of zoster, 122 cases of varicella, and 5 cases of MS in 5601 Hutterites compared to 76 cases of zoster ($P < 0.001$), 172 cases of varicella ($P < 0.001$), and 17 cases of MS ($P < 0.014$) in 5601 non-Hutterite controls (Ross et al., 1995). These findings raised the question of whether the significantly lower rates of zoster, varicella, and MS were related. In a retrospective mail survey in Manitoba, 16.8% patients of 633 MS reported a history of zoster compared to 5.4% of 3534 general practice patients and 6.8% of 616 patients with neurological disorders other than MS (Ross et al., 1999). No cases of MS were observed in 590 zoster patients over 9389 person-years of follow-up in the Rochester, MN as opposed to the expected number of 0.2 cases. This cohort study was probably inadequately powered to detect a difference (Ragozzino and Kurland, 1983).

In a case control study of multiple risk factors for SLE (Strom et al., 1994), a significant association was found between SLE and a history of shingles (adjusted odds ratio, 6.4, 95% CI, 1.4–28.0). Because the investigators could not determine when the immunological deficits of SLE began in these cases, these results probably confirm the association of zoster and the cell mediated immune deficits of SLE. In a case control study of risk factors for glioma in the San Francisco Bay Area Adult Glioma study (Wrensch et al., 1997), a history of shingles was significantly less likely in cases than controls (odds ratio, 0.5, 95% CI, 0.3–0.8). This interesting observation will need confirmation in cohort studies.

2.7. Transmission of herpes zoster

Zoster epidemiology is ultimately determined by the transmission and spread of VZV in populations. The most important condition in the spread of VZV is primary varicella (chickenpox) infection but latent and reactivated VZV infections also play important roles in maintaining VZV infection in populations (Arvin, 1996). Latently infected elderly adults and immunosuppressed patients are important reservoirs of virus because VZV is more likely to reactivate in these groups. When zoster does occur, VZV can be transmitted during the vesicular phase of the rash and cause primary varicella infection when the zoster exposure consists of person-to-person contact with a seronegative individual. A zoster exposure with a seropositive, latently-infected individual may result in a subclinical reinfection and boost of humoral and cellular VZV immunity, but it is unlikely to cause varicella or herpes zoster (Arvin, 1996). Investigators have reported clusters of zoster cases over a short period of time in the workplace and have reported zoster after prior exposure to varicella (Berlin and Campbell, 1970; Palmer et al., 1985). It is not clear whether these episodes are coincidence, a clinical manifestation of exogenous reinfection, or stimulation of endogenous VZV reactivation. It is clear that the great majority of exposures of latently infected individuals with zoster or varicella do not result in zoster or varicella. However, zoster or varicella exposure in latently infected individuals may possibly prevent zoster as a consequence of the boosting of VZV immunity.

What impact will varicella vaccination have on the incidence and morbidity rates of zoster (Halloran et al., 1994)? One hypothesis is that varicella vaccination of children will change varicella exposure rates in populations, reduce immune boosting and shift the age of onset of zoster in latently infected adults. Another hypothesis is that vaccination of children may reduce zoster incidence or complications by preventing primary wild type infection, assuming latent vaccine virus is less likely to reactivate or cause zoster complications when it does reactivate. It will be several decades before the data become available to test these hypotheses. Finally, varicella vaccination of elderly adults may reduce the incidence of zoster or its complications, an hypothesis now being tested in clinical trials (Oxman, 1995; Levin et al., 1998).

Epidemiologists can track the spread of infectious agents by detecting genetic differences in organisms. The VZV genome is remarkably stable but Hawrami et al. (1997) raised the possibility of the existence of VZV strains in one genetic marker. They examined the presence or absence of the *Bgl*I restriction site in gene 54 in VZV samples from cases of varicella and zoster from 1971 to 1995 in a multiethnic area of London. The *Bgl*I restriction site was present in 63% of zoster cases who had chickenpox in countries with lower adult immunity to varicella (mostly non-white individuals) compared to 10% who had chickenpox in countries with higher adult immunity to varicella (mostly white individuals). The results suggested that a geographically distinct, *Bgl*I-positive viral strain of VZV was carried to London by immigrants from countries with lower adult immunity to varicella.

3. Postherpetic neuralgia

In a considerable percentage of patients with herpes zoster, pain persists following healing of the rash. Persisting herpes zoster pain is termed postherpetic neuralgia (PHN), a chronic pain syndrome that can last for years and cause substantial suffering and reduction in quality of life. As is true of other chronic pain syndromes, PHN patients can develop depression and other types of psychological distress as well as physical, occupational, and social disability as a consequence of their unremitting pain (Portenoy et al., 1986; Schmader, 1995, 1998). In one recent study, it was reported that 59% of a sample of PHN patients attending a pain clinic in Liverpool had taken time off from their usual activities and that these patients had been prevented from pursuing these activities for up to 16 years, with the average being 1.4 years (Davies et al., 1994). In another study of the psychosocial impact of PHN, patients who had PHN for longer than 6 months were found

to have greater disability and psychological distress than patients who had PHN for less than 6 months (Graff-Radford et al., 1986). The results of this study suggest that increases in psychosocial distress may occur as a result of the chronic pain of PHN (as discussed below, it is also possible that prolonged pain is a consequence of greater distress).

Not surprisingly, there is evidence of substantial utilization of a variety of health care resources by patients with PHN. For example, Davies et al. (1994) reported that PHN patients in a pain clinic sample had visited their general physicians an average of 19 times (range 0–69 visits) and had required visits by home health aides an average of 16 times (range 0 507 visits).

Until recently, it was believed that there were no pain-free intervals in patients with PHN. However, there is now evidence that pain in PHN can be discontinuous, with pain-free intervals of varying durations occurring (Watson et al., 1991; Huff et al., 1993; McKendrick and Wood, 1995). In a study of 156 patients with PHN, Watson et al. (1991) noted that "25% of patients with a poor outcome said that they could recall a time after the rash when they had little or no pain for a period of weeks to as much as 12 months." Consistent with these findings are the results of a long-term follow-up study of patients originally enrolled in an antiviral trial conducted in the United Kingdom; 16 of 132 patients who had reported no pain upon completion of participation in the trial 9 years earlier reported pain within the preceding year (McKendrick and Wood, 1995). Moreover, in an antiviral trial conducted in the United States, 4 of 187 patients first reported pain at 1 month after zoster onset and continued to report pain until the final follow-up assessment seven months later (Huff et al., 1993). The data from these four patients suggest that PHN can develop even in herpes zoster patients who have not had acute pain.

The quality of pain in zoster and PHN has been examined in two studies (Bhala et al., 1988; Bowsher, 1993; see also Dubuisson and Melzack, 1976). Sharp, stabbing pain was found to be more common in patients with zoster than in patients with PHN, whereas burning pain was more common in PHN patients and much less likely to be reported by patients with zoster. The investigators noted that the word tender was chosen by both groups of patients to describe allodynia (i.e. pain in response to a stimulus that does not normally provoke pain). These adjectives reflect the three different types of pain that have been distinguished in research on PHN: a steady throbbing or burning pain, an intermittent sharp or shooting pain, and allodynia. The results of a recent study, however, suggest that throbbing and burning pain should be examined separately. In a sample of patients with established PHN, those who had received antiviral therapy during their acute infection were found to be much less likely to report burning pain than those who had not been treated with an antiviral agent; reports of throbbing pain in these two groups, however, did not differ (Bowsher, 1992, 1993).

3.1. Definitions of PHN

As discussed elsewhere (Dworkin and Portenoy, 1996; Dworkin et al., 1997a), a variety of approaches have been used to define PHN and to examine prolonged pain in zoster. Some authors have defined PHN as any pain persisting after the zoster rash has healed (Burgoon et al., 1957; Bamford and Boundy, 1968). Others have defined it as pain persisting beyond a specified interval following rash onset — for example, 4 weeks (Rogers and Tindall, 1971), 6 weeks (Brown, 1976), 3 months (Max et al., 1988), or 6 months (Harding et al., 1987) after rash onset. Yet another approach is to define PHN as any pain persisting beyond a specified interval following rash healing — for example, 1 month (Rowbotham et al., 1995) or 3 months (Baron and Saguer, 1993) after rash healing.

Because the differences in the definitions of PHN that have been used have important implications for the interpretation of research findings, the use of a diagnosis of PHN has recently been challenged. It has been suggested that pain in herpes zoster be considered "as a continuum, rather than distinguishing acute pain from an arbitrary definition of postherpetic neuralgia" (Huff et al., 1993). Several recent

studies have used this approach to examine the efficacy of various medications in reducing the duration of zoster pain (e.g. Degreef, 1994; Beutner et al., 1995; Whitley et al., 1996; Wood et al., 1996). In these trials, the primary endpoint used in evaluating treatment efficacy was the time from enrolment in the trial to complete cessation of all herpes zoster associated pain. When pain is examined in this manner, no distinction is made between acute pain and PHN (Wood, 1995).

Such analyses of herpes zoster pain considered as a continuum can provide a worthwhile overview of factors associated with pain duration, not only in studies of the efficacy of treatments for reducing pain duration, but also in research on risk factors for prolonged pain. One important advantage of examining zoster pain as a continuum is that no assumption is required regarding the point at which PHN begins. However, to the extent that acute pain in zoster and PHN differ clinically and have different pathophysiologies, examining pain only as a continuum would be misleading and could impede progress in understanding both acute and chronic pain.

The available data provide considerable support for the validity and importance of examining acute pain in zoster and PHN separately (Dworkin et al., 1997a). However, making a diagnosis of PHN and examining pain as a continuum are not mutually exclusive approaches to studying the persistence of zoster pain; pain data collected on multiple occasions beginning during the acute infection and continuing for several months thereafter can be examined by using a continuum of pain duration as well as by analyzing the incidence and duration of PHN. Accordingly, in the following discussion of prolonged pain in patients with herpes zoster, findings based on a diagnosis of PHN, however defined, will be considered together with findings based on analyses in which zoster pain is examined as a continuum of overall pain duration.

3.2. Incidence and prevalence of PHN

The number of herpes zoster patients with pain declines with time, and estimates of the proportion of

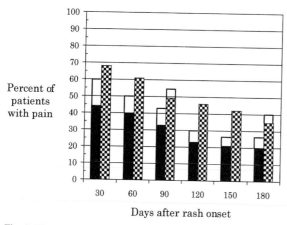

Percent of patients with pain

Days after rash onset

Fig. 1. The percent of placebo-treated herpes zoster patients with pain at monthly intervals from 1 to 6 months after rash onset in the major antiviral trials. Solid bars are all patients enrolled in the trials, checked bars are the subgroups of patients 50 years of age and older, and unshaded areas above the bars denote the range of values reported from different studies. All values reflect the results of one or more studies reporting follow-up data at these intervals.

patients who develop PHN have therefore varied depending on the definition of PHN used. In clinic and community studies, 9–24% of adult zoster patients have been reported to have PHN defined as pain persisting after rash healing (Burgoon et al., 1957; De Moragas and Kierland, 1957; Hope-Simpson, 1975; Molin, 1969; Ragozzino et al., 1982a); 34% were reported to have PHN defined as pain at 6 weeks (Brown, 1976) and 13% at 2 months (Molin, 1969) after rash onset. In a clinic study of patients over 60 years of age, 47% had pain at 1 month after rash onset (Rogers and Tindall, 1971). In two recent community studies in which some patients were treated with antiviral agents, 8% (Choo et al., 1997) and 19% (Helgason et al., 1996) of adult zoster patients had PHN defined as pain persisting after 1 month from rash onset, decreasing to 4.5% at 2 months (Choo et al., 1997) and 8% at 3 months (Helgason et al., 1996) after rash onset. The variability among the results of these studies must be at least partially explained by differences in samples, methods, and proportions of patients treated with antiviral agents.

Fig. 1 summarizes estimates of the proportion of patients reporting pain from 1 to 6 months after

rash onset in zoster patients who were enrolled in the placebo groups of the major antiviral trials that reported data at monthly follow-up intervals (Morton and Thomson, 1989; Harding and Porter, 1991; Huff et al., 1993; Wood et al., 1996; Dworkin et al., 1998). As can be seen from the figure, the percentage of herpes zoster patients with persisting pain declines with time in all patients enrolled in these trials, who were typically 18 years of age and older. There is a similar decline in persisting pain in the subgroup of placebo-treated patients enrolled in these trials who were 50 years of age and older (Wood et al., 1996; Dworkin et al., 1998).

The likelihood of persisting pain in the placebo groups in these antiviral trials is greater than what has been reported in most of the clinic and community studies (Cunningham and Dworkin, 2000). The explanation for this may be that patients with more severe herpes zoster infections — which are more likely to lead to the development of prolonged pain (see below) — are more likely to enroll in clinical trials. These differences might also be explained by more systematic and sensitive assessment of pain in the clinical trials than in many of the clinic and community studies.

Fig. 2 summarizes estimates of the proportion of patients reporting pain from 1 to 6 months after rash onset in zoster patients who were treated with either acyclovir, famciclovir, or valaciclovir in the major antiviral trials that reported data at monthly follow-up intervals. Estimates are provided for patients 18 years of age and older (Morton and Thomson, 1989; Harding and Porter, 1991; Huff et al., 1993; Wood et al., 1996; Dworkin et al., 1998) and for patients 50 years of age and older (Beutner et al., 1995; Wood et al., 1996; Dworkin et al., 1998). As in the placebo-treated patients, the risk of pain declines with time in all patients as well as in the older subgroup.

As can be seen by comparing Figs. 1 and 2, treating zoster patients with the antiviral agents acyclovir, famciclovir, and valacyclovir reduces the risk of developing PHN and the overall duration of pain, (Beutner et al., 1995; Tyring et al., 1995; Wood et al., 1996; Jackson et al., 1997; Dworkin et al., 1998;

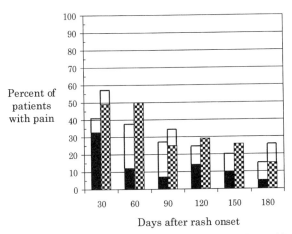

Fig. 2. The percent of antiviral-treated herpes zoster patients with pain at monthly intervals from 1 to 6 months after rash onset in the major antiviral trials. Solid bars are all patients enrolled in the trials, checked bars are the subgroups of patients 50 years of age and older, and unshaded areas above the bars denote the range of values reported from different studies. All values reflect the results of one or more studies reporting follow-up data at these intervals.

Tyring et al., 2000). Although the results of each of these studies taken singly can be challenged, the consistency of the findings provides strong support for the efficacy of antiviral therapy in reducing the risk of PHN. Because antiviral therapy in treating patients with zoster has become widespread in many areas, it is likely that the risk of prolonged pain has decreased over the past decade. The magnitude of any reduction in PHN in a population is difficult to estimate and would depend on several factors, including the percentage of zoster patients prescribed adequate antiviral treatment, patient compliance in completing an adequate course of treatment, and, if antiviral medications differ in efficacy, the proportions of patients administered different medications.

There have been no systematic attempts to investigate the prevalence of PHN. Bennett (1997) estimated that 500,000 individuals in the United States have PHN, but did not discuss how this figure was determined. It is possible, however, that the prevalence of PHN is higher than this. Based on a survey of community dwelling elders in the United Kingdom, Bowsher (1999) estimated that "the number of ongoing cases of PHN in the elderly population in the U.K. at any one time must be about 200,000; and would be of the order of one million in the United States" and observed that "these are very conservative estimates ..."

3.3. Risk factors for PHN

There are a considerable number of recent studies in which risk factors for PHN have been investigated. The impetus for these studies has come from several sources, including attempts to identify risk factors as a means of increasing understanding of the natural history and pathogenesis of PHN (Dworkin and Banks, 1999). In addition, studies of the role of covariates in clinical trials of antiviral agents and other drugs in herpes zoster have also identified risk factors for PHN (Dworkin et al., 1997a, 1998; Whitley et al., 1998, 1999). Furthermore, knowledge of risk factors can be used to design interventions intended to prevent the development of PHN (Dworkin et al., 2000b). Finally, studies of risk factors for PHN make it possible to identify those zoster patients who have the greatest need for preventive efforts because of their increased risk of chronic pain (Johnson, 1995).

3.3.1. Greater age
Until recently, age was the only factor that had been consistently associated with an increased risk of PHN (Burgoon et al., 1957; De Moragas and Kierland, 1957; Hope-Simpson, 1975; Brown, 1976; Ragozzino et al., 1982a; Harding et al., 1987; Choo et al., 1997). In children with herpes zoster, the risk of PHN approaches zero (Rogers and Tindall, 1972; Hope-Simpson, 1975; Guess et al., 1985; Petursson et al., 1998). An early investigation reported that persisting pain was infrequent in herpes zoster patients under 40 years of age, but that the proportion of patients with pain lasting 1 year or more approached 50% in those over the age of 70 years (De Moragas and Kierland, 1957). In Cirencester, England, the prevalence of pain one or more months after rash onset was 3–4% in age groups 30–49 years but 21, 29, and 34% in the age groups 60–69, 70–79, and greater than 80 years, respectively (Hope-Simpson, 1975). In Rochester, MN, the average age of zoster

patients with pain persisting after rash healing was 67 years compared to an average age of 46 years in the remainder of the cohort (Ragozzino et al., 1982a). In a recent study conducted in Boston, patients aged 50 years or older had a 14.7-fold higher prevalence (95% CI, 6.8–32.0) of pain 30 days after rash onset compared to patients younger than 50 years old (Choo et al., 1997). In Iceland, 2, 15, and 41% of zoster patients aged 0–39, 40–59 and 60 years and older, respectively, had pain 1 month after rash onset (Helgason et al., 1996).

Perhaps the most interesting unanswered question about risk factors for PHN is why older age is a risk factor (Wall, 1993). It has been hypothesized that age is associated with the development of PHN because older patients have more severe zoster infections (Higa et al., 1988, 1997), but the results of the studies reviewed above do not provide uniform support for a relationship between greater age and more severe acute infection. Moreover, the results of several recent studies suggest that age and acute pain and rash severity make independent contributions to identifying which zoster patients develop PHN (Beutner et al., 1995; Wood et al., 1996; Dworkin et al., 1997b, 1998; Whitley et al., 1998). To the extent that acute pain and rash severity reflect a more severe infection, these findings suggest that the increased risk of PHN in the elderly is not completely accounted for by more severe infections, and that this increased risk reflects an additional pathophysiologic process. Indeed, Hope-Simpson (1967) recognized that although severe zoster infections are frequently associated with the development of PHN, even mild cases are sometimes followed by PHN.

One pathophysiologic process which might contribute to an increased risk of PHN in the elderly involves nervous system senescence. The results of a recent study, discussed below, in which large fiber polyneuropathy in zoster patients predicted the development of PHN is consistent with this possibility (Baron et al., 1997). A second process that might explain the increased risk of PHN in the elderly involves immunopathogenesis. It has been hypothesized that autoimmune phenomena and age-associated disturbances in cytokine production, possi-

bly involving cytokine neurotoxicity, may result in nerve damage and contribute to the development of prolonged pain in zoster patients (Weksler, 1994; Dworkin and Portenoy, 1996). The contribution of immunopathological processes to the development of PHN has not been examined directly. However, this hypothesis is consistent not only with the greater risk of PHN in the elderly, but also with several other recent findings, including the existence of pain-free intervals in PHN, evidence of inflammation in patients with well-established PHN, and apparently equivalent risks of PHN in immunocompromised and immunocompetent patients (Dworkin and Johnson, 1999).

3.3.2. Greater acute pain severity

The possibility that "there may be a correlation between the duration of pain and the severity of pain on presentation" in herpes zoster was proposed as a hypothesis in need of further investigation only several years ago (Wood et al., 1994). However, as summarized in Table II, there are now a considerable

TABLE II

Studies of the relationship between acute pain severity in herpes zoster and the development of prolonged pain

Authors and date	Sample size
Molin, 1969	706
Riopelle et al., 1984	72
Harding et al., 1987	71
Dworkin et al., 1992	19
Leijon et al., 1993	52
Cioni et al., 1994	52
Beutner et al., 1995	1141
Bruxelle, 1995	301
McKendrick and Wood, 1995	160
Whitley et al., 1996	208
Wood et al., 1996	316
Dworkin et al., 1997b	129
Dworkin et al., 1998	419
Meister et al., 1998	635
Söltz-Szöts et al., 1998	511
Harrison et al., 1999	170
Decroix et al., 2000	1897
Haanpää et al., 2000	113
Tyring et al., 2000	597

number of independent studies that have reported that patients with more severe acute pain are at greater risk for both prolonged zoster pain assessed as a continuum and for PHN. In addition, acute pain severe enough to interfere with activities of daily living has also been found to be a risk factor for PHN (Choo et al., 1997; Galil et al., 1997). The majority of these studies examined the persistence of pain using a 6-month follow-up period. However, greater acute pain severity has also been reported to predict greater duration of pain in patients with pain resolving before rash healing (Bamford and Boundy, 1968) as well as the presence of PHN 9 years after acute zoster (McKendrick and Wood, 1995).

Although a variety of research designs, pain measures, and approaches to examining prolonged pain have been used in these studies, all but one (Molin, 1969) studied patients prospectively. In addition, the relationship between acute pain severity and prolonged pain has been found in immunocompromised patients (Harrison et al., 1999) as well as immunocompetent patients. Given the uniformity of the findings, greater acute pain severity can now be considered an established risk factor, one which may have implications for the prevention of PHN (Dworkin et al., 2000b). The focus of future research should, therefore, become the identification of mechanisms accounting for this relationship. In pursuing this task, a priority should be to conduct a careful examination of the specific aspects of acute zoster pain that predict the development of chronic pain (Dworkin, 1997).

Few of the studies that have reported a relationship between the severity of acute pain and PHN have examined the different types of pain associated with zoster. For example, is the predominant quality of pain in zoster — whether burning, throbbing, stabbing, or allodynia — associated with the risk of developing PHN? As discussed above, burning pain is more common in PHN patients than in zoster patients, who are more likely to report sharp, stabbing pain. Burning pain, however, was much less likely to be reported by PHN patients whose zoster had been treated with acyclovir than by PHN patients who had not been treated with an antiviral drug (Bowsher, 1992, 1993). Antiviral drugs inhibit VZV replication

and may thereby limit neural damage contributing to the development of PHN (Mondelli et al., 1996). Considered together, the greater prevalence of burning pain in PHN compared to zoster and the reduced burning pain in PHN patients treated with acyclovir suggest that burning pain may reflect an important pathophysiologic mechanism in the development of prolonged pain.

It could, therefore, be hypothesized that zoster patients with prominent burning pain are at greater risk for the development of PHN. Preliminary reports of the results of recent studies, however, suggested that patients who described their zoster pain as sharp (Johnson et al., 1995) and who had allodynia (Shukla et al., 1996; Haanpää et al., 2000) were more likely to have persisting pain. Allodynia is associated with greater acute pain (Haanpää et al., 1999, 2000), and so it is possible that such relationships reflect the relationship between acute pain severity and PHN. Additional prospective studies are needed to clarify the relationship between pain quality in zoster and the development of PHN.

3.3.3. Greater rash severity

Several studies have reported that greater severity of the zoster cutaneous eruption is associated with prolonged pain and the development of PHN (Wildenhoff et al., 1979, 1981; Wilson, 1986; Higa et al., 1988, 1992, 1997; Marsh and Cooper, 1993; Whitley et al., 1996, 1999; Choo et al., 1997; Dworkin et al., 1998; Meister et al., 1998; Harrison et al., 1999). The severity of the zoster rash has been assessed using a variety of methods in these studies, including counts of the number of vesicles and ratings of the proportion of the dermatome affected. In addition, the duration of time until the occurrence of various aspects of rash healing has been examined, including assessments of time to cessation of new vesicle formation and time to complete crusting. Few studies, however, have reported assessments of rash severity on multiple occasions, which would allow rash progression from onset to healing to be examined. Even fewer studies have evaluated the interrater reliability of their ratings of rash severity, which involve judgments with a subjective component.

Although scarring in the affected dermatome is common in patients following healing of the zoster rash, no studies have examined the relationship between rash severity and the development of scarring. Three studies, however, have examined the relationship between scarring and PHN and have reported that presence (Battock et al., 1990; Nurmikko and Bowsher, 1990; Bowsher, 1999) and greater extent (Battock et al., 1990) of scarring distinguished patients with PHN from zoster patients whose pain did not persist. Because it is likely that scarring is a consequence of a more severe rash during the acute infection, these findings are consistent with the data suggesting that greater rash severity is a risk factor for PHN. It has also been reported that scarring is less severe in PHN patients with prominent allodynia (Rowbotham and Fields, 1989), which suggests that zoster patients with a less severe rash are more likely to suffer from allodynia if they develop PHN.

3.3.4. Greater neurological abnormalities

A fourth risk factor for PHN that has been identified by several groups of investigators is the presence of greater neurological abnormalities during acute zoster. Herpes zoster patients with greater sensory abnormalities in the affected dermatome, compared to the contralateral unaffected dermatome, were found to be at greater risk for PHN in several studies (Noda et al., 1987; Nurmikko et al., 1990; Leijon et al., 1993; Bruxelle, 1995). Evaluations of sensory dysfunction in the affected dermatome included clinical assessments of hypoesthesia as well as quantitative sensory testing (e.g. elevated thermal and vibration thresholds).

Thermal and tactile thresholds, however, did not predict PHN in the largest prospective study of sensory risk factors (Haanpää and Nurmikko, 1997; T.J. Nurmikko, personal communication, March 17, 1999). In this sample of 113 patients, however, dynamic and static mechanical allodynia (and pinprick hypoesthesia) were associated with the later development of PHN (Haanpää et al., 2000).

In an MRI study of zoster, abnormalities in the brainstem and cervical cord assessed within 2 weeks of rash onset predicted PHN defined as pain lasting more than 3 months after rash onset (Haanpää et al., 1998). Although a relationship was also found between EMG motor abnormalities assessed during zoster and PHN (Haanpää et al., 1997), this trend was not statistically significant.

Interestingly, Baron et al. (1997) recently reported that elevated vibration thresholds outside the affected dermatome (i.e. in the hands and feet) in zoster patients predicted PHN. These investigators concluded that a generalized subclinical large fiber polyneuropathy is a risk factor for PHN. Indirect support for this conclusion is provided by the report of an almost two-fold greater risk of PHN in patients who developed zoster after the onset of diabetes compared to patients who developed zoster before they developed diabetes, which suggests that diabetic polyneuropathy may render the individual more susceptible to PHN (McCulloch et al., 1982). As noted above, on the basis of the results of these studies it may be hypothesized that the relationship between greater age and increased risk of PHN is explained by an age-associated generalized large fiber loss.

It has also been reported that there is greater sensory dysfunction in the affected dermatome in patients with PHN than in zoster patients whose pain did not persist (Wildenhoff et al., 1979, 1981; Nurmikko and Bowsher, 1990; Leijon et al., 1993). The results of these studies indicate that sensory dysfunction can persist well beyond the acute phase of zoster and that it is a frequent concomitant of prolonged pain. This sensory dysfunction seems to be associated with ipsilateral (Rowbotham et al., 1996) as well as bilateral (Oaklander et al., 1998) loss of cutaneous innervation.

3.3.5. Presence of a prodrome

In recent studies, the presence of prodromal pain and symptoms was found to be associated with prolonged pain and the development of PHN (Beutner et al., 1995; Choo et al., 1997; Meister et al., 1998; Whitley et al., 1998). The zoster prodrome is often accompanied by other symptoms — including fatigue, dysesthesias, and headache — and some patients may have these prodromal symptoms in the absence of pain. In futures studies of risk factors for

PHN, it will be necessary to carefully distinguish prodromal dermatomal pain from other prodromal symptoms. Because there is also variability in the duration of the zoster prodrome and in the severity of prodromal pain, it will be important to examine prodrome duration and pain intensity in future research.

3.3.6. More pronounced immune response

Greater magnitude and duration of the humoral and cell-mediated immune response in zoster patients has been reported to predict prolonged pain (Dan et al., 1983; Higa et al., 1988, 1992). Significant relationships were found between the immune response measures and rash severity, suggesting that a more pronounced VZV-specific immune response during zoster may predict prolonged pain because it reflects a more severe acute infection (Dan et al., 1983; Higa et al., 1988, 1992).

Several other findings are consistent with this hypothesis. VZV-specific cell-mediated immune responses reach their maximum 1–2 weeks after the onset of zoster, which is usually the time of maximal infection (Arvin et al., 1978). In addition, measures of both humoral and cell-mediated immunity were found to be lower in acyclovir-treated compared to placebo-treated zoster patients (Mitchell et al., 1986). These group differences were not statistically significant, but the dose of acyclovir used was only half of what is now accepted as adequate antiviral treatment for zoster. In discussing their results, the investigators suggested that the reduced immune response may have reflected a reduced antigenic burden resulting from the inhibition of viral replication associated with acyclovir treatment (Mitchell et al., 1986).

3.3.7. Fever

In a single study, fever greater than 38°C during zoster was reported to predict the development of PHN (Wildenhoff et al., 1981).

3.3.8. Gender

Several investigators have examined whether there is a relationship between the patient's gender and the risk of prolonged pain, and the majority of these studies have found that men and women are equally likely to develop PHN (Hope-Simpson, 1975; Brown, 1976; Wildenhoff et al., 1979, 1981; Harding et al., 1987; Beutner et al., 1995; Wood et al., 1996; Choo et al., 1997; Dworkin et al., 1998; Whitley et al., 1998).

3.3.9. Dermatome

The relationship between the specific dermatome affected in zoster and the risk of prolonged pain has been examined in a number of studies (Burgoon et al., 1957; De Moragas and Kierland, 1957; Hope-Simpson, 1975; Wildenhoff et al., 1979, 1981; Ragozzino et al., 1982a; Choo et al., 1997; Higa et al., 1997). Although the results of several of these studies suggested that the likelihood of prolonged pain is greater in patients with ophthalmic or trigeminal zoster, this relationship has not been found consistently.

The results of recent analyses of a large sample of patients indicated that pain at 6 months after rash onset was present in a higher proportion of patients with ophthalmic zoster (12%) than in patients with zoster in other dermatomes (7%); this difference, however, was not statistically significant (Decroix et al., 2000). Considered together with the results of previous research, these results suggest that any increased risk of PHN in patients with ophthalmic zoster is not substantial.

3.3.10. Psychosocial risk factors

The risk factors for PHN discussed to this point have consisted of demographic and biomedical characteristics of zoster patients. It has also been suggested that psychosocial factors might play a role in determining which patients will have pain that persists. Pilowsky (1977) proposed that the herpes zoster patients who develop PHN are characterized by a constellation of certain premorbid personality traits and stressful life events. Although this hypothesis was based on psychiatric interviews with patients who had suffered from PHN for as long as 15 years, the results of recent cross-sectional, retrospective, and prospective studies suggest that psychosocial factors play a role in the development of PHN.

In a cross-sectional study in which patients with PHN were compared with individuals with a history of zoster who did not have persisting pain, the PHN patients had more symptoms of anxiety and rated their past experiences of pain as more intense (Rose et al., 1992). PHN patients had also experienced fewer stressful life events in the preceding year in this study, a finding that the authors attributed to the withdrawal from activities that characterizes chronic pain patients. The results of a second cross-sectional study that attempted to identify predictors of PHN found a higher frequency of 'psychopathological impairment' in patients with PHN than in patients with a history of zoster who did not develop chronic pain (Leplow et al., 1990).

In a retrospective study, patients who reported having other diseases and/or psychosocial stress at the time they developed zoster were significantly more likely to have PHN, changed daily activities, and lower levels of well-being than individuals who reported no other diseases or psychosocial stress at the onset of their zoster (Engberg et al., 1995). Bowsher (1999), in a recent retrospective survey of an elderly population, found that living alone at the time of a zoster infection significantly predicted an increased risk of PHN defined as pain persisting for 3 or more months after rash onset.

The results of these studies are consistent with the existence of psychosocial risk factors for PHN. However, the use of cross-sectional and retrospective methods makes it impossible to determine whether psychosocial distress is a risk factor for PHN or whether the recollection of such distress being present at the time of acute zoster is simply one of the consequences of PHN. Prospective studies are necessary to determine whether variables that may plausibly be either antecedents or consequences of chronic pain are risk factors (Dworkin, 1997). In a prospective study of a small sample of zoster patients, those who developed PHN had lower life satisfaction and greater depression, anxiety, and disease conviction during their acute infection than patients who did not develop PHN (Dworkin et al., 1992). Preliminary analyses of the data from a recent prospective study of a larger sample have

provided additional evidence that psychosocial factors, including disease conviction and somatosensory amplification, are associated with an increased risk of PHN independently of age and acute pain severity (Dworkin et al., 1997b). Two chronic stressors — poor physical health and financial resources — also predicted PHN in this study, but these variables did not remain significant when age and acute pain severity were controlled (Dworkin et al., 1997b).

In a large sample of zoster patients 50 years of age and older enrolled in a recent antiviral trial, Mauskopf et al. (1995) examined whether the scales of a health-related quality of life measure predicted zoster pain duration assessed as a continuum after taking into account demographic and clinical variables. Measures of physical mobility and energy made an independent contribution to predicting overall pain duration, but sleep, social isolation, and emotional reaction did not. It is likely that physical mobility and energy during zoster reflect not only the severity of the infection but also psychosocial factors, which are known to have an important impact on disability and activity level.

Considered together with the research discussed above on psychosocial risk factors for acute zoster, the results of these studies suggest that psychological distress and stressful life events play a role in the onset of herpes zoster and also in the development of PHN. This conclusion is consistent with the evidence suggesting that psychosocial factors contribute to the onset and course of other herpes virus infections (Glaser and Kiecolt-Glaser, 1994).

3.3.11. Future research directions on PHN risk factors

Except for age and psychosocial variables, the risk factors for PHN that have been identified — acute pain severity, rash severity, neurological abnormalities, presence of a prodrome, more pronounced immune responses, and fever — can all be considered concomitants of a more severe infection. Several of these risk factors have been identified by independent groups of investigators, and they provide appreciable support for the conclusion that there is a greater risk of PHN in patients with more severe zoster. Indeed, over 30 years ago Hope-Simpson (1967) proposed that patients with more severe infections are more likely to develop PHN. More severe zoster infections are accompanied by greater neural damage, and it has been proposed that this neural damage contributes prominently to the development of PHN (Bennett, 1994; Dworkin and Portenoy, 1996). However, few studies have attempted to systematically examine the damage to neural tissue caused by severe zoster infections, whether by skin punch biopsy or by detailed sensory testing.

Another important question about risk factors for PHN involves the nature of the associations among the risk factors that have been identified. Although a number of studies, discussed above, have examined the relationships between acute pain severity and age and rash severity, little is known about the relationships between these risk factors and neurological abnormalities, humoral and cellular immune responses, and psychosocial distress during herpes zoster. In addition, interactions among the risk factors for PHN have rarely been examined. For example, is greater acute pain severity a risk factor for PHN irrespective of age and rash severity, or is this relationship limited to, or stronger in, certain groups of patients? The results of such research on herpes zoster will be important in evaluating single-factor (e.g. Higa et al., 1997), multifactorial (Dworkin and Banks, 1999), and multiple-mechanism (Rowbotham et al., 1998) approaches to understanding the pathogenesis of PHN.

One of the goals of research on risk factors discussed above is to identify which zoster patients have the greatest risk of PHN. Accurate identification of such patients would make it possible to aggressively attempt to prevent chronic pain in those patients most likely to develop it. A recent study by Whitley et al. (1999) is an important demonstration of the value of combining risk factors to identify patients with a high risk of prolonged pain. These investigators categorized zoster patients over the age of 50 years by degree of acute pain and number of lesions assessed within 72 h of rash onset. Patients who rated their acute pain as severe and who had 47 or more lesions were very likely to continue to have pain throughout the follow-up period. Approximately 70% of these patients still had pain 6 months after rash onset, a very high rate of identification given the use of only two risk factors.

4. PHN in the immunocompromised patient

Unfortunately, there have been few studies that have specifically examined acute zoster pain and PHN in immunocompromised patients. On the basis of clinical observations and a limited number of studies, several investigators have suggested that there seem to be equivalent risks of PHN in immunocompromised and immunocompetent patients (Balfour, 1988; Rusthoven et al., 1988a; Wood, 1991; Gershon, 1993). Because immunocompromised patients are more likely to have severe zoster — with greater cutaneous and visceral dissemination — this apparent absence of an increased risk of PHN further suggests that the severity of the acute infection does not fully account for PHN, as noted above. In a recent study, however, herpes zoster patients with HIV infection, connective tissue diseases, and organ transplants had a higher risk of developing PHN (Choo et al., 1997).

Harrison et al. (1999) recently reported the results of a study of pain in AIDS patients with zoster enrolled in an antiviral trial. These investigators found that pain intensity at enrolment and rash severity and duration predicted the severity of acute pain, defined as pain during the first month after rash onset. The severity of chronic pain, defined as pain from 1 to 12 months after rash onset, was predicted by pain and rash severity at enrolment. Because these two risk factors for PHN have also been found in numerous studies of immunocompetent patients, these results suggest that the natural history and mechanisms of PHN in immunocompromised and immunocompetent patients may be similar. Certainly, additional research on the epidemiology and natural history of zoster pain in immunocompromised patients (ideally matched to immunocompetent patients for age) is greatly needed.

5. Conclusions

As discussed previously, there is some evidence that the incidence of zoster has increased in recent decades. Regardless of whether this has occurred, it is likely that the number of patients suffering from herpes zoster and PHN will increase substantially in the future. As Weller (1995) has observed, zoster can be expected to "increase as the mean age of our population increases, reflecting both the age-related decay of cellular immunity and the enhanced propensity for malignancy in the elderly." PHN will become more prevalent not only because of this increased incidence of zoster but also because PHN is more likely to develop in the older individuals whose numbers are increasing (Schmader, 1995, 1998). Because PHN patients suffer from physical and social disability and psychological distress and have greatly increased health care utilization as a result of their chronic pain, this substantial increase in the prevalence of PHN will have a major impact on public health.

References

Antonelli, M.A., Moreland, L.W. and Brick, J.E. (1991) Herpes zoster in patients with rheumatoid arthritis treated with weekly, low-dose methotrexate. Am. J. Med., 90: 295–298.

Arvin, A.M. (1996) Varicella-zoster virus. In: B.N. Fields, D.M. Knipe, P.M. Howley, R.M. Chanock, J.L. Melnick, T.P. Monath, B. Roizman and S.E. Straus (Eds.), Fields Virology, 3rd edn., Lippincott-Raven, Philadelphia, PA, pp. 2547–2587.

Arvin, A.M., Pollard, R.B., Rasmussen, L.E. and Merigan, T.C. (1978) Selective impairment of lymphocyte reactivity to varicella-zoster virus antigen among untreated patients with lymphoma. J. Infect. Dis., 137: 531–540.

Baba, K., Yabuuchi, H., Takahashi, M. and Ogra, P.L. (1986) Increased incidence of herpes zoster in normal children infected with varicella zoster virus during infancy: community-based follow-up study. J. Pediatr., 108: 372–377.

Balfour, H.H. Jr. (1988) Varicella zoster virus infections in immunocompromised hosts: a review of the natural history and management. Am. J. Med., 85 (Suppl. 2A): 68–73.

Bamford, J.C. and Boundy, C.P. (1968) The natural history of herpes zoster (shingles). Med. J. Aust., 13: 524–528.

Baron, R. and Saguer, M. (1993) Postherpetic neuralgia: are C-nociceptors involved in signalling and maintenance of tactile allodynia? Brain, 116: 1477–1496.

Baron, R., Haendler, G. and Schulte, H. (1997) Afferent large fiber polyneuropathy predicts the development of postherpetic neuralgia. Pain, 73: 231–238.

Battock, T.M., Finn, R. and Barnes, R.M.R. (1990) Observations on herpes zoster: 1. residual scarring and post-herpetic neuralgia; 2. handedness and the risk of infection. Br. J. Clin. Pract., 44: 596–598.

Bean, B., Deamant, C. and Aeppli, D. (1993) Acute zoster: course, complications, and treatment in the immunocompetent host. In: C.P.N. Watson (Ed.), Herpes Zoster and Postherpetic Neuralgia. Elsevier, Amsterdam, pp. 37–58.

Bennett, G.J. (1994) Hypotheses on the pathogenesis of herpes zoster-associated pain. Ann. Neurol., 35 (Suppl.): S38–S41.

Bennett, G.J. (1997) Neuropathic pain: an overview. In: D. Borsook (Ed.), Molecular Neurobiology of Pain. IASP Press, Seattle, pp. 109–113.

Berlin, B.S. and Campbell, T. (1970) Hospital-acquired herpes zoster following exposure to chickenpox. J. Am. Med. Assoc., 211: 1831–1832.

Beutner, K.R., Friedman, D.J., Forszpaniak, C., Andersen, P.L. and Wood, M.J. (1995) Valaciclovir compared with acyclovir for improved therapy for herpes zoster in immunocompetent adults. Antimicrob. Agents Chemother., 39: 1546–1553.

Bhala, B.B., Ramamoorthy, C., Bowsher, D. and Yelnoorker, K.N. (1988) Shingles and postherpetic neuralgia. Clin. J. Pain, 4: 169–174.

Boon, R.J. and Griffin, D.R.J. (1996) Famciclovir: efficacy in zoster and issues in the assessment of pain. In: J. Mills, P.A. Volberding and L. Corey (Eds.), Antiviral Chemotherapy 4: New Directions for Clinical Application and Research. Plenum Press, New York, pp. 17–31.

Bower, J.H., Hammack, J.E., McDonnell, S.K. and Tefferi, A. (1997) The neurologic complications of B-cell chronic lymphocytic lymphoma. Neurology, 48: 407–412.

Bowsher, D. (1992) Acute herpes zoster and postherpetic neuralgia: effects of acyclovir and outcome of treatment with amitriptyline. Br. J. Gen. Pract., 42: 244–246.

Bowsher, D. (1993) Sensory change in postherpetic neuralgia. In: C.P.N. Watson (Ed.), Herpes Zoster and Postherpetic Neuralgia. Elsevier, Amsterdam, pp. 97–107.

Bowsher, D. (1999) The lifetime occurrence of herpes zoster and prevalence of postherpetic neuralgia: a retrospective survey in an elderly population. Eur. J. Pain, 3: 335–342.

Brown, G.R. (1976) Herpes zoster: correlation with age, sex, distribution, neuralgia, and associated disorders. South. Med. J., 69: 576–578.

Brunell, P.A., Miller, L.H. and Lovejoy, F. (1968) Zoster in children. Am. J. Dis. Child., 115: 432–437.

Bruxelle, J. (1995) Prospective epidemiologic study of painful and neurologic sequelae induced by herpes zoster in patients treated early with oral acyclovir. Neurology, 45 (Suppl. 8): S78–S79.

Buchbinder, S.P., Katz, M.H., Hessol, N.A., Liu, J.Y., O'Malley, P.M., Underwood, R. and Holmberg, R. (1992) Herpes zoster and human immunodeficiency virus infection. J. Infect. Dis., 166: 1153–1156.

Burgoon, C.F., Burgoon, J.S. and Baldridge, G.D. (1957) The natural history of herpes zoster. J. Am. Med. Assoc., 164: 265–269.

Choo, P.W., Galil, K., Donahue, J.G., Walker, A.M., Spiegelman, D. and Platt, R. (1997) Risk factors for postherpetic neuralgia. Arch. Intern. Med., 157, 1217–1224.

Cioni, R., Giannini, F., Passero, S., Paradiso, C., Rossi, S., Fimiani, M. and Battistini, N. (1994) An electromyographic evaluation of motor complications in thoracic herpes zoster. Electromyogr. Clin. Neurophysiol., 34: 125–128.

Cobo, L.M., Foulks, G.N., Liesegang, T., Lass, J., Sutphin, J.E., Wilhelmus, K., Jones, D.B., Chapman, S., Segreti, A.C. and King, D.H. (1986) Oral acyclovir in the treatment of acute herpes zoster ophthalmicus. Ophthalmology, 93: 763–770.

Colebunders, R., Mann, J.M., Francis, H., Bila, K., Izaley, L., Ilwaya, M., Kakonde, N., Quinn, T.C., Curran, J.W. and Piot, P. (1988) Herpes zoster in African patients: a clinical predictor of human immunodeficiency virus infections. J. Infect. Dis., 157: 314–318.

Cooper, M. (1987) The epidemiology of herpes zoster. Eye, 1: 413–421.

Cunningham, A.L. and Dworkin, R.H. (2000) The challenge of postherpetic neuralgia. Br. Med. J., 321: 778–779.

Dan, K., Higa, K., Tanaka, K. and Mori, R. (1983) Herpetic pain and cellular immunity. In: T. Yokota and R. Dubner (Eds.), Current Topics in Pain Research and Therapy. Excerpta Medica, Amsterdam, pp. 293–305.

Davies, L., Cossins, L., Bowsher, D. and Drummond, M. (1994) The cost of treatment for post-herpetic neuralgia in the UK. PharmacoEconomics, 6: 142–148.

Decroix, J., Partsh, H., Gonzalez, R., Mobacken, H., Goh, C.L., Walsh, L., Shukla, S. and Naisbett, B. (2000) Factors influencing pain outcome in herpes zoster: an observational study with valaciclovir. J. Eur. Acad. Dermatol. Venereol., 14: 22–33.

De Moragas, J.M. and Kierland, R.R. (1957) The outcome of patients with herpes zoster. Am. Med. Assoc. Arch. Dermatol., 75: 193–196.

Degreef, H. (1994) Famciclovir, a new oral antiherpes drug: results of the first controlled clinical study demonstrating its efficacy and safety in the treatment of uncomplicated herpes zoster in immunocompetent patients. Int. J. Antimicrob. Agents, 4: 241–246.

Dehne, K.L., Dhlakama, D.G., Richter, C., Mawadza, M., Mc-Clean, D. and Huss, R. (1992) Herpes zoster as an indicator of HIV infection in Africa. Trop. Doct., 22: 68–70.

Dolin, R., Reichman, R.C., Mazur, M.H. and Whitley, R.J. (1978) Herpes zoster-varicella infections in immunosuppressed patients. Ann. Intern. Med., 89: 375–388.

Donahue, J.G., Choo, P.W., Manson, J.E. and Platt, R. (1995) The incidence of herpes zoster. Arch. Intern. Med., 155: 1605–1609.

Dubuisson, D. and Melzack, R. (1976) Classification of clinical

pain descriptions by multiple group discriminant analysis. Exp. Neur., 51: 480–487.

Dworkin, R.H. (1996) Racial differences in herpes zoster and age at onset of varicella. J. Infect. Dis., 174: 239–241.

Dworkin, R.H. (1997) Which individuals with acute pain are most likely to develop a chronic pain syndrome? Pain Forum, 6: 127–136.

Dworkin, R.H. and Banks, S.M. (1999) A vulnerability-diathesis-stress model of chronic pain: herpes zoster and the development of postherpetic neuralgia. In: R.J. Gatchel and D.C. Turk (Eds.), Psychosocial Factors in Pain: Critical Perspectives. Guilford, New York, pp. 247–269.

Dworkin, R.H. and Johnson, R.W. (1999) A belt of roses from hell: pain in herpes zoster and postherpetic neuralgia. In: A.R. Block, E.F. Kremer and E. Fernandez (Eds.), Handbook of Pain Syndromes: Biopsychosocial Perspectives. Erlbaum, Hillsdale, NJ, pp. 371–402.

Dworkin, R.H. and Portenoy, R.K. (1996) Pain and its persistence in herpes zoster. Pain, 67: 241–251.

Dworkin, R.H., Hartstein, G., Rosner, H.L., Walther, R.R., Sweeney, E.W. and Brand, L. (1992) A high-risk method for studying psychosocial antecedents of chronic pain: the prospective investigation of herpes zoster. J. Abnorm. Psychol., 101: 200–205.

Dworkin, R.H., Carrington, D., Cunningham, A., Kost, R., Levin, M., McKendrick, M., Oxman, M., Rentier, B., Schmader, K.E., Tappeiner, G., Wassilew, S.W. and Whitley, R.J. (1997a) Assessment of pain in herpes zoster: lessons learned from antiviral trials. Antiviral Res., 33: 73–85.

Dworkin, R.H., Cooper, E.M., Walther, R.R. and Sweeney, E.W. (1997b) Risk factors for postherpetic neuralgia: a prospective study of acute herpes zoster patients. Third International Conference on the Varicella-Zoster Virus, Palm Beach, FL.

Dworkin, R.H., Boon, R.J., Griffin, D.R.G. and Phung, D. (1998) Postherpetic neuralgia: impact of famciclovir, age, rash severity, and acute pain in herpes zoster patients. J. Infect. Dis., 178 (Suppl. 1), S76–S80.

Dworkin, R.H., Johnson, R.W. and Griffin, D.R.J. (2000a) Acute pain in herpes zoster. In: M. Devor, M.C. Rowbotham and Z. Wiesenfeld-Hallin (Eds.), Proceedings of the 9th World Congress on Pain, IASP Press, Seattle, pp. 725–731.

Dworkin, R.H., Perkins, F.M. and Nagasako, E.M. (2000b) Prospects for the prevention of postherpetic neuralgia in herpes zoster patients. Clin. J. Pain, 16: S90–S100.

Dworsky, M., Whitely, R. and Alford, C. (1980) Herpes zoster in early infancy. Am. J. Dis. Child., 134: 618–619.

Engberg, I.B., Gröndahl, G. and Thibom, K. (1995) Patients' experiences of herpes zoster and postherpetic neuralgia. J. Adv. Nurs., 21: 427–433.

Engels, E.A., Rosenberg, P.S. and Biggar, R.J. (1999) Zoster incidence in human immunodeficiency virus-infected hemophiliacs and homosexual men, 1984–1997: District of Columbia Gay Cohort Study, Multicenter Hemophilia Cohort Study. J. Infect. Dis., 180: 1784–1789.

Fueyo, M.A. and Lookingbill, D.P. (1984) Herpes zoster and occult malignancy. J. Am. Acad. Dermatol., 11: 480–482.

Friedman-Kien, A.E., Lafleur, F.L., Gendler, E., Hennessey, N.P., Montagna, R., Halbert, S., Rubinstein, P., Krasinski, K., Zang, E. and Poiez, B. (1986) Herpes zoster: a possible early clinical sign for development of acquired immunodeficiency syndrome in high-risk individuals. J. Am. Acad. Dermatol., 14: 1023–1028.

Galil, K., Choo, P.W., Donahue, J.G. and Platt, R. (1997) The sequelae of herpes zoster. Arch. Intern. Med., 157: 1209–1213.

Gershon, A.A. (1993) Zoster in immunosuppressed patients. In: C.P.N. Watson (Ed.), Herpes Zoster and Postherpetic Neuralgia, Elsevier, Amsterdam, pp. 73–86.

Gershon, A.A., Mervish, N., LaRussa, P., Steinberg, S., Lo, S.H., Hodes, D., Fikrig, S., Bonagura, V. and Bakshi, S. (1997) Varicella-zoster virus infection in children with underlying human immunodeficiency virus infection. J. Infect. Dis., 176: 1496–1500.

Gilden, D.H., Dueland, A.N., Cohrs, R., Martin, J.R., Kleinschmidt-DeMasters, B.K. and Mahalingam, R. (1991) Preherpetic neuralgia. Neurology, 41: 1215–1218.

Gilden, D.H., Dueland, A.N., Devlin, M.E., Mahalingam, R. and Cohrs, R. (1992) Varicella-zoster virus reactivation without rash. J. Infect. Dis., 166 (Suppl. 1), S30–S34.

Gilden, D.H., Wright, R.R., Schneck, S.A., Gwaltney, J.M. and Mahalingam, R. (1994) Zoster sine herpete, a clinical variant. Ann. Neurol., 35: 530–533.

Glaser, R. and Kiecolt-Glaser, J.K. (1994) Stress-associated immune modulation and its implications for reactivation of latent herpesviruses. In: R. Glaser and J.F. Jones (Eds.), Herpesvirus Infections, Dekker, New York, pp. 245–270.

Glesby, M., Moore, R.D. and Chaisson, R.E. (1995) Clinical spectrum of herpes zoster in adults with HIV. Clin. Infect. Dis., 21: 370–375.

Graff-Radford, S.B., Kames, L.D. and Naliboff, B.D. (1986) Measures of psychological adjustment and perception of pain in postherpetic neuralgia and trigeminal neuralgia. Clin. J. Pain, 2: 55–58.

Guess, H.A., Broughton, D.D., Melton, L.J. III and Kurland, L.T. (1985) Epidemiology of herpes zoster in children and adolescents: a population-based study. Pediatrics, 76: 512–517.

Guinee, V.F., Guido, J.J., Pfalzgraf, K.A., Giacco, G.G., Lagarde, C., Durand, M., van der Velden, J.W., Lowenberg, B., Jereb, B., Bretsky, S., Meilof, J., Hamersma, E.A.M., Dische, S. and Anderson, P. (1985) The incidence of herpes zoster in patients with Hodgkin's disease. Cancer, 56: 642–648.

Haanpää, M. and Nurmikko, T. (1997) Sensory thresholds, allodynia and pain in acute herpes zoster and their association with postherpetic neuralgia. Third International Conference on the Varicella-Zoster Virus, Palm Beach, FL.

Haanpää, M., Häkkinen, V. and Nurmikko, T. (1997) Motor involvement in acute herpes zoster. Muscle Nerve, 20: 1433–1438.

Haanpää, M., Dastidar, P., Weinberg, A., Levin, M., Miettinen, A., Lapinlampi, A., Laippala, P. and Nurmikko, T. (1998) CSF and MRI findings in patients with acute herpes zoster. Neurology, 51: 1405–1411.

Haanpää, M., Laippala, P. and Nurmikko, T. (1999) Pain and somatosensory dysfunction in acute herpes zoster. Clin. J. Pain, 15: 78–84.

Haanpää, M., Laippala, P. and Nurmikko, T. (2000) Allodynia and pinprick hypesthesia in acute herpes zoster, and the development of postherpetic neuralgia. J. Pain Symptom Manage., 20: 50–58.

Halloran, M.E., Cochi, S.L., Lieu, T.A., Wharton, M. and Fehrs, L. (1994) Theoretical epidemiologic and morbidity effects of routine varicella immunization of preschool children in the United States. Am. J. Epidemiol., 140: 81–104.

Hamaguchi, T., Kotani, Y., Imanaka, S., Morito, S. and Kawamura, Y. (1970) Lupus erythematosus and herpes zoster. Mie Med. J., 19: 189–192.

Han, C.S., Miller, W., Haake, R. and Weisdorf, D. (1994) Varicella zoster infection after bone marrow transplantation: incidence, risk factors and complications. Bone Marrow Transplant., 13: 277–283.

Harding, S. and Porter, S. (1991) Oral acyclovir in herpes zoster ophthalmicus. Curr. Eye Res., 10: 177–182.

Harding, S.P., Lipton, J.R. and Wells, J.C.D. (1987) Natural history of herpes zoster ophthalmicus: predictors of postherpetic neuralgia and ocular involvement. Br. J. Ophthalmol., 71: 353–358.

Harrison, R.A., Soong, S., Weiss, H.L., Gnann, J.W. Jr. and Whitley, R.J. (1999) A mixed model for factors predictive of pain in AIDS patients with herpes zoster. J. Pain Sympt. Manage., 17: 410–417.

Hawrami, K., Hart, I.J., Pereira, F., Argent, S., Bannister, B., Bovill, B., Carrington, D., Ogilvie, M., Rawstorne, S., Tryhorn, Y. and Breuer, J. (1997) Molecular epidemiology of varicella-zoster virus in East London, England, between 1971 and 1995. J. Clin. Microbiol., 35: 807–809.

Helgason, S., Sigurdsson, J.A. and Gudmundsson, S. (1996) The clinical course of herpes zoster: a prospective study in primary care. Eur. J. Gen. Pract., 2: 12–16.

Higa, K., Dan, K., Manabe, H. and Noda, B. (1988) Factors influencing the duration of treatment of acute herpetic pain with sympathetic nerve block: importance of severity of herpes zoster assessed by the maximum antibody titers to varicella-zoster virus in otherwise healthy patients. Pain, 32: 147–157.

Higa, K., Noda, B., Manabe, H., Sato S and Dan, K. (1992) T-lymphocyte subsets in otherwise healthy patients with herpes zoster and relationships to the duration of acute herpetic pain. Pain, 51: 111–118.

Higa, K., Mori, M., Hirata, K., Hori, K., Manabe, H. and Dan, K. (1997) Severity of skin lesions of herpes zoster at the worst phase rather than age and involved region most influences the duration of acute herpetic pain. Pain, 69: 245–253.

Holmberg, S.D., Buchbinder, S.P., Conley, L.J., Wong, L.C., Katz, M.H., Penley, K.A., Hershow, R.C. and Judson, F.N. (1995) The spectrum of medical conditions and symptoms before acquired immunodeficiency syndrome in homosexual and bisexual men infected with the immunodeficiency virus. Am. J. Epidemiol., 141: 395–404.

Hope-Simpson, R.E. (1954) Studies on shingles: is the virus ordinary chicken pox virus? Lancet, ii: 1299–1302.

Hope-Simpson, R.E. (1965) The nature of herpes zoster: a long-term study and a new hypothesis. Proc. R. Soc. Med., 58: 9–20.

Hope-Simpson, R.E. (1967) Herpes zoster in the elderly. Geriatrics, 22: 151–159.

Hope-Simpson, R.E. (1975) Postherpetic neuralgia. J. R. Coll. Gen. Pract., 25: 571–575.

Huff, J.C., Drucker, J.L., Clemmer, A., Laskin, O.L., Connor, J.D., Bryson, Y.J. and Balfour, H.H. Jr. (1993) Effect of oral acyclovir on pain resolution in herpes zoster: a reanalysis. J. Med. Virol., 93–96.

Jackson, J.L., Gibbons, R., Meyer, G. and Inouye, L. (1997) The effect of treating herpes zoster with oral acyclovir in preventing postherpetic neuralgia: a meta-analysis. Arch. Intern. Med., 157: 909–912.

Johnson, R.W. (1995) The future of predictors, prevention, and therapy in postherpetic neuralgia. Neurology, 45 (Suppl. 8), S70–S72.

Johnson, R.W., Shukla, S. and Fletcher, P. (1995) Qualitative aspects of zoster-associated pain: evaluation of a new approach. European Federation of IASP Chapters, Verona, Italy.

Kahl, L.E. (1994) Herpes zoster infections in systemic lupus erythematosus: risk factors and outcomes. J. Rheumatol., 21: 84–86.

Kakourou, T., Theodoridou, M., Mostrou, G., Syriopoulou, V., Papadogeorgaki, H. and Constantopoulos, A. (1998) Herpes zoster in children. J. Am. Acad. Dermatol., 39: 207–210.

Keiser, P., Jockus, J., Horton, H. and Smith, J.W. (1996) Prednisone therapy is not associated with increased risk of herpetic infections in patients infected with human immunodeficiency virus. Clin. Infect. Dis., 23: 201–202.

Kurtzke, J.F. (1984) Neuroepidemiology. Ann. Neurol, 16: 265–277.

Latif, R. and Shope, T.C. (1983) Herpes zoster in normal and immunocompromised children. Am. J. Dis. Child., 137: 801–802.

Leijon, G., Boivie, J., Roberg, M. and Forsberg, P. (1993) Sensory abnormalities accompanying herpes zoster and post-herpetic neuralgia. Abstracts: 7th World Congress on Pain, IASP Publications, Seattle, pp. 184–185.

Lenman, J.A. and Peters, T.J. (1969) Herpes zoster and multiple sclerosis. Br. Med. J., 2: 218–220.

Leplow, B., Lamparter, U., Risse, A. and Wassilev, S.W. (1990) Die postherpetische Neuralgie: Klinische Prädiktoren und psychopathologischer Befund. Nervenarzt, 61: 46–51.

Levin, M., Barber, D., Goldblatt, E., Jones, M., LaFleur, B., Chan, C., Stinson, D., Zerbe, G. and Hayward, A. (1998) Use of a live attenuated varicella vaccine to boost varicella-specific immune responses in seropositive people 55 years of age and older: duration of booster effect. J. Infect. Dis., 178: S109–S112.

Lewis, G.W. (1958) Zoster sine herpete, Br. Med. J., 2: 418–421.

Lo, C.Y. and Cheng, I.K. (1996) Varicella-zoster infection in cyclosporine A-treated renal transplant. Transplant. Proc., 28: 1511–1512.

Luby, J.P., Ramierez-Ronda, C., Rinner, S., Hull, A. and Vergne-Marini, P. (1977) A longitudinal study of varicella-zoster virus infections in renal transplant recipients. J. Infect. Dis., 135: 659–663.

Lydick, E., Epstein, R., Himmelberger, D. and White, C.J. (1995a) Area under the curve: a metric for patient subjective responses in episodic diseases. Qual. Life Res., 4: 41–45.

Lydick, E., Epstein, R., Himmelberger, D. and White, C.J. (1995b) Herpes zoster and quality of life: a self-limited disease with severe impact. Neurology, 45 (Suppl. 8), S52–S53.

Manzi, S., Kuller, L.H., Kutzer, J., Pazin, G.J., Sinacore, J., Medsger, T.A. and Ramsey-Goldman, R. (1995) Herpes zoster in systemic lupus erythematosus. J. Rheumatol., 22: 1254–1258.

Marsh, R.J. and Cooper, M. (1993) Ophthalmic herpes zoster. Eye, 7: 350–370.

Mauskopf, J., Austin, R., Dix, L. and Berzon, R. (1994) The Nottingham Health Profile as a measure of the quality of life in zoster patients: convergent and discriminant validity. Qual. Life Res., 3: 431–435.

Mauskopf, J., Austin, R., Dix, L. and Berzon, R. (1995) Estimating the value of a generic quality-of-life measure. Med. Care, 33: 4: AS195–AS202.

Max, M.B., Schafer, S.C., Culnane, M., Dubner, R. and Gracely, R.H. (1988) Association of pain relief with drug side effects in postherpetic neuralgia: a single-dose study of clonidine, codeine, ibuprofen, and placebo. Clin. Pharmacol. Ther., 43: 363–371.

Mazur, M.H. and Dolin, R. (1978) Herpes zoster at the NIH: A 20 year experience. Am. J. Med., 65: 738–743.

McCulloch, D.K., Fraser, D.M. and Duncan, L.P.J. (1982) Shingles in diabetes mellitus. Practitioner, 226: 531–532.

McGregor, R.M. (1957) Herpes zoster, chicken pox and cancer in general practice. Br. Med. J., 1: 84–87.

McKendrick, M.W. and Wood, M.J. (1995) Acyclovir and postherpetic neuralgia. Br. Med. J., 310: 1005.

McNulty, A., Li, Y., Radtke, U., Kaldor, J., Rohrsheim, R., Cooper, D.A. and Donovan, B. (1997) Herpes zoster and the stage and prognosis of HIV-1 infection. Genitourin. Med., 73: 467–470.

Meister, W., Neiß, A., Gross, G., Doerr, H.W., Höbel, W., Malin,

J.P., von Essen, J., Reimann, B.Y., Witke, C. and Wutzler, P. (1998) A prognostic score for postherpetic neuralgia in ambulatory patients. Infection, 26: 359–363.

Melbye, M., Grossman, R.J., Goedert, J.J., Eyster, M.E. and Biggar, R.J. (1987) Risk of AIDS after herpes zoster. Lancet, 1: 728–731.

Miller, E., Vurdien, J. and Farrington, P. (1993) Shift in age in chickenpox. Lancet, 1: 308–309.

Mitchell, C.D., Gehrz, R.C. and Balfour, H.H. Jr. (1986) Vari-cella-zoster-specific immune responses in acute herpes zoster during a placebo-controlled trial of oral acyclovir therapy. Diagn. Microbiol. Infect. Dis., 5: 113–126.

Moga, I., Formiga, F., Canet, R., Pac, M., Mitjavila, F. and Pujol, R. (1995) Herpes-zoster virus infection in patients with systemic lupus erythematosus. Rev. Clin. Esp., 195: 530–533.

Molin, L. (1969) Aspects of the natural history of herpes zoster. A follow-up investigation of outpatient material. Acta Dermatol. Venereol., 49: 569–583.

Mondelli, M., Romano, C., Passero, S., Della Porta, P. and Rossi, A. (1996) Effects of acyclovir on sensory axonal neuropathy, segmental motor paresis and postherpetic neuralgia in herpes zoster patients. Eur. Neurol., 36: 288–292.

Moore, R.D. and Chaisson, R.E. (1996) Natural history of oppor-tunistic disease in an HIV-infected urban clinical cohort. Ann. Intern. Med., 124: 633–642.

Morton, P. and Thomson, A. (1989) Oral acyclovir in the treat-ment of herpes zoster in general practice. New Zealand Med. J., 102: 93–95.

Moutsopoulos, H.M., Gallagher, J.D., Decker, J.L. and Steinberg, A.D. (1978) Herpes zoster in patients with systemic lupus erythematosus. Arthritis Rheum., 21: 789–802.

Nagaoka, S., Tani, K., Ishigatsubo, Y., Chiba, J., Kato, K., Mat-sunaga, K., Narita, M., Igarashi, T. and Okubo, T. (1990) Her-pes zoster in patients with polymyositis and dermatomyositis. Kansenshogaku Zasshi, 64: 1394–1399.

Naraqi, S., Jackson, G.G., Jonasson, O. and Yamashiroya, H.M. (1977) Prospective study of prevalence, incidence and source of herpes virus infections in patients with renal allografts. J. Infect. Dis., 136: 531–540.

Noda, B., Dan, K., Manabe, H. and Higa, K. (1987) Prognostic clinical signs in herpes zoster pain. Pain, Suppl. 4: S382.

Nurmikko, T.J. and Bowsher, D. (1990) Somatosensory findings in postherpetic neuralgia. J. Neurol. Neurosurg. Psychiatry, 53: 135–141.

Nurmikko, T.J., Rasanen, A. and Hakkinen, V. (1990) Clinical and neurophysiological observations on acute herpes zoster. Clin. J. Pain, 6: 284–290.

Oaklander, A.L., Romans, K., Horasek, S., Stocks, A., Hauer, P. and Meyer, R.A. (1998) Unilateral postherpetic neuralgia is as-sociated with bilateral sensory neuron damage. Ann. Neurol., 44: 789–795.

Oxman, M. (1995) Immunization to reduce the frequency and severity of herpes zoster and its complications. Neurology, 45 (Suppl. 8), S41–S46.

Palmer, S.R., Caul, E.O., Donald, D.E., Kwantes, W. and Tillett, H. (1985) An outbreak of shingles? Lancet, 2: 1108–1111.

Panda, S., Sarkar, S., Mandal, B.K., Singh, T.B.K., Singh, K.L., Mitra, D.K., Sarkar, K., Tripathy, S.P. and Deb, B.C. (1994) Epidemic of herpes zoster following HIV epidemic in Ma-nipur. Indian J. Infect., 28: 167–173.

Paul, E. and Thiel, T. (1996) Epidemiology of varicella zoster infection: results of a prospective study in the Ansbach area. Hautarzt, 47: 604–649.

Petursson, G., Helgason, S., Gudmundsson, S. and Sigurdsson, J.A. (1998) Herpes zoster in children and adolescents. Pediatr. Infect. Dis. J., 17: 905–908.

Pilowsky, I. (1977) Psychological aspects of post-herpetic neu-ralgia: some clinical observations. Br. J. Med. Psychol., 50: 283–288.

Portenoy, R.K., Duma, C. and Foley, K.M. (1986) Acute her-petic and postherpetic neuralgia: clinical review and current management. Ann. Neurol., 20: 651–664.

Preiksaitis, J.K., Rosno, S., Grumet, C. and Merigan, T.C. (1983) Infections due to herpes viruses in cardiac transplant recipi-ents: role of the donor heart and immunosuppressive therapy. J. Infect. Dis., 147: 974–981.

Ragozzino, M.W. and Kurland, L.T. (1982) Subsequent risk of rheumatoid arthritis in patients diagnosed with herpes zoster. Lancet, 2: 884.

Ragozzino, M.W. and Kurland, L.T. (1983) Epidemiologic inves-tigation of the association between herpes zoster and multiple sclerosis. Neurology, 33: 648–649.

Ragozzino, M.W., Melton, L.F. III and Kurland, L.T. (1982a) Population-based study of herpes zoster and its sequelae. Medicine, 61: 310–316.

Ragozzino, M.W., Melton, L.J. III, Kurland, L.T., Chu, C.P. and Perry, H.O. (1982b) Risk of cancer after herpes zoster: a population-based study., New Engl. J. Med., 307: 393–397.

Ragozzino, M.W., Melton, L.J. III and Kurland, L.T. (1983) Herpes zoster and diabetes mellitus: an epidemiological inves-tigation. J Chron. Dis., 36: 501–505.

Rand, K.H., Rasmussen, L.E., Pollard, R.B., Arvin, A. and Merigan, T.C. (1977) Cellular immunity and herpes virus infection in cardiac-transplant patients. New Engl. J. Med., 296: 1372–1377.

Rifkind, D. (1966) The activation of varicella-zoster virus infec-tions by immunosuppressive therapy. J. Lab. Clin. Med., 68: 463–474.

Riopelle, J.M., Naraghi, M. and Grush, K.P. (1984) Chronic neuralgia incidence following local anesthetic therapy for herpes zoster. Arch. Dermatol., 120: 747–750.

Rogers, R.S. III and Tindall, J.P. (1971) Geriatric herpes zoster. J. Am. Geriatr. Soc., 19: 495–504.

Rogers, R.S. III and Tindall, J.P. (1972) Herpes zoster in chil-dren. Arch. Dermatol., 106: 204–207.

Rogues, A., Dupon, M., Ladner, J., Ragnaud, J.M., Pellegrin, J.L. and Dabis, F. (1993) Herpes zoster and human immunodeficiency virus infection: a cohort study of 101 coinfected patients. J. Infect. Dis., 168: 245.

Rose, M.J., Klenerman, L., Atchison L and Slade, P.D. (1992) An application of the fear avoidance model to three chronic pain conditions. Behav. Res. Ther., 30: 359–365.

Ross, R.T., Nicolle, L.E. and Cheang, M. (1995) Varicella zoster virus and multiple sclerosis in a Hutterite population. J. Clin. Epidemiol., 48: 1319–1324.

Ross, R.T., Nicolle, L.E., Dawood, M.R., Cheang, M. and Feschuk, C. (1997) Varicella zoster antibodies after herpes zoster, varicella and multiple sclerosis. Can. J. Neurol. Sci., 24: 137–139.

Ross, R.T., Cheang, M., Landry, G., Klassen, L. and Doerksen, K. (1999) Herpes zoster and multiple sclerosis. Can. J. Neurol. Sci., 26: 29–32.

Rowbotham, M.C. and Fields, H.L. (1989) Post-herpetic neuralgia: the relation of pain complaint, sensory disturbance, and skin temperature. Pain, 39: 129–144.

Rowbotham, M.C., Davies, P.S. and Fields, H.S. (1995) Topical lidocaine gel relieves postherpetic neuralgia. Ann. Neurol., 37: 246–253.

Rowbotham, M.C., Yosipovitch, G., Connolly, M.K., Finlay, D., Forde, G. and Fields, H.L. (1996) Cutaneous innervation density in the allodynic form of posthereptic neuralgia. Neurobiol. Dis., 3: 205–214.

Rowbotham, M.C., Petersen, K.L. and Fields, H.L. (1998) Is postherpetic neuralgia more than one disorder? Pain Forum, 7: 231–237.

Rusthoven, J.J. (1994) The risk of varicella-zoster infections in different patient populations: a critical review. Transfusion Med. Rev., 8: 96–116.

Rusthoven, J.J., Ahlgren, P., Elhakim, T., Pinfold, P., Reid, J., Stewart, L. and Feld, R. (1988a) Varicella-zoster infection in adult cancer patients: a population study, Arch. Intern. Med., 148: 1561–1566.

Rusthoven, J.J., Ahlgren, P., Elhakim, T., Pinfold, P., Stewart, L. and Feld, R. (1988b) Risk factors for varicella zoster disseminated infection among adult cancer patients with localized zoster. Cancer, 62: 1641–1646.

Sandor, E.V., Millman, A., Corxson, T.S. and Mildvan, D. (1986) Herpes zoster ophthalmicus in patients at risk for the acquired immune deficiency syndrome (AIDS) Am. J. Ophthalmol., 101: 153–155.

Schimpff, S.S., Serpick, A., Stoler, B., Rumack, B., Mellin, H., Joseph, J.M. and Block, J. (1972) Varicella-zoster infection in patients with cancer. Ann. Intern. Med., 76: 241–254.

Schmader, K. (1995) Management of herpes zoster in elderly patients. Infect. Dis. Clin. Pract., 4: 293–299.

Schmader, K. (1998) Postherpetic neuralgia in immunocompetent elderly people. Vaccine, 16: 1768–1770.

Schmader, K. (2000) Herpes zoster epidemiology. In: A. Arvin and A. Gershon (Eds.), Varicella-Zoster Virus. Cambridge University Press, Cambridge, pp. 2220–2246.

Schmader, K., Studenski, S., MacMillan, J., Grufferman, S. and Cohen, H.J. (1990) Are stressful life events risk factors for herpes zoster?, J. Am. Geriatr. Soc., 38: 1188–1195.

Schmader, K., George, L.K., Newton, B. and Hamilton, J.D. (1994) The accuracy of self-reports of herpes zoster. J. Clin. Epidemiol., 47: 1271–1276.

Schmader, K., George, L.K. and Hamilton, J.D. (1995) Racial differences in the occurrence of herpes zoster. J. Infect. Dis., 171: 701–704.

Schmader, K., George, L.K., Burchett, B.M., Hamilton, J.D. and Pieper, C.F. (1998) Race and stress in the incidence of herpes zoster in the elderly. J. Am. Geriatr. Soc., 46: 973–977.

Schuchter, L.M., Wingard, J.R., Piantadosi, S., Burns, W., Santos, G.W. and Saral, R. (1989) Herpes zoster infection after autologous bone marrow transplantation. Blood, 74: 1424–1427.

Shukla, S., Johnson, R. and Fletcher, P. (1996) Qualitative aspects of zoster-associated pain: evaluation of a new approach. Abstracts: 8th World Congress on Pain, IASP Press, Seattle, p. 270.

Smith, C.G. and Glaser, D.A. (1996) Herpes zoster in childhood: case report and review of the literature. Pediatr. Dermatol., 13: 226–229.

Söltz-Szöts, J., Tyring, S., Andersen, P.L., Lucht, R.F., McKendrick, M.W., Diaz-Perez, J.L., Shukla, S. and Fiddian, A.P. (1998) A randomized controlled trial of acyclovir versus netivudine for treatment of herpes zoster. J. Antimicrob. Chemother., 41: 549–556.

Straus, S.E. (1993) Shingles: sorrows, salves, and solutions. J. Am. Med. Assoc., 269: 1836–1839.

Straus, S.E., Reinhold, W., Smith, H.A., Ruyechan, W.T., Henderson, D.K., Blaese, R.M. and Hay, J. (1984) Endonuclease analysis of viral DNA from varicella and subsequent zoster infections in the same patient. New Engl. J. Med., 311: 1362–1364.

Strom, B.L., Reidenberg, M.M., West, S., Snyder, E.S., Freundlich, B. and Stolley, P.D. (1994) Shingles, allergies, family medical history, oral contraceptives and other potential risk factors for systemic lupus erythematosus. Am. J. Epidemiol., 140: 632–642.

Terada, K., Kawano, S., Yoshihiro, K., Miyashima, H. and Morita, T. (1993) Characteristics of herpes zoster in otherwise normal children. Pediatr. Infect. Dis. J., 12: 960–961.

Timothy, D.J. and Williams, M.L. (1979) Herpes zoster in infancy. Scand. J. Infect. Dis., 11: 185–186.

Tyndall, M.W., Nasio, J., Agoki, E., Malisa, W., Ronald, A.R., Ndinya-Achola, J.O. and Plummer, F.A. (1995) Herpes zoster as the initial presentation of human immunodeficiency virus type 1 infection in Kenya. Clin. Infect. Dis., 21: 1035–1037.

Tyring, S., Barbarash, R.A., Nahlik, J.E., Cunningham, A., Marley, J., Heng, M., Jones, T., Rea, T., Boon, R. and Saltzman, R. (1995) Famciclovir for the treatment of acute herpes zoster: effects on acute disease and postherpetic neuralgia: a randomized, double-blind, placebo-controlled trial. Ann. Intern. Med., 123: 89–96.

Tyring, S.K., Beutner, K.R., Tucker, B.A., Anderson, W.C. and Crooks, R.J. (2000) Antiviral therapy for herpes zoster: randomized, controlled clinical trial of valacyclovir and famciclovir therapy in immunocompetent patients 50 years and older. Arch. Fam. Med., 9: 863–869.

Tzeng, C.H., Liu, J.H., Fan, S., Wang, S.Y., Wang, S.R., Chen, K.Y., Hsieh, R.K., Yung, C.H. and Chen, P.M. (1995) Varicella zoster virus infection after allogeneic or autologous hemopoietic stem cell transplantation. Taiwan I Hsueh Hui Tsa Chih, 94: 313–317.

Van de Perre, P., Bakkers, E., Batungwanayo, J., Kestelyn, P., Lepage, P., Nzaramba, D., Bogaerts, J., Serufilira, A., Rouvroy, D., Uwimana A and Butzler, J.P. (1988) Herpes zoster in African patients: an early manifestation of HIV infection. Scand. J. Infect. Dis., 20: 277–282.

Veenstra, J., Krol, A., van Praag, R.M., Frissen, P.H., Schellekens, P.T., Lange, J.M., Coutinho, R.A. and van der Meer, J.T. (1995) Herpes zoster, immunological deterioration and disease progression in HIV-1 infection. AIDS, 9: 1153–1158.

Veenstra, J., van Praag, R.M., Krol, A., Wertheim van Dillen, P.M., Weigel, H.M., Schellekens, P.T., Lange, J.M., Coutinho, R. and van der Meer, J.T. (1996) Complications of varicella-zoster virus reactivation in HIV-infected homosexual men. AIDS, 10: 393–399.

Wacker, P., Hartmann, O., Benhamou, E., Salloum, E. and Lemerle, J. (1989) Varicella-zoster virus infections after autologous bone marrow transplantation in children. Bone Marrow Transplant., 4: 191–194.

Wall, P.D. (1993) An essay on the mechanisms which may contribute to the state of postherpetic neuralgia. In: C.P.N. Watson (Ed.), Herpes Zoster and Postherpetic Neuralgia, Elsevier, Amsterdam, pp. 123–138.

Watson, C.P.N., Watt, V.R., Chipman, M., Birkett, N. and Evans, R.T., The prognosis with postherpetic neuralgia. Pain, 46: 195–199.

Weksler, M.E. (1994) Immune senescence. Ann. Neurol., 35: S35–S37.

Weller, T.H. (1983) Varicella and herpes zoster: changing concepts of the natural history, control, and importance of a not-so-benign virus., New Engl. J. Med., 309: 1362–1368: 1434–1440.

Weller, T.H. (1995) Varicella-zoster virus: history, perspectives, and evolving concerns. Neurology, 45 (Suppl. 8): S9–S10.

Weller, T.H. (1997) Varicella-herpes zoster virus. In: A.S. Evans and R.A. Kaslow (Eds.), Viral Infections of Humans: Epidemiology and Control, 4th edn., Plenum, New York, p. 866.

Weller, T.H., Witton, H.M. and Bell, E.J. (1958) The etiologic agents of varicella and herpes zoster: isolation, propagation, and cultural characteristics in vitro. J. Exp. Med., 108: 843–868.

Whitley, R.J., Weiss, H., Gnann, J.W. Jr., Tyring, S., Mertz, G.J. Pappas, P.G., Schleupner, C.J., Hayden, F., Wolf, J. and Soong, S.J. (1996) Acyclovir with and without prednisone for the treatment of herpes zoster: a randomized, placebo-controlled trial. Ann. Intern. Med., 125: 376–383.

Whitley, R.J., Shukla, S. and Crooks, R.J. (1998) The identification of risk factors associated with persistent pain following herpes zoster. J. Infect. Dis., 178 (Suppl. 1), S71–S75.

Whitley, R.J., Weiss, H.L., Soong, S.J. and Gnann, J.W. (1999) Herpes zoster: risk categories for persistent pain. J. Infect. Dis., 179: 9–15.

Wildenhoff, K.E., Ipsen, J., Esmann, V., Ingemann-Jensen, J. and Poulsen, J.H. (1979) Treatment of herpes zoster with idoxuridine ointment, including a multivariate analysis of symptoms and signs. Scand. J. Infect. Dis., 11: 1–9.

Wildenhoff, K.E., Esmann, V., Ipsen, J., Harving, H., Peterslund, N.A. and Schonheyder, H. (1981) Treatment of trigeminal and thoracic zoster with idoxuridine. Scand. J. Infect. Dis., 13: 257–262.

Wilson, J.B. (1986) Thirty one years of herpes zoster in a rural practice. Br. Med. J., 293: 1349–1351.

Wood, M.J. (1991) Herpes zoster and pain. Scand. J. Infect. Dis., Suppl. 78: 53–61.

Wood, M.J. (1995) For debate: how should zoster trials be conducted?, J. Antimicrob. Chemother., 36: 1089–1101.

Wood, M.J., Johnson, R.W., McKendrick, M.W., Taylor, J., Mandal, B.K. and Crooks, J. (1994) A randomized trial of acyclovir for 7 days or 21 days with and without prednisolone for treatment of acute herpes zoster. New Engl. J. Med., 330: 896–900.

Wood, M.J., Kay, R., Dworkin, R.H., Soong, S.J. and Whitley, R.J. (1996) Oral acyclovir therapy accelerates pain resolution in patients with herpes zoster: a meta-analysis of placebo-controlled trials. Clin. Infect. Dis., 22: 341–347.

Wrensch, M., Weinberg, A., Wiencke, J., Masters, H., Miike, R., Barger, G. and Lee, M. (1997) Does prior infection with varicella-zoster virus influence risk of adult glioma? Am. J. Epidemiol., 145: 594–597.

Wurzel, C.L., Kahan, J., Heitler, M. and Rubin, L.G. (1986) Prognosis of herpes zoster in healthy children. Am. J. Dis. Child., 140: 477–478.

Herpes Zoster and Postherpetic Neuralgia, 2nd Revised and Enlarged Edition
Pain Research and Clinical Management, Vol. 11
Edited by C.P.N. Watson and A.A. Gershon

CHAPTER 6

Herpes zoster: natural history, diagnosis and therapy

Richard J. Whitley [*]

Departments of Pediatrics, Microbiology, and Medicine, University of Alabama at Birmingham,
Birmingham, AL 35233, USA

1. Introduction

Herpes zoster is a disease that occurs at all ages, but it will afflict about 20% or more of the population overall, mainly the elderly (Hope-Simpson, 1965; Ragozzino et al., 1982). Herpes zoster occurs in persons who are seropositive for varicella-zoster virus (VZV), namely those who have had chicken pox. Reactivation appears to be dependent on a balance between virus and host factors. Most patients who develop herpes zoster have no history of exposure to other persons with VZV infection at the time of the appearance of lesions. The highest incidence of disease varies between 5 and 10 cases per 1000 for persons older than 60 years of age. In a 7-year study performed by McGregor the annualized rate of herpes zoster was 4.8 cases per 1000 patients, three fourths of those patients being older than 45 years of age (McGregor, 1957). It has been suggested that approximately 4% of patients will suffer a second episode of herpes zoster; however, recurrences of dermatomal lesions are usually caused by herpes simplex virus. Persons who are immunocompromised have a higher incidence of both chicken pox and shingles (Feldman et al., 1975; Arvin et al., 1980; Whitley, 1984; Locksley et al., 1985).

Herpes zoster can occur within the first 2 years of life in children born to women who have had chicken pox during pregnancy. These cases probably reflect in-utero chicken pox with reactivation early in life.

2. Pathogenesis

Histopathologic findings of VZV infections, whether chicken pox or herpes zoster, are virtually identical. The vesicles involve the corium and dermis. As viral replication progresses, the epithelial cells undergo degenerative changes characterized by ballooning, with the subsequent appearance of multinucleated giant cells and prominent eosinophilic intranuclear inclusions. Under unusual circumstances, necrosis and hemorrhage may appear in the upper portion of the dermis. As the vesicle evolves, the collected fluid becomes cloudy as a consequence of the appearance of polymorphonuclear leukocytes, degenerated cells, and fibrin. Ultimately, either the vesicles rupture and release infectious fluid, or the fluid gradually becomes reabsorbed.

Varicella-zoster virus characteristically becomes latent after chicken pox. The virus establishes latency within the dorsal root ganglia. Reactivation of

[*] Correspondence to: Dr. Richard J. Whitley, Suite 616, ACC, The Children's Hospital of Alabama, 1600 Seventh Avenue South, Birmingham, AL 35233, USA. Phone: +1 (205) 939-9594; Fax: +1 (205) 934-8559; E-mail: rwhitley@peds.uab.edu

latent virus leads to herpes zoster or shingles, as noted is a sporadic disease. Histopathologic examination of the nerve root after infection with VZV demonstrates characteristics indicative of infection, namely satellitosis, lymphocytic infiltration in the nerve root, and degeneration of the ganglia cells (Bastian et al., 1974; Esiri and Tomlinson, 1974). Intranuclear inclusions can be found within the ganglia cells. The molecular mechanism by which VZV establishes latency remains unknown.

3. Clinical manifestations of herpes zoster

Herpes zoster is characterized by a unilateral vesicular eruption with a dermatomal distribution (Fig. 1). Thoracic and lumbar dermatomes are most commonly involved. Herpes zoster may involve the eyelids when the first or second branch of the fifth cranial nerve is affected, but keratitis heralds a sight-threatening condition, herpes zoster ophthalmicus. Although lesions on the tip of the nose are said to presage corneal lesions, absence of such skin lesions does not guarantee corneal sparing. Keratitis may be followed by iridocyclitis, secondary glaucoma, or neuroparalytic keratitis. Ophthalmologic consultation should be requested for any patient with suspected herpes zoster ophthalmicus. Generally, the onset of disease is heralded by pain within the dermatome that precedes the lesions by 48 to 72 h. Early in the disease course, erythematous, macropapular lesions appear that rapidly evolve into a vesicular rash. Vesicles may coalesce to form bullous lesions. In the normal host, these lesions continue to form over a period of 3 to 5 days, with the total duration of disease being 10 to 15 days. However, it may take as long as 1 month before the skin returns to normal. Some patients experience unilateral pain characteristic of herpes zoster but never develop a pathognomic rash. Serologic evidence of infection can be demonstrated. This entity is known as zoster sin herpetica.

Unusual cutaneous manifestations of herpes zoster, in addition to ophthalmic disease, include the involvement of the maxillary or mandibular branch of the trigeminal nerve, which results in intraoral in-

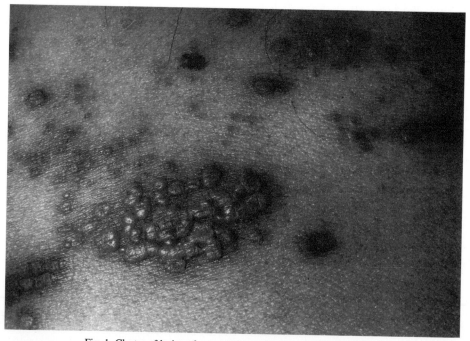

Fig. 1. Cluster of lesions from a patient with herpes zoster infection.

volvement with lesions on the palate, tonsillar fossa, floor of the mouth, and tongue. When the geniculate ganglion is involved, a Ramsay–Hunt syndrome may occur, with pain and vesicles in the external auditory meatus, loss of taste on the anterior two thirds of the tongue, and ipsilateral facial palsy.

No known factors are responsible for the precipitation of the episodes of herpes zoster. If herpes zoster occurs in children, the course is generally benign and not associated with progressive pain or discomfort. In adults, systemic manifestations are mainly those associated with pain, as noted below.

The most significant clinical manifestations of herpes zoster are associated acute neuritis and, subsequently, post-herpetic neuralgia. Post-herpetic neuralgia, although uncommon in young people, may occur in as many as 25 to 50% of persons older than 50 years of age even with therapy (Demorgas and Kierland, 1957; Watson and Evans, 1986; Esmann et al., 1987) depending upon factors noted below. In the absence of antiviral therapy, 50% of persons older than 50 years of age have debilitating pain that persists for more than 1 month. Post-herpetic neuralgia may cause constant pain in the involved dermatome, burning, intermittent stabbing pain or altered cutaneous sensations. Pain may be worse at night or on exposure to temperature changes. At its worst, the neuralgia can be incapacitating, as recently reviewed (Kost and Straus, 1996).

Extracutaneous sites of involvement include the central nervous system, as manifested by meningoencephalitis or encephalitis. The clinical manifestations are similar to those of other viral infections of the central nervous system (CNS). However, a rare manifestation of CNS involvement is granulomatous cerebral angiitis. Involvement of the CNS following cutaneous herpes zoster probably is more common than is recognized clinically. Frequently, patients who undergo cerebrospinal fluid examination for other reasons during episodes of shingles can have pleocytosis without elevated cerebrospinal fluid protein levels. These patients arc without signs of meningeal irritation and, infrequently, complain of headaches.

Shingles involves dorsal root ganglia. As a conse-quence, motor paralysis can occur as a consequence of the involvement of the anterior horn cells, in a manner similar to that encountered with polio. Patients with involvement of the anterior horn cells are particularly likely to experience excruciating pain. Other neuromuscular disorders associated with herpes zoster include the Guillain–Barré syndrome, transverse myelitis (Hogan and Krigman, 1973) and myositis (Rubin and Fusfeld, 1965; Norris et al., 1969).

Herpes zoster in the immunocompromised patient is more severe than in the normal person. In the absence of therapy, lesion formation continues for up to 2 weeks, and scabbing may not take place until 3 to 4 weeks into the disease course (Whitley, 1984). Patients with lymphoproliferative malignancies are at risk for cutaneous dissemination and visceral involvement, including varicella pneumonitis, hepatitis, and meningoencephalitis. However, even in the immunocompromised patient, disseminated herpes zoster is rarely fatal.

In recent years, herpes zoster has been recognized as a frequent infection in persons with human immunodeficiency virus (HIV) infection, occurring in 8 to 11% of patients. Although the occurrence of cutaneous dissemination is infrequent, complications such as VZV retinitis, acute retinal necrosis, and chronic progressive encephalitis have been reported (Gnann and Whitley, 1991).

Chronic herpes zoster may also occur in immunocompromised patients, particularly those persons with a diagnosis of HIV infection. These patients experience new lesion formation with an absence of healing of the existing lesions that continues over weeks and even months. These syndromes can be particularly debilitating and, of interest, have been associated with the isolation of VZV isolates resistant to acyclovir.

4. Diagnosis

The diagnosis of shingles is usually made by history and physical examination. The unilateral localization and distribution of a vesicular rash makes the diagnosis of herpes zoster highly likely; however, other viral exanthems can occasionally be confused with the disease.

Unilateral vesicular lesions in a dermatomal pattern should immediately lead the clinician to suspect a diagnosis of shingles. Herpes simplex virus infections and coxsackievirus infections can also cause dermatomal vesicular lesions. In such situations, diagnostic viral cultures remain the best method of establishing the cause of infection. Confirmation of the diagnosis is possible through the isolation of VZV in susceptible tissue culture cell lines or by the demonstration of either seroconversion or serologic antibody rises using standard assays on acute and convalescent sera. A Tzanck smear, performed by scraping the base of the lesion, can demonstrate multinucleated giant cells; however, the sensitivity of this test is no better than 60%. Commercially available reagents are useful for direct fluorescent antibody staining of smears obtained from scraping vesicular lesions. Useful antibody assays include immune adherence hemagglutination assay, fluorescence antibody to membrane antigen (FAMA) assay, or enzyme-linked immunosorbent assay (ELISA) (Forghani et al., 1978).

The application of PCR to the cerebrospinal fluid can be used to detect VZV DNA and, therefore, infections of the central nervous system. It has also been applied to the evaluation of skin lesions in research laboratories

5. Therapeutic agents

Clinical trials with vidarabine in the late 1970s provided a successful proof-of-concept for antiviral therapy of VZV infections. Over the last 20 years, a series of effective and well-tolerated antiviral compounds have been licensed for treatment of herpes zoster (Balfour, 1999). Three oral antiviral drugs (acyclovir, valaciclovir, and famciclovir) are currently approved in the United States for treatment of herpes zoster in the immunocompetent host. Intravenous acyclovir and foscarnet are also available for therapy of complicated or disseminated VZV

infections, including herpes zoster in immunocompromised individuals.

5.1. Acyclovir and valaciclovir

Acyclovir (Zovirax®) was the first oral antiviral compound marketed for treatment of herpes zoster. While widely and successfully prescribed, the efficacy of acyclovir for herpes zoster is somewhat limited by its poor oral bioavailability. Valaciclovir (Valtrex®), the L-valine ester prodrug of acyclovir has been developed to provide an orally administered drug with an improved pharmacokinetic profile.

5.1.1. Chemistry, mechanism of action, and antiviral activity

Acyclovir (9-{2-hydroxyethoxymethyl}guanine) is a synthetic acyclic purine nucleoside analogue which is a selective inhibitor of herpes simplex virus (HSV types 1 and 2) and VZV replication (Elion et al., 1977; Schaeffer et al., 1978). Acyclovir is converted by virus-encoded thymidine kinase (TK) to its monophosphate derivative, an event that does not occur to any significant extent in uninfected cells (Fyfe et al., 1978). Subsequent di- and tri-phosphorylation steps are catalyzed by cellular enzymes, resulting in acyclovir-triphosphate concentrations 40- to 100-fold higher in HSV- and VZV-infected cells. Acyclovir triphosphate inhibits viral DNA synthesis by competing with the deoxyguanosine triphosphate as a substrate for viral DNA polymerase (Derse et al., 1981). Because acyclovir triphosphate lacks the $3'$ hydroxyl group required for DNA chain elongation, viral DNA synthesis is terminated. Viral DNA polymerase is tightly associated with the terminated DNA chain and is functionally inactivated (Furman et al., 1984). In addition, the viral polymerase has greater affinity for acyclovir triphosphate than does cellular DNA polymerase, resulting in little incorporation of acyclovir into cellular DNA. In vitro, acyclovir is most active against HSV-1 (EC_{50} = 0.04 μg/ml), HSV-2 (EC_{50} = 0.3 μg/ml), and VZV (Collins and Bauer, 1979).

Valaciclovir is cleaved to acyclovir by valine hydrolase, which then is metabolized in infected cells to the active triphosphate of acyclovir (Soul-Lawton et al., 1995). Because it is converted to acyclovir, it has the same in vitro spectrum of activity as the parent compound.

5.1.2. Absorption, distribution and elimination

For the treatment of herpes zoster, acyclovir is available in oral and intravenous formulations. Absorption of acyclovir after oral administration is slow and incomplete, with bioavailability of about 15–30% (DeMiranda and Blum, 1983). After multidose oral administration of 200 mg or 800 mg of acyclovir, the mean steady-state levels are about 0.57 and 1.57 μg/ml, respectively (Laskin, 1984). Acyclovir plasma concentrations following intravenous doses of 5 mg/kg or 10 mg/kg every 8 h are about 9.9 and 20.0 μg/ml, respectively. Acyclovir penetrates most body tissues well, including the brain. The terminal plasma half-life is 2 to 3 h in adults with normal renal function. Acyclovir is minimally metabolized and about 85% of the administered dose is excreted unchanged in the urine via renal tubular secretion and glomerular filtration. Acyclovir is readily removed by hemodialysis, but not by peritoneal dialysis. Acyclovir dosage adjustment is required in patients with impaired renal function. For herpes zoster patients with a creatinine clearance (CrCl) of >25 ml/min the dose of acyclovir is 800 mg orally every 4 h (5 times daily). For CrCl of 10–25 or <10 ml/min, the acyclovir is given as 800 mg orally every 8 or 12 h, respectively.

Valaciclovir is only available as a tablet formulation. It is metabolized nearly completely to acyclovir within minutes after absorption (Soul-Lawton et al., 1995). The subsequent oral bioavailability of acyclovir is about 54% (Perry and Faulds, 1996). Notably, plasma area-under-the-curve (AUC) levels of acyclovir which are achieved following 2 g of valaciclovir dosed orally three times daily approximate those achieved with acyclovir 10 mg/kg administered every 8 h intravenously Weller et al., 1993). The recommended dose of valaciclovir for the treatment of herpes zoster is 1000 mg orally every 8 h. Dosage reduction is required in patients with CrCl < 50 ml/min.

5.2. Penciclovir and famciclovir

5.2.1. Chemistry, mechanism of action and in vitro activity

Penciclovir, 9-(4-hydroxy-3-hydroxymethylbut-1-yl)guanine, is an acyclic guanine derivative that is similar to acyclovir in structure, mechanism of action, and spectrum of antiviral activity (Boyd et al., 1987). There are, however, differences between acyclovir and penciclovir in terms of activation and intracellular concentrations (Earnshaw et al., 1992). In HSV or VZV-infected cells, penciclovir is first monophosphorylated by virally encoded TK and then further phosphorylated to the triphosphate moiety by cellular enzymes. Penciclovir triphosphate blocks viral DNA synthesis through competitive inhibition of viral DNA polymerase (Vere Hodge, 1993). Unlike acyclovir triphosphate, penciclovir triphosphate is not an obligate chain terminator and can be incorporated into the extending DNA chain. Compared with acyclovir triphosphate, intracellular concentrations of penciclovir triphosphate are much higher. However, this potential advantage is offset by a much lower affinity of penciclovir triphosphate for viral DNA polymerase (Vere Hodge, 1993). The in vitro activity of penciclovir against HSV-1, HSV-2 and VZV is similar to that of acyclovir, with median EC_{50} values of 0.4, 1.5, and 4.0 μg/ml, respectively, in MRC-5 cells (Boyd et al., 1993). Compared with acyclovir triphosphate, penciclovir triphosphate has a much longer intracellular half-life in virus-infected cells (Earnshaw et al., 1992). For example, the half-life values for penciclovir triphosphate and acyclovir triphosphate in HSV-1-infected cells are 10 h and 0.7 h, respectively. The clinical significance (if any) of the prolonged intracellular half-life is not known.

5.2.2. Absorption, distribution, and elimination

Penciclovir is very poorly absorbed (less than 5%) after oral administration. Intravenous infusion of a penciclovir dose of 10 mg/kg over 1 h yields a peak plasma concentration of 12.1 μg/ml (Pue and Benet, 1993). Plasma protein binding of penciclovir is <20%. The drug is cleared by renal tubular secretion and passive filtration. The plasma elimination half-life of penciclovir is about 2 h and approximately 70% of the administered dose is recovered unchanged in the urine (Fowles et al., 1992; Pue et al., 1994). The intravenous preparation of penciclovir has not yet been approved or commercially released.

Just as valaciclovir is a prodrug of acyclovir, famciclovir is a prodrug of penciclovir. Because penciclovir is very poorly absorbed, famciclovir (the diacetyl ester of 6-deoxy-penciclovir) was developed as the oral formulation (Vere Hodge, 1993). Famciclovir is well absorbed after oral administration. The first acetyl side chain is cleaved by esterases found in the intestinal wall. On first pass through the liver, the second acetyl group is removed and oxidation catalyzed by aldehyde oxidase occurs at the six position, yielding penciclovir, the active antiviral compound. When administered as the famciclovir prodrug, the bioavailability of penciclovir is about 77% (Pue and Benet, 1993). Following a single oral dose of 250 mg or 500 mg of famciclovir, peak plasma penciclovir concentrations of 1.9 and 3.5 µg/ml are achieved at 1 h (Pue et al., 1994). The pharmacokinetics of penciclovir are linear and dose-independent over a famciclovir dosing range of 125–750 mg. Food slows famciclovir absorption and lowers the peak plasma penciclovir concentration, but does not alter the AUC value.

6. Clinical effectiveness of antiviral therapy of herpes zoster

The goals of therapy of herpes zoster in immunocompetent adults are to accelerate the events of cutaneous healing, reduce the severity of acute neuritis, and, most importantly, to reduce the incidence, severity, and duration of chronic pain. Three oral antiviral drugs are currently approved in the United States for treatment of herpes zoster. Acyclovir, valaciclovir, and famciclovir have all been demonstrated to reduce the duration of viral shedding, promote resolution of skin lesions, and limit the duration of pain when antiviral therapy is initiated within 72 h of shingles' onset (Huff et al., 1988; Beutner et al.,

1995; Tyring et al., 1995; Wood et al., 1996). In the immunocompromised host, the goals are identical; however, none of these compounds is licensed for oral therapy. Regardless, two, valaciclovir and famciclovir, are employed in many circumstances.

Oral acyclovir (800 mg 5 times daily for 7 days) accelerates cutaneous healing and reduces the severity of acute neuritis in immunocompetent adults with herpes zoster (Huff et al., 1988; Wood et al., 1988; Morton and Thomson, 1989). In placebo-controlled trials, acyclovir therapy reduced new vesicle formation by approximately 1.5 days and time to crusting by 2 days. Benefits are maximized when therapy is initiated within 48 h of appearance of lesions. Acyclovir therapy is also highly effective for prevention of ocular complications of herpes zoster ophthalmicus, including keratitis and uveitis (Cobo et al., 1986; Harding and Porter, 1991). Acyclovir does not alter the incidence of post-herpetic neuralgia, but can accelerate the resolution of acute pain (Jackson et al., 1997). A meta-analysis of all of the placebo-controlled trials of acyclovir for herpes zoster demonstrated a significant reduction of zoster-associated pain among acyclovir recipients (Table I). Zoster-associated pain (ZAP) defines pain as a continuous variable rather than a discontinuous one, as occurs with the assessment of post-herpetic neuralgia.

Valaciclovir (1000 mg 3 times daily for 7 days) was compared with acyclovir (800 mg 5 times daily for 7 days) in a study of 1141 immunocompetent patients over 50 years of age with herpes zoster (Beutner et al., 1995). The progression of cutaneous healing was similar in the two treatment groups. However, patients in the valaciclovir treatment group had a shorter duration of zoster-associated pain (median: 38 days versus 51 days; $P = 0.001$). Extending valaciclovir therapy to 14 days did not result in any additional benefit (Table II).

Famciclovir has also been evaluated for treatment of dermatomal herpes zoster in immunocompetent patients (De Greef and Famciclovir Herpes Zoster Clinical Study Group, 1994; Tyring et al., 1995). In a placebo-controlled clinical trial, famciclovir accelerated cutaneous healing and reduced the duration of both viral shedding and post-herpetic neuralgia

TABLE I

Efficacy of acyclovir in herpes zoster (Wood et al., 1996)

	Acyclovir versus placebo Hazard ratio[2] (95% confidence interval)	P[1]	Studies analyzed
Time to complete cessation of zoster-associated pain:			Morton and Thomson (1989); Huff et al. (1988); Harding and Porter (1991)
All patients	1.79 (1.34, 2.39)	<0.001	
Patients >50 years	2.13 (1.42, 3.19)	<0.001	
Time to complete cessation of moderate/severe zoster-associated pain	1.46 (1.11, 1.93)	0.007	Morton and Thomson (1989); Huff et al. (1988); Harding and Porter (1991)
Time to first pain-free period	1.31 (1.08, 1.60)	0.007	Morton and Thomson (1989); Huff et al. (1988); Harding and Porter (1991); Wood et al. (1988)

[1] Statistical calculations determined by Cox logistic regression analyses.
[2] Hazard ratio: ratio of risk for achieving cessation of pain between treatment groups.

TABLE II

Accelerated resolution of zoster associated pain (Beutner et al., 1995)

	Intent-to-treat analysis hazard ratio[1]	P[2]
Valaciclovir 7 days vs. acyclovir	1.34 (1.12, 1.60)	0.001
Valaciclovir 14 days vs. acyclovir	1.22 (1.03, 1.46)	0.03
Valaciclovir 7 days vs. valaciclovir 14 days	1.10 (0.92, 1.30)	NS

[1] Intent-to-treat analysis: analysis utilizes all subjects randomized.
[2] Statistical calculations determined by Cox logistic regression analyses.

(Tyring et al., 1995). In a subset of subjects over 50 years of age, the duration of post-herpetic neuralgia was reduced from a median of 163 days to 63 days in the placebo and famciclovir treatment groups, respectively ($P = 0.004$) (Tyring et al., 1995). Successful treatment with famciclovir at a dose of 750 mg once daily for 7 days has also been claimed (Ashton, 1996). In the United States, the recommended dose of famciclovir for uncomplicated herpes zoster is 500 mg 3 times daily, while doses of 250 mg 3 times daily and 750 mg once daily are approved in Europe and the United Kingdom. The effects of famciclovir on pain are summarized in Table III.

6.1. Therapy of herpes zoster in the immunocompromised host

Both vidarabine (Whitley et al., 1976, 1992) and acyclovir have been proven efficacious for the treat-ment of herpes zoster in the immunocompromised host. However, vidarabine is no longer available as an intravenous formulation. Both drugs accelerate cutaneous healing, and decrease both cutaneous dissemination and visceral complications. Acyclovir therapy is administered intravenously at 500 mg/m² for 7–10 days. Intravenous therapy is reserved for the most severely immunocompromised hosts, i.e. bone marrow and solid organ transplant recipients. In spite of the lack of controlled clinical trials in the immunocompromised host, many physicians resort to the oral administration of valaciclovir or famciclovir since plasma levels are equivalent to that achieved following efficacious intravenous therapy. Indeed, even acyclovir was satisfactorily tolerated in three therapeutic trials in the immunosuppression host (two HIV and one cancer) (Gnann et al., 1995, 1998; Bodsworth et al., 1997). These patients did not develop progressive cutaneous or visceral disease.

TABLE III

Hazard ratios (De Greef and Famciclovir Herpes Zoster Clinical Study Group, 1994; Tyring et al., 1995)

	Zoster-associated pain (intent-to-treat analysis of patients treated within 72 hours of rash onset)	Zoster-associated pain (efficacy evaluable subgroup, treated within 48 hours of rash onset with age as a continuous covariate)	Post-herpetic neuralgia
500 mg famciclovir vs. placebo	–	–	1.7 (1.1, 2.7) $P = 0.02$
750 mg famciclovir vs. placebo	–	–	1.9 (1.2, 2.9) $P = 0.005$
250 mg famciclovir [1]	1.4 (na) $P = 0.086$	1.62 (1.06, 2.46) $P = 0.025$	–
500 mg famciclovir [1]	1.8 (na) $P = 0.003$	1.51 (0.99, 2.29) $P = 0.053$	–
750 mg famciclovir [1] vs. 800 mg acyclovir [2]	1.4 (na) $P = 0.05$	1.39 (0.925, 2.09) $P = 0.113$	–

– = not analyzed in publication; na = confidence intervals not provided.
[1] 3 × per day.
[2] 5 × per day.

7. Adjunctive therapies

Appropriate supportive care will help make patients with herpes zoster more comfortable. Skin lesions should be kept clean and dry to reduce the risk of bacterial superinfection. Astringent soaks (e.g. Domeboro solution) may be soothing. Most patients with acute herpes zoster will have very significant pain and require symptomatic therapy with narcotic analgesics. Clinicians should not underestimate the requirement for potent, narcotic analgesics in older patients with herpes zoster.

The controversial issue of corticosteroid therapy for herpes zoster has recently been addressed in two large controlled clinical trials (Wood et al., 1994; Whitley et al., 1996). The only placebo-controlled study demonstrated that the combination of acyclovir plus corticosteroids accelerated healing of skin lesions, reduced requirements for analgesic use, and accelerated the times for return to usual activity and uninterrupted sleep. Despite these benefits on the acute symptoms of herpes zoster, neither study demonstrated any reduction in the incidence of PHN. In the study of acyclovir plus prednisone for herpes zoster conducted in the United States by the NIAID Collaborative Antiviral Study Group (CASG), the clinical trial was based on a randomized 2 × 2 factorial design (Whitley et al., 1996). Pain was assessed

serially during the first month of study enrollment (acute neuritis) and also as a continuum extending from study enrollment through 6 months of follow-up (zoster-associated pain). In the study population of relatively healthy patients over 50 years of age, pain and quality-of-life endpoints (which included return to usual activities, ability to sleep uninterrupted, and cessation of analgesic use) were evaluated as functions of treatment and other covariates. Based on a step-wise Cox regression model, two covariates predicted the times to resolution of acute neuritis and ZAP. These symptoms resolved significantly faster in patients with no or mild pain at baseline, compared with those with severe or incapacitating pain. Furthermore, patients who had the fewest number of lesions at enrollment had accelerated rates of resolution of acute and long-term pain. These variables significantly predicted resolution of herpes zoster pain independent of the effects of treatment (Table IV) and are discussed in more detail below.

Thus, a tapering dose of corticosteroids should be considered in older individuals who do not otherwise have contraindications to corticosteroid administration. Because of potential complications of corticosteroid administration, the use of prednisone in this setting is considered controversial by some physicians and should be limited to those older indi-

TABLE IV

Disease resolution according to Cox regression model [1] (Whitley et al., 1996)

Dependent variable	Risk ratio [2] (95% CI) acyclovir plus prednisone compared with placebo
One-month evaluation of cutaneous healing	
Time to total crusting	2.27 [3] (1.46, 3.55)
Time to total healing	2.07 [3] (1.26, 3.38)
One-month evaluation of quality of life	
Time to cessation of acute neuritis	3.02 [3] (1.42, 6.41)
Time to uninterrupted sleep	2.12 [3] (1.25, 3.58)
Time to return to 100% usual activity	3.22 [3] (1.92, 5.40)
Time to no use of analgesics agents	3.15 [3] (1.69, 5.89)
Six-month evaluation of pain	
Time to cessation of zoster-associated pain	1.56 (0.92, 2.66)

[1] Prognostic variables included in the model were: sex, race, age, number and duration of lesions prior to enrollment surface area of lesions, and severity of pain at baseline.

[2] Risk ratio: ratio of the risk for achieving cessation of pain between treatment groups. Three times daily for 7 to 10 days. Both medications are well tolerated.

[3] $P < 0.05$; statistical calculations determined by Cox logistic regression analyses.

viduals at greatest risk for pain which are those with significant pain and large surface area involvement at the time of presentation (Whitley et al., 1996, 1998). No data are available to support combination therapy of prednisone with famciclovir or valaciclovir, but these regimens should theoretically be as efficacious as prednisone with acyclovir.

Treatments which will consistently and reliably reduce the risk of chronic pain remain an unmet need in herpes zoster management. Drugs such as tricyclic antidepressants (Watson et al., 1992) and gabapentin (Rowbotham et al., 1998) have beneficial effects for treatment of established post-herpetic neuralgia. The potential utility of these drugs in patients with acute herpes zoster has not yet been investigated.

8. Factors which influence outcome

From the therapeutic trials, three dominant factors have been shown to influence the outcome of pain. These are: severity of pain at presentation, age of the patient, and the extent of dermatomal disease. While the first two observations are intuitive, the last is less so; however, all three warrant elaboration. As

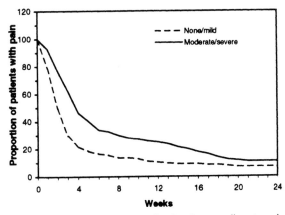

Fig. 2. Duration of zoster-associated pain according to pain severity at presentation.

illustrated in Fig. 2 (Whitley et al., 1998), patients who present with moderate or severe disease at diagnosis are more likely to experience post-herpetic neuralgia. This observation is supported by studies performed by the NIAID CASG, as well, and as illustrated in Table V. A second dominant variable is the age of the patient at presentation, as indicated in Table VI. There is a direct relationship between the age of the patient and the probability of persistent pain. Those specific host factors responsible for this

TABLE V

Significant prognostic variables (first month) Cox regression model (Whitley et al., 1996)

Dependent variable	Risk ratio (95% confidence interval)	
	severity of pain at baseline [1]	number of lesions prior to enrollment [2]
One-month evaluation		
Time to cessation of acute neuritis	1.82 (1.34, 2.47)	2.02 (1.50, 2.72)
Uninterrupted sleep	1.61 (1.27, 2.03)	1.48 (1.20, 1.84)
Perform usual activity	1.94 (1.54, 2.43)	1.47 (1.20, 1.80)
No use of analgesics	1.76 (1.35, 2.29)	1.65 (1.29, 2.11)
Six-month evaluation		
Time to cessation of zoster-associated pain	1.89 (1.48, 2.40)	1.54 (1.24, 1.92)

[1] Severe/incapacitating pain coded as reference level.
[2] Category with largest number of lesions coded as reference level.

TABLE VI

Influence of age on resolution of zoster-associated pain (Whitley et al., 1998)

Age group comparison	Median zoster-associated pain duration (days)	Hazard ratio (95% confidence interval)	*P*-value for hazard ratio
vs. patients < 30 years old			
30–40 years	19 vs. 16	0.97 (0.66, 1.41)	0.87
40–50 years	22 vs. 16	0.74 (0.51, 1.09)	0.13
50–60 years	31 vs. 16	0.59 (0.42, 0.82)	0.002
60–70 years	47 vs. 16	0.48 (0.35, 0.66)	0.0001
>70 years	50 vs. 16	0.40 (0.29, 0.56)	0.0001
>60 years vs. 50–60 years			
Trial 5	50 vs. 31	0.70 (0.60, 0.83)	0.0001
Trial 6	45 vs. 27	0.66 (0.52, 0.83)	0.0005

observation, other than 'aging', are unknown. Lastly, the extent of disease, as measured by the number of lesions within the dermatome, can be modeled for pain severity. This observation is best illustrated in Fig. 3 (Whitley et al., 1999).

The recognition of these factors is important for several reasons. First, it guides the clinician in a treatment approach. For example, older patients who present with severe pain and extensive dermatomal disease warrant the most aggressive therapy, including antivirals, analgesics and corticosteroids, in the absence of contraindications. Conversely, young patients (<50 years) who are without pain at presentation and otherwise immune competent can simply be observed and managed with analgesics, if necessary.

9. Summary of treatment of herpes zoster

Acyclovir, valaciclovir, and famciclovir are currently available for treatment of uncomplicated herpes zoster in immunocompetent patients. These drugs are all well tolerated and appear to be approximately comparable in clinical efficacy. Because of their improved pharmacokinetic profiles and simpler dosing regimens, valaciclovir and famciclovir have emerged as the drugs of choice for this indication. Immunocompetent individuals under 50 years of age who develop herpes zoster tend to have relatively benign courses and are at low risk for chronic pain. Many physicians elect to manage these patients with analgesics alone and consider antiviral therapy op-

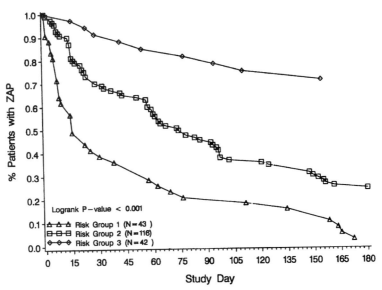

Fig. 3. Time to cessation of zoster-associated pain by severity of pain and number of lesions at baseline. Risk group 1 includes those patients who have ≤20 lesions and no or mild pain at clinical presentation. Risk group 2 includes those patients who had 21–46 lesions and moderate pain at presentation. Risk group 3 represents those patients with most extensive cutaneous disease (≥47 lesions) and severe or incapacitating pain at the onset of disease.

tional. Older patients, however, are at increased risk for more severe disease and long-term complications and should be more aggressively treated with antiviral drugs. The subpopulation of herpes zoster patients most likely to benefit from antiviral therapy are those over the age of 60 who present with significant pain at onset and who have a large number of lesions within the involved dermatome. Administration of an antiviral drug should be considered mandatory for patients presenting with active herpes zoster involving the first division of the trigeminal nerve, primarily to prevent ocular complications that are potentially sight-threatening.

Physicians frequently encounter patients who present beyond the 48-to-72-h window that is considered the optimal time for initiation of antiviral therapy for herpes zoster. Very little information from clinical trials is currently available to support the value of these drugs for herpes zoster that has been clinically apparent for >72 h. One clue that clinicians may find useful is to examine the cutaneous eruption carefully for evidence of ongoing new vesicle formation. The presence of new vesicles

(that is, those that are clear and not yet pustular) correlates well with ongoing VZV replication and may suggest that the patient would still benefit from antiviral drug therapy.

Finally, as with all infectious diseases, prevention is preferable to treatment. Investigators have hypothesized that administration of a live VZV vaccine to older adults (who are already latently infected with VZV) may stimulate the waning cellular immune responses, thereby preventing herpes zoster during the last decades of life when patients are at highest risk for shingles (Levin et al., 1994). Controlled clinical trials are currently ongoing to determine whether administration of a VZV vaccine can reduce the frequency or severity of herpes zoster in older adults.

Acknowledgements

Studies performed by the author and reported herein are funded in whole or in part with funds from the National Institutes for Allergy and Infectious Diseases (NIAID), National Institutes of Health, under

Contract No. N01-AI-65306, the National Cancer Institute (NCI) CA RO-1-13148, Division of Research Resources (DRR) RR-032, and a grant from the State of Alabama.

References

Arvin, A.M., Pollard, R.B., Rasmussen, L.E. and Merigan, T.C. (1980) Cellular and humoral immunity in the pathogenesis of recurrent herpes viral infection in patients with lymphoma. J. Clin. Invest., 65: 869–878.

Ashton, R.E. (1996) Efficacy of once and twice daily famciclovir in the treatment of acute zoster. European Congress of Chemotherapy, Glasgow.

Balfour, H.H., Jr. (1999) Antiviral drugs. N. Engl. J. Med., 340: 1255–1268.

Bastian, F.O., Rabson, A.S., Yee, C.L. and Tralka, T.S. (1974) Herpes virus varicella: isolated from human dorsal root ganglia. Arch. Pathol., 97: 331–336.

Beutner, K.R., Friedman, D.J., Forszpaniak, C., Andersen, P.L. and Wood, M.J. (1995) Valaciclovir compared with acyclovir for improved therapy for herpes zoster in immunocompetent adults. Antimicrob. Agents Chemother., 39: 1546–1553.

Bodsworth, N.J., Boag, F., Burdge, D., Genereux, M., Borleffs, J.C.C., Evans, B.A., Modai, J., Colebunders, R., Thomis, J. and The Multinational Sorivudine Study Group (1997) Evaluation of sorivudine (BV-araU) versus acyclovir in the treatment of acute localized herpes zoster in human immunodeficiency virus-infected adults. J. Infect. Dis., 176: 103–111.

Boyd, M.R., Bacon, T.H., Sutton, D. and Cole, M. (1987) Antiherpesvirus activity of 9-(4-hydroxy-3-hydroxy-methylbut-1-yl) guanine (BRL 39123) in cell structure. Antimicrob. Agents Chemother., 31: 1238–1242.

Boyd, M.R., Safrin, S. and Kern, E.R. (1993) Penciclovir: a review of its spectrum of activity, selectivity, and cross-resistance pattern. Antiviral Chem. Chemother., 4 (Suppl. 1): 3–11.

Cobo, L.M., Foulks, G.N. and Liesegang, T. (1986) Oral acyclovir in the treatment of acute herpes zoster ophthalmicus. Ophthalmology, 93: 763–770.

Collins, P. and Bauer, D.J. (1979) The activity in vitro against herpes virus of 9-(2-hydroxyethoxymethyl) guanine (acycloguanosine), a new antiviral agent. J. Antimicrob. Chemother., 5: 432–436.

De Greef, H. and Famciclovir Herpes Zoster Clinical Study Group (1994) Famciclovir, a new oral antiherpes drug: Results of the first controlled clinical study demonstrating its efficacy and safety in the treatment of uncomplicated herpes zoster in immunocompetent patients. Int. J. Antimicrob. Agents, 4: 241–246.

DeMiranda, P. and Blum, M.R. (1983) Pharmacokinetics of acyclovir after intravenous and oral administration. J. Antimicrob. Chemother., 12: 29–37.

Demorgas, J.M. and Kierland, R.R. (1957) The outcome of patients with herpes zoster. Arch. Dermatol., 75: 193–196.

Derse, D., Chang, Y.-C., Furman, P.A. and Elion, G.B. (1981) Inhibition of purified human and herpes simplex virus-induced DNA polymerase by 9-(2-hydroxyethoxy methyl)guanine [acyclovir] triphosphate: effect on primer-template function. J. Biol. Chem., 256: 11447–11451.

Earnshaw, D.L., Bacon, T.H., Darlison, S.J., Edmonds, K., Perkins, R.M. and Vere Hodge, R.A. (1992) Mode of antiviral action on penciclovir in MRC-5 cells infected with herpes simplex virus type 1, HSV-2, and varicella-zoster virus. Antimicrob. Agents Chemother., 36: 2747–2757.

Elion, G.B., Furman, P.A., Fyfe, J.A., de Miranda, P., Beauchamp, L. and Schaffer, H.J. (1977) Selectivity of action of an antiherpetic agent, 9-(2-hydroxyethoxymethyl) guanine. Proc. Natl. Acad. Sci. U.S.A., 74: 5716–5720.

Esiri, M.M. and Tomlinson, A.H. (1974) Herpes zoster: demonstration of virus in trigeminal and nerve ganglion by immunofluorescence and electron microscopy. J. Neurol. Sci., 15: 35–48.

Esmann, V., Kroon, S., Peterslund, N.A., Ronne-Rasmussen, J.O., Geil, J.P., Fogh, H., Petersen, C.S. and Danielsen, L. (1987) Prednisolone does not prevent post-herpetic neuralgia. Lancet, 2: 126–129.

Feldman, S., Hughes, W.T. and Daniel, C.B. (1975) Varicella in children with cancer: seventy-seven cases. Pediatrics, 56: 388–399.

Forghani, B., Schmidt, N.J. and Dennis, J. (1978) Antibody assays for varicella-zoster virus: Comparison of enzyme immunoassay with neutralization, immune adherence hemagglutination, and complement fixation. J. Clin. Microbiol., 8: 545–552.

Fowles, S.E., Pierce, D.M. and Prince, W.T. (1992) The tolerance to and pharmacokinetics of penciclovir (BRL 39123A), a novel antiherpes agent, administered by intravenous infusion to healthy subjects. Eur. J. Clin. Pharmacol., 43: 513–516.

Furman, P.A., St. Clair, M.H. and Spector, T. (1984) Acyclovir triphosphate is a suicide inactivator of the herpes simplex virus DNA polymerase. J. Biol. Chem., 259: 9575–9579.

Fyfe, J.A., Keller, P.M., Furman, P.A., Miller, R.A. and Elion, G.B. (1978) Thymidine kinase from herpes simplex virus phosphorylates the new antiviral compound, 9-(2-hydroxyethoxymethyl)guanine. J. Biol. Chem., 253(24): 8721–8727.

Gnann, J.W. and Whitley, R.J. (1991) Natural history and treatment of varicella-zoster in high risk populations. J. Hosp. Infect., 18: 317–329.

Gnann, J., Whitley, R.J., Weiss, H., Tyring, S., Wolf, J., Pollard, R., Mertz, G., Pappas, P., Laughlin, C., Sherrill, L., Hayden, F., Schlupner, C., Soong, S.-J. and the National Institute of Allergy and Infectious Diseases Collaborative Antiviral Study Group (1995) Sorivudine (BV-araU) versus acyclovir for herpes zoster in HIV-infected patients; Results of a multi-center controlled trial, San Diego, California.

Gnann, J.W., Crumpacker, C.S., Lalezari, J.P., Smith, J.A., Tyring, S.K., Baum, K.F., Borucki, M.J., Joseph, W.P., Mertz, G.J., Steigbigel, R.T., Cloud, G.A., Soong, S.-J., Sherrill, L.C., DeHertogh, D.A., Whitley, R.J. and The Collaborative Antiviral Study Group/AIDS Clinical Trials Group and Herpes Zoster Study Group (1998) Sorivudine versus acyclovir for treatment of dermatomal herpes zoster in human immunodeficiency virus-infected patients: results from a randomized, controlled clinical trial. Antimicrob. Agents Chemother., 42: 1139–1145.

Harding, S.P. and Porter, S.M. (1991) Oral acyclovir in herpes zoster ophthalmicus. Curr. Eye Res., 10: 177–182.

Hogan, E.L. and Krigman, M.R. (1973) Herpes zoster myelitis. Arch. Neurol., 29: 309–313.

Hope-Simpson, R.E. (1965) The nature of herpes zoster: a long-term study and a new hypothesis. Proc. R. Soc. Med., 58: 9–20.

Huff, J.C., Bean, B., Balfour, H.H., Jr., Laskin, O.L., Connor, J.D., Corey, L., Bryson, Y.J. and McGuirt, P.W. (1988) Therapy of herpes zoster with oral acyclovir. Am. J. Med., 85: 84–89.

Jackson, J.L., Gibbons, R., Meyer, G. and Inouye, L. (1997) The effect of treating herpes zoster with oral acyclovir in preventing postherpetic neuralgia. Arch. Intern. Med., 157: 909–912.

Kost, R.G. and Straus, S.E. (1996) Drug therapy: Postherpetic neuralgia — pathogenesis, treatment, and prevent. N. Engl. J. Med., 335: 32–42.

Laskin, O.L. (1984) Acyclovir: Pharmacology and clinical experience. Arch. Intern. Med., 144: 1241–1246.

Levin, M.J., Murray, M., Zerbe, G.O., White, C.J. and Hayward, A.R. (1994) Immune response of elderly persons four years after receiving a live attenuated varicella vaccine. J. Infect. Dis., 170: 522–526.

Locksley, R.M., Flournoy, N., Sullivan, K.M. and Myers, J.D. (1985) Infection with varicella-zoster virus after marrow transplantation. J. Infect. Dis., 152: 1172–1181.

McGregor, R.M. (1957) Herpes zoster, chickenpox, and cancer in general practice. Br. Med. J., 1: 84–87.

Morton, P. and Thomson, A.N. (1989) Oral acyclovir in the treatment of herpes zoster in general practice. N. Z. Med. J., 102: 93–95.

Norris, F.H., Jr., Dramov, B., Calder, C.D. and Hohnson, S.G. (1969) Virus-like particles in myositis accompanying herpes zoster. Arch. Neurol., 21: 25.

Perry, C.M. and Faulds, D. (1996) Valaciclovir: a review of its antiviral, pharmacokinetic properties and therapeutic efficacy in herpesvirus infections. Drugs, 52: 754–772.

Puc, M.A. and Benet, L.Z. (1993) Pharmacokinetics of famciclovir. Antiviral Chem. Chemother., 4 (Suppl. 1): 47–56.

Pue, M.A., Pratt, S.K., Fairless, A.J., Fowles, S., Laroche, J., Georgiou, P. and Prince, W. (1994) Linear pharmacokinetics

of penciclovir following administration of single oral doses of famciclovir 125, 250, 500 and 750 mg to healthy volunteers. J. Antimicrob. Chemother., 33: 119–127.

Ragozzino, M.W., Melton, L.J. III., Kurland, L.T., Chu, C.P. and Perry, H.O. (1982) Populations-based study of herpes zoster and its sequelae. Medicine, 61: 310–316.

Rowbotham, M., Harden, N., Stacey, B., Bernstein, P. and Magnus-Miller, L. (1998) Gabapentin for the treatment of postherpetic neuralgia. A randomized controlled trial. JAMA, 280: 1837–1842.

Rubin, D. and Fusfeld, R.D. (1965) Muscle paralysis in herpes zoster. Calif. Med., 103: 261–266.

Schaeffer, H.J., Beauchamp, L., deMiranda, P., Elion, G.B., Bauer, D.J. and Collins, P. (1978) 9-(2-hydroxyethoxymethyl) guanine activity against viruses of the herpes group. Nature, 272: 583–585.

Soul-Lawton, J., Seaber, E., On, N., Wootton, R., Rolan, P. and Posner, J. (1995) Absolute bioavailability and metabolic disposition of valaciclovir, the L-valyl ester of acyclovir, following oral administration to humans. Antimicrob. Agents Chemother., 39: 2759–2764.

Tyring, S., Barbarash, R.A., Nahlik, J.E., Cunningham, A., Marley, J., Heng, M., Jones, T., Rea, T., Boon, R., Saltzman R. and the Collaborative Famciclovir Herpes Zoster Study Group (1995) Famciclovir for the treatment of acute herpes zoster. Effects on acute disease and postherpetic neuralgia: A randomized, double-blind, placebo-controlled trial. Ann. Intern. Med., 123: 89–96.

Vere Hodge, R.A. (1993) Famciclovir and penciclovir. The mode of action of famciclovir including its conversion to penciclovir. Antiviral Chem. Chemother., 4: 67–84.

Watson, C.P.N., Chipman, M., Reed, K., Evans, R.J. and Birkett, N. (1992) Amitriptyline versus maprotiline in postherpetic neuralgia: a randomized, double-blind, crossover trial. Pain, 48: 29–36.

Watson, P.N. and Evans, R.J. (1986) Postherpetic neuralgia: A review. Arch. Neurol., 43: 836–840.

Weller, S., Blum, R., Doucette, M., Burnette, T., Cederberg, D.M., de Miranda, P. et al. (1993) Pharmacokinetics of the acyclovir prodrug valaciclovir after escalating single- and multiple-dose administration to normal volunteers. Clin. Pharmacol. Ther., 54: 595–605.

Whitley, R.J. (1984) Varicella-zoster virus infections. In: G.J. Galasso, T.C. Merigan and R.A. Buchanan (Eds.), Antiviral Agents and Viral Diseases of Man. Raven Press, New York, pp. 517–541.

Whitley, R.J., Chien, L.T., Dolin, R., Galasso, G.J., Alford, C.A. and the National Institute of Allergy and Infectious Diseases Collaborative Antiviral Study Group (1976) Adenine arabinoside therapy of herpes zoster in the immunosuppressed. N. Engl. J. Med., 294: 1193–1199.

Whitley, R.J., Gnann, J.W., Hinthorn, D., Chein, L., Pollard, R.B., Hayden, F., Mertz, G.J., Oxman, M., Soong, S.-J. and the National Institute of Allergy and Infectious Diseases Collaborative Antiviral Study Group (1992) Disseminated herpes zoster in the immunocompromised host: A comparative trial of acyclovir and vidarabine. J. Infect. Dis., 165: 450–455.

Whitley, R.J., Weiss, H., Gnann, J.W., Tyring, S., Mertz, G.J., Pappas, P., Schleupner, C.C., Hayden, F., Wolf, J., Soong. S.-J. and National Institute of Allergy and Infectious Diseases Collaborative Antiviral Study Group (1996) A randomized, placebo-controlled trial of acyclovir with and without steroids for the treatment of herpes zoster. Ann. Intern. Med., 125: 376–383.

Whitley, R.J., Shukla, S. and Crooks, R.J. (1998) The identification of risk factors associated with persistent pain following herpes zoster. J. Infect. Dis., 178 (Suppl. 1): S71–S75.

Whitley, R.J., Weiss, H.L., Soong, S.J. and Gnann, J.W. (1999) Herpes zoster: risk categories for persistent pain. J. Infect. Dis., 179: 9–15.

Wood, M.J., Ogan, P.H., McKendrick, M.W., Care, C.D., McGill, J.I. and Webb, E.M. (1988) Efficacy of oral acyclovir treatment of acute herpes zoster. Am. J. Med., 85: 79–83.

Wood, M.J., Johnson, R.W., McKendrick, M.W., Taylor, J., Mandal, B.K. and Crooks, J. (1994) A randomized trial of acyclovir for 7 days or 21 days with and without prednisolone for treatment of acute herpes zoster. N. Engl. J. Med., 330: 896–900.

Wood, M.J., Kay, R., Dworkin, R.H., Soong, S.-J. and Whitley, R.J. (1996) Oral acyclovir accelerates pain resolution in herpes zoster: A meta-analysis of placebo-controlled trials. Clin. Infect. Dis., 22: 341–347.

Herpes Zoster and Postherpetic Neuralgia, 2nd Revised and Enlarged Edition
Pain Research and Clinical Management, Vol. 11
Edited by C.P.N. Watson and A.A. Gershon

CHAPTER 7

Latency and neurologic aspects of zoster

James J. LaGuardia, Randall J. Cohrs and Donald H. Gilden [*]

Department of Neurology, University of Colorado Health Sciences Center, 4200 East 9th Avenue, Mail Stop B182,
Denver, CO 80262, USA

1. Introduction

After primary infection, varicella-zoster virus (VZV) becomes latent in cranial and dorsal root ganglia and reactivates with increasing age or immunosuppression. Reactivation produces both peripheral and central nervous system (CNS) disease (Gilden et al., 2000). The peripheral manifestations are herpes zoster, commonly known as shingles, and postherpetic neuralgia. Severe sharp, lancinating, radicular pain and rash characterize zoster. Postherpetic neuralgia is defined as pain persisting more than 4–6 weeks after rash. Additionally, zoster sine herpete may occur, consisting of dermatomal distribution pain without antecedent rash. Uncommonly, a postinfectious polyneuritis (Guillain–Barré syndrome) may follow zoster.

In immunocompetent and especially in immunocompromised patients, CNS complications can occur after VZV reactivation when virus spreads to the spinal cord, brain or arteries. Immunocompetent individuals may develop myelitis or large-vessel encephalitis/granulomatous arteritis, while immunocompromised patients develop small-vessel encephalitis, meningoencephalitis, or ventriculitis. Some patients develop both large- and small-vessel disease, although one form usually predominates (Gilden et al., 1996).

The biologic mechanisms underlying the transition from latency to active viral replication are unknown. Because of the high incidence of zoster and the seriousness of its sequelae, an understanding of VZV latency is important. Many laboratories have devoted major efforts to determining the physical state of the virus during latency as a key to understanding VZV reactivation mechanism(s). Such information is essential in predicting and preventing the often serious neurological complications produced by reactivation. The remainder of this chapter is devoted to a review of the pathogenesis and physical state of VZV during latency.

2. Pathology and pathogenesis

Despite the ubiquitous nature and frequency of VZV infection, the pathogenesis of zoster remains largely unknown. Our present understanding of virus spread, localization and replication is based on in vitro studies of infected human or primate cells in tissue culture, correlation of the presence of VZV in human tissues with pathologic changes in different

---
[*] Correspondence to: Dr. Donald H. Gilden, Department of Neurology, University of Colorado Health Sciences Center, 4200 East 9th Avenue, Mail Stop B182, Denver, CO 80262, USA. Phone: +1 (303) 315-8281; Fax: +1 (303) 315-8720; E-mail: don.gilden@uchsc.edu

clinical situations, and attempts to produce disease experimentally.

The histologic features of zoster are typically confined to dorsal root ganglia and adjacent nerves. Pathologic changes in ganglia corresponding to the segmental distribution of rash were first noted by Von Barensprung (1863) and more extensively detailed by Head and Campbell (1900) and Denny-Brown et al. (1944). Lesions described were localized and occurred in immunocompetent individuals, except perhaps in arsenic-treated syphilis patients. The cardinal pathologic features were inflammation and hemorrhagic necrosis of dorsal root ganglia often associated with neuritis, localized leptomeningitis in adjacent spinal cord, unilateral segmental poliomyelitis, and degeneration of related motor and sensory roots. Demyelination was also seen in areas of mononuclear cell infiltration and microglial proliferation. Much later, intranuclear inclusions (Cheatham et al., 1956; Ghatak and Zimmerman, 1973), viral antigen and herpesvirus particles (Esiri and Tomlinson, 1972; Nagashima et al., 1975) were detected in ganglia. VZV was first isolated from ganglia by Bastian et al. (1974). However, those studies were performed on ganglia from patients with underlying malignancies or other immune dysfunction who developed disseminated zoster just before death. There is a single report of VZV antigen detection and virus isolation from ganglia of a fatal case of bacterial pneumonitis, with acute thoracic zoster superimposed (Shibuta et al., 1974).

Zoster is presumed to reflect reactivation and retrograde transport of virus from ganglia to skin in a host partially immune to VZV. Viremia has also been demonstrated in otherwise immunocompetent individuals with acute zoster (Gilden et al., 1987a). Although the significance of viremia in zoster patients remains to be determined, VZV DNA was detected by in situ hybridization (ISH) in blood mononuclear cells (MNCs) of 4 uncomplicated zoster patients for 3–7 weeks after rash (Gilden et al., 1988), coinciding with the period during which these patients experienced pain.

In immunocompromised patients with localized and disseminated zoster, VZV can also be isolated from blood (Gold, 1966; Feldman and Epp, 1976; Feldman et al., 1977; Gershon et al., 1978; Myers, 1979), suggesting a role for hematogenous spread in the pathogenesis of zoster in such individuals. VZV in blood is cell-associated (Myers, 1979) and has been detected by electron microscopy in monocytes (Twomey et al., 1974). A loss of cell-mediated immunity to VZV may be responsible for the increased risk of zoster in immunocompromised patients (Rand et al., 1977; Arvin et al., 1978; Hardy et al., 1991). Such a notion is supported by an increased detection of VZV DNA in blood of bone marrow transplant recipients with or without zoster (Wilson et al., 1992).

VZV has been detected in macrophages (Arbeit et al., 1982), in B cells (Leventon-Kriss et al., 1979; Cauda et al., 1986), and in T cells (Gilden et al., 1987a), particularly in activated T lymphocytes (Koropchak et al., 1989). Initial nucleic acid hybridization studies revealed no replication of VZV DNA in human MNCs (Gilden et al., 1987a), a finding confirmed by Koropchak et al. (1989). However, Mainka et al. (1998) found evidence of active VZV replication in MNCs of zoster patients, at least during the first few days after the onset of rash. Annunziato et al. (2000) also found active VZV replication in epithelial cells, endothelial cells, nerves, and $CD43^+/CD68^+$ inflammatory cells in the epidermis and dermis of zoster patients. Thus, while replication of VZV in various types of blood MNCs may occur, productive viral infection appears to be transient.

3. Latent VZV infection

Analysis of latent VZV is difficult for several reasons. VZV is exclusively a human pathogen. Although inoculation of rodents with VZV will result in viral DNA in ganglia and other tissues, disease does not develop, and there is no evidence of reactivation. VZV is latent only in human ganglia (Gilden et al., 1983, 1987b; Mahalingam et al., 1990), a tissue not accessible in living individuals. Thus, analysis of latent VZV has been restricted to human ganglia obtained at autopsy. Difficulties associated with the use of such human samples include differences in initial VZV inoculation during primary infection, and in time from primary infection to death, as well as the possibility of subclinical reinfection and/or reactivation, and the potential for reactivation between the time of death and autopsy. Although efforts have been made to avoid procuring samples from individuals who were immunocompromised before death or with a recent history of zoster or evident skin rash, or where there was a long delay between death and autopsy, these factors may account for some of the variability seen in studies described below.

3.1. Configuration of latent VZV DNA

Clarke et al. (1995) exploited the fact that the U_L segment of the VZV genome rarely inverts with respect to the U_S segment (Straus et al., 1982; Kinchington et al., 1985; Hayakawa and Hyman, 1987; Davison, 1991) and showed by PCR analysis that the ends of the VZV DNA molecule are covalently connected. The simplest interpretation of these results, obtained using PCR primers that amplified across the termini of the VZV genome, is that the genome assumes a circular, episomal state during latency, similar to that identified in ganglia latently infected with HSV-1 (Rock and Fraser, 1983, 1985; Efstathiou et al., 1986).

3.2. Site of latent VZV DNA

Identification of the cell type harboring latent VZV is important, since the pathogenesis of initial infection and reactivation may depend on the number and type of cells initially infected (Croen and Straus, 1991; Meier and Straus, 1992; Kennedy and Steiner, 1994; Steiner, 1996). Several studies have attempted to identify latently infected cells using in situ hybridization (ISH), with or without PCR amplification. These techniques require careful attention to tissue fixation, slide preparation, probe sensitivity and specificity, hybridization and post-hybridization conditions, signal development, and maintenance of nuclease-free conditions. Further, when ISH is used without PCR amplification, sensitivity is limited and is also dependent on the number of copies of target DNA or RNA per cell. As the technique of ISH evolved, PCR amplification of the target DNA was added before hybridizing with a probe sequence ('indirect' in situ PCR), or hybridization was replaced with direct incorporation of tagged nucleotides during PCR ('direct' in situ PCR).

Table I lists the site of latent VZV as detected by various ISH and/or PCR techniques in multiple studies. Using ISH with a radioactive DNA probe made by nick-translation of the entire VZV genome, which hybridized to any and all VZV RNA transcripts, Hyman et al. (1983) detected VZV exclusively in ganglionic neurons at an abundance of 0 to 0.3% of neurons from the trigeminal ganglia of five subjects. ISH with a radioactive RNA probe (specific activity $> 10^8$ cpm/μg) transcribed from the *Sal*I-P VZV DNA fragment to detect VZV DNA and RNA also identified neurons as the site of latency in an analysis of four thoracic ganglia of a single subject (Gilden et al., 1987b). However, cytoplasmic ^{32}P signal was also noted in both of these studies, instead of the ex-

TABLE I

Site of VZV latency

Site	Technique	Reference
Neurons (0–0.3%)	ISH for any VZV RNA transcripts	Hyman et al. (1983)
Neurons (many)	ISH for VZV DNA	Gilden et al. (1987b)
Satellite cells (few)	ISH for VZV RNA (ORFs 29 and 62)	Croen et al. (1988); Meier et al. (1993)
Neurons and satellite cells (5–31%)	ISH for VZV DNA in ORF 54	Lungu et al. (1995)
Neurons	indirect in situ PCR for VZV DNA ORF 40	Dueland et al. (1995)
Neurons (2–5%) and satellite cells (<0.1%)	ISH, direct in situ PCR, and indirect in situ PCR	Kennedy et al. (1998)
Neurons (2–5%) and some satellite cells	ISH and direct in situ PCR	Kennedy et al. (1999)
Neurons and some non-neuronal cells	separation of cell types, liquid PCR	LaGuardia et al. (1999)

pected predominant nuclear signal seen with HSV-1 DNA and its latency-associated transcript. There was also a significant discrepancy between the two studies in the numbers of positive neurons, perhaps due to differences in the amount of initial VZV inocula of the subjects. Transcripts corresponding to VZV genes 29 and 62 were detected by ISH, primarily in a small number of non-neuronal satellite cells, but not in neurons (Croen et al., 1988; Meier et al., 1993). However, the subjectivity associated with localization of silver grains over smaller satellite cells makes these studies difficult to interpret. Using ISH to detect VZV DNA mapping to ORF 54, Lungu et al. (1995) reported a positive signal in 5–30% of both neurons and non-neuronal cells in latently infected ganglia from two individuals, and in the majority of neurons and non-neuronal cells in ganglia corresponding to the distribution of zoster from an individual with clinical reactivation. Combined in situ PCR with ISH (indirect in situ PCR) identified an amplified product from VZV gene 40, exclusively in neurons, albeit with some leakage of signal into the cytoplasm (Dueland et al., 1995). In a well-designed and carefully controlled study in which several investigators studying VZV latency submitted latently infected human ganglia for analysis by a single laboratory, latent VZV DNA was detected almost exclusively in the nuclei of neurons, with 2–5% of neurons and less than 0.1% of non-neuronal cells showing a positive signal, by ISH alone (genes 29 and 63), direct in situ PCR (genes 21 and 29), and indirect in situ PCR (gene 29) (Kennedy et al., 1998). A second report from the same laboratory again found 2–5% of neurons and only occasional non-neuronal cells positive for VZV DNA and RNA (genes 4, 21, 29 and 63) in normal individuals (Kennedy et al., 1999). Given the differences in the techniques used, the studies by Kennedy et al. (1998, 1999) appear to be the most convincing, since all three techniques showed consistent results. Our laboratory adopted a strategy using semi-quantitative PCR analysis to study neurons and non-neuronal cells from postmortem ganglion cells sorted by size. This approach also revealed VZV DNA primarily in neurons (LaGuardia et al., 1999). Overall, most

data indicate that VZV is latent primarily in neurons (Hyman et al., 1983; Gilden et al., 1987b; Dueland et al., 1995; Kennedy et al., 1998, 1999; LaGuardia et al., 1999), analogous to other alphaherpesviruses (Stevens et al., 1987; Mitchell et al., 1990; Kutish et al., 1990; Priola et al., 1990; Croen et al., 1991; Bratanich et al., 1992).

3.3. Copy number of latent VZV DNA

Analysis of animal models of HSV-1 latency suggests that the likelihood of clinical reactivation depends on the copy number of latent virus (Lekstrom-Himes et al., 1998; Sawtell et al., 1998). Accurate quantitation of virus DNA content depends on the technique used. Initially, Southern blot analysis detected VZV DNA in human ganglia (Gilden et al., 1983), but the amount of virus DNA present was not determined. With the advent of PCR, it became possible to quantitate latent VZV DNA in human ganglia. Three PCR-based methods have been developed to quantitate rare DNA sequences. Semi-quantitative PCR uses samples of known copy numbers of viral DNA to generate a standard curve to which experimental samples are compared. Drawbacks of this technique include the requirements for standard and experimental samples in separate PCR tubes, and the transfer of PCR products to nylon membranes to be probed with radioactive oligonucleotides. Potential errors in quantitation rest in variations during PCR, DNA transfer and immobilization, or probing under conditions where the radiolabeled oligonucleotide is not in excess, and the need to detect the signal within a linear response. In competitive quantitative PCR, samples of known copy numbers of a mutated viral sequence are added to aliquots of an experimental sample, and the copy number is estimated from samples in which mutant and wild-type viral sequences compete equally for PCR reagents. This technique has the advantage of known and experimental samples in the same tube, but still requires transfer to membranes and subsequent probing. In addition, the mutated viral DNA fragment is cloned into a vector sequence, and this fragment may not amplify with the same efficiency as native viral DNA. Real-time

TABLE II

Number of latent VZV genomes

Copies/10^5 cells	Technique	Reference
10^3–10^5	Semi-quantitative PCR	Clarke et al. (1995)
6–31	Competitive, quantitative PCR	Mahalingam et al. (1993)
5.5	Semi-quantitative PCR	LaGuardia et al. (1999)
258 ± 38	Real-time quantitative PCR	Pevenstein et al. (1999)

quantitative PCR is the most recent advance, wherein viral DNA in samples of known and unknown copy number are assessed during the actual PCR cycling by detecting products that emit fluorescence, thus ensuring that copy numbers are quantitated during exponential amplification. Although no probing is required, this technique does require separate tubes for known and unknown samples.

Table II summarizes the results of studies to quantitate latent VZV copy number using various PCR techniques. Semi-quantitative PCR showed that 10^3–10^5 copies of latent VZV DNA were present in 10^5 ganglionic cells (Clarke et al., 1995), similar to the amount of latent HSV-1 found in human ganglia by Southern blot analysis (Efstathiou et al., 1986). Using competitive, quantitative PCR, Mahalingam et al. (1993) detected 6–31 copies of the VZV genome per 10^5 cells in ganglia at all levels of the neuraxis. Semi-quantitative PCR using neurons separated from a liquid suspension of human trigeminal ganglia cells revealed 2–5 copies of VZV DNA in 4 of 20 lots of 100 neurons each; assuming 100 non-neuronal cells per neuron, these data average to approximately 5.5 copies of VZV DNA per 10^5 cells (LaGuardia et al., 1999). Real-time quantitative PCR analysis detected 258 ± 38 copies of VZV DNA per 10^5 ganglionic cells (Pevenstein et al., 1999). The large range of VZV DNA molecules reported in these studies might reflect differences in the natural history of the infection in the individuals from whom the samples were obtained or differences in the techniques used to estimate copy numbers. If discrepancies in copy numbers were due to the techniques used, the real-time PCR quantitation data of Pevenstein et al. (1999) may be the most valid although those data need to be confirmed.

3.4. Latently transcribed VZV genes

While alphaherpesviruses share similar biological features during latency (cell type harboring latent virus and configuration of latent virus DNA), the transcriptional pattern of latent virus DNA differs. A single latent HSV-1 transcriptional unit has been consistently detected in human ganglia and in animal models. This latency-associated transcript (LAT) accumulates in the nuclei of latently infected neurons (Stevens et al., 1987; Mitchell et al., 1990; Zwaagstra et al., 1990; Wagner, 1994; Zabolotny et al., 1997). However, during VZV latency in human ganglia, at least 5 VZV transcripts have been detected (Cohrs et al., 1996; Kennedy et al., 1999). 'Reverse Northern' analysis showed that a transcript mapping to the *Sal*I fragment C of the VZV genome was present during latency (Cohrs et al., 1992). VZV gene 21, which maps to this region, was then detected in a cDNA library constructed from poly[A]$^+$ RNA extracted from a pool of latently infected human trigeminal ganglia (Cohrs et al., 1994). Meier et al. (1993) detected VZV gene 29 and 62 transcripts in Northern blots of poly[A]$^+$ RNA extracted from hundreds of pooled human ganglia. In a cDNA library constructed from latently infected human trigeminal ganglia enriched for VZV transcripts by hybridization selection, VZV gene 21, 29, 62 and 63 transcripts were found (Cohrs et al., 1996). Using ISH and direct in situ PCR, Kennedy et al. (1999) confirmed and extended these data by detecting transcripts for genes 4, 21, 29 and 63 in normal human dorsal root ganglia. Overall, VZV genes 21, 29, 62, 63, and 4 are actively transcribed during latency.

3.5. Latently translated VZV proteins

Although no protein has been reproducibly identified that corresponds to the HSV-1 LAT transcript, proteins have been identified that correspond to latent VZV transcripts. The use of rabbit antisera raised against VZV gene 63 protein (Debrus et al., 1995) identified the protein only in neurons of latently infected human ganglia (Mahalingam et al., 1996). Another study identified the protein products of VZV genes 4, 21, 29, 62, and 63, but not genes 10, 14, or 67, primarily in the cytoplasm of neurons from latently infected individuals, and in both the cytoplasm and nucleus of an individual with zoster at the time of death (Lungu et al., 1998). These VZV-specific proteins are normally seen in the nuclei of productively infected cells in tissue culture. The investigators speculated that the aberrant localization might provide a mechanism to maintain VZV in a latent state, namely by restricting regulatory proteins from the nucleus. Confirmation of this work may lead to a better understanding of VZV latency.

3.6. Reactivation from latency after VZV vaccination

The effect of childhood VZV vaccination on the subsequent development of zoster in elderly adults remains an important issue. Because such vaccination efforts in Japan preceded those in the United States, the answer will be known first in Japan. Nevertheless, some information about VZV reactivation in children is available. In a study to determine whether children immunized with live varicella vaccine were at greater risk of developing zoster than children who had varicella, the incidence of zoster was compared in children with acute lymphocytic leukemia who had had varicella vs. those children who had been vaccinated with live varicella. During a 5-year observation period, 15 of 73 children who had had varicella developed zoster compared to none of 34 vaccinated children (Brunell et al., 1986). Hardy et al. (1991) confirmed a lower incidence of zoster in another group of leukemic children after immunization with live attenuated VZV vaccine compared with children who had naturally occurring

VZV infection. These well-controlled studies suggest that zoster in the future elderly population might be less frequent in vaccinees than in those who had naturally occurring chicken pox. However, studies by Krause and Klinman (2000) suggested that the vaccine (Oka) strain of VZV frequently reactivates, particularly in individuals with low anti-VZV titers after vaccination in whom the frequency of clinical infection and immunological boosting substantially exceeded the 13% per year rate after exposure to wild-type varicella. Those findings suggest that Oka VZV persists in vivo and may reactivate as serum antibody titers decrease after vaccination. These studies have not been substantiated by PCR data, however, which indicate that disseminated rashes months to years after vaccination are caused by the wild-type strain and not Oka (LaRussa et al., 2000). Because anti-VZV immunity is weaker in vaccinees than in individuals infected with wild-type VZV, the long-term effect of frequent Oka VZV reactivation on the development of clinical zoster in the elderly will not be known for decades. To date, however, development of clinical zoster after immunization of healthy individuals is exceedingly rare (Sharrar et al., 2000). Although it is unclear how Oka VZV reactivation will affect individuals in whom anti-VZV immunity wanes or who become immunosuppressed as adults, results of a controlled study in immunocompromised children indicated that Oka VZV vaccination is safer than wild-type VZV infection (Hardy et al., 1991). Nevertheless, it will be important to monitor the rates of zoster in childhood vaccine recipients as they become 60 years or older. Thus, current trials to boost immunity in middle-aged individuals may be valuable, since vaccination of prior vaccine recipients or of individuals with a history of childhood chicken pox may extend the duration of immunity.

4. Summary

Reactivation of VZV from latency can produce serious peripheral and CNS complications, including the severe pain of herpes zoster lesions. Much effort has been focused on elucidating the mechanisms that underlie VZV latency. During latency in human ganglia, VZV maintains a circular state, primarily in the nuclei of neurons within the trigeminal and dorsal root ganglia, and transcribes at least 5 genes. Discovery of the functions and interactions of these gene transcripts and their protein products may prove to be fundamental in understanding the maintenance of VZV latency, as well as in targeting therapy to prevent reactivation.

References

Annunziato, P., Lungu, O., Panagiotidis, C., Zhang, J.G., Silvers, D., Gershon, A. and Silverstein, S. (2000) Varicella-zoster virus proteins in skin lesions: implications for a novel role of ORF29p in chickenpox. J. Virol., 74: 2005–2010.

Arbeit, R.D., Zaia, J.A., Valerio, M.A. and Levin, M.J. (1982) Infection of human peripheral blood mononuclear cells by varicella-zoster virus. Intervirology, 18: 56–65.

Arvin, A.M., Pollard, R.B., Rasmussen, L. and Merigan, T. (1978) Selective impairment in lymphocyte reactivity to varicella-zoster antigen among untreated lymphoma patients. J. Infect. Dis., 137: 531–540.

Bastian, F.O., Rabson, A.S., Yee, C.L. and Tralka, T.S. (1974) Herpesvirus varicellae: Isolated from human dorsal root ganglia. Arch. Pathol., 97: 331–332.

Bratanich, A.C., Hanson, N.D. and Jones, C.J. (1992) The latency-related gene of bovine herpesvirus 1 inhibits the activity of immediate-early transcription unit 1. Virology, 191: 988–991.

Brunell, P.A., Taylor-Wiedeman, J., Geiser, C.F., Frierson, L. and Lydick, E. (1986) Risk of herpes zoster in children with leukemia: Varicella vaccine compared with history of chickenpox. Pediatrics, 77: 53–56.

Cauda, R., Chatterjee, S., Tiden, A.B., Grossi, C.E. and Whitley, R.J. (1986) Replication of varicella zoster virus in Raji cells. Virus Res., 4: 337–342.

Cheatham, W.J., Weller, T.H., Dolan, T.F. and Dower, J.C. (1956) Varicella: Report on two fatal cases with necropsy, virus isolation, and serologic studies. Am. J. Pathol., 32: 1015–1035.

Clarke, P., Beer, T., Cohrs, R. and Gilden, D.H. (1995) Configuration of latent varicella-zoster virus DNA. J. Virol., 69: 8151–8154.

Cohrs, R., Mahalingam, R., Dueland, A.N., Wolf, E., Wellish, M. and Gilden, D.H. (1992) Restricted transcription of varicella-zoster virus in latently infected human trigeminal and thoracic ganglia. J. Infect. Dis., 166(Suppl. 1): 24–29.

Cohrs, R.J., Srock, K., Barbour, M.B., Owens, G., Mahalingam, R., Devlin, M.E., Wellish, M. and Gilden, D.H. (1994) Varicella-zoster virus (VZV) transcription during latency in human ganglia: construction of a cDNA library from latently infected human trigeminal ganglia and detection of a VZV transcript. J. Virol., 68: 7900–7908.

Cohrs, R., Barbour, M.B. and Gilden, D.H. (1996) Varicella-zoster virus (VZV) transcription during latency in human ganglia: detection of transcripts mapping to genes 21, 29, 62 and 63 in a cDNA library enriched for VZV RNA. J. Virol., 70: 2789–2796.

Croen, K.D. and Straus, S.E. (1991) Varicella-zoster virus latency. Annu. Rev. Microbiol., 45: 265–282.

Croen, K.D., Ostrove, J.M., Dragovic, L.J. and Straus, S.E. (1988) Patterns of gene expression and sites of latency in human nerve ganglia are different for varicella-zoster and herpes simplex viruses. Proc. Natl. Acad. Sci. U.S.A., 85: 9773–9777.

Croen, K.D., Dragovic, L., Ostrove, J.M. and Straus, S.E. (1991) Characterization of herpes simplex virus type 2 latency associated transcription in human sacral ganglia and in cell culture. J. Infect. Dis., 163: 23–28.

Davison, A.J. (1991) Varicella-zoster virus: The Fourteenth Fleming Lecture. J. Gen. Virol., 72: 475–486.

Debrus, S., Sadzot-Delvaux, C., Nikkels, A.F., Piette, J. and Rentier, B. (1995) Varicella-zoster virus gene 63 encodes an immediate-early protein that is abundantly expressed during latency. J. Virol., 69: 3240–3245.

Denny-Brown, D., Adams, R.D. and Fitzgerald, P.J. (1944) Pathologic features of herpes zoster: A note on 'geniculate herpes'. Arch. Neurol. Psychiatry, 51: 216–231.

Dueland, A.N., Ranneberg-Nilsen, T. and Degre, M. (1995) Detection of latent varicella zoster virus DNA and human gene sequences in human trigeminal ganglia by in situ amplification combined with in situ hybridization. Virology, 140: 2055–2066.

Efstathiou, S., Minson, A.C., Field, H.J., Anderson, J.R. and Wildy, P. (1986) Detection of herpes simplex virus-specific sequences in latently infected mice and in humans. J. Virol., 57: 446–455.

Esiri, M.M. and Tomlinson, A.H. (1972) Herpes zoster: Demonstration of virus in trigeminal nerve and ganglion by immunofluorescence and electron microscopy. J. Neurol. Sci., 15: 35–48.

Feldman, S. and Epp, E. (1976) Isolation of varicella-zoster virus from blood. J. Pediatr., 88: 265–267.

Feldman, S., Chaudary, S., Ossi, M. and Epp, E. (1977) A viremic phase for herpes zoster in children with cancer. J. Pediatr., 91: 597–600.

Gershon, A.A., Steinberg, S. and Silber, R. (1978) Varicella-zoster viremia. J. Pediatr., 92: 1033–1034.

Ghatak, N.R. and Zimmerman, H.M. (1973) Spinal ganglion in herpes zoster. Arch. Pathol., 95: 411–415.

Gilden, D.H., Vafai, A., Shtram, Y., Becker, Y., Devlin, M. and Wellish, M. (1983) Varicella-zoster virus DNA in human sensory ganglia. Nature, 306: 478–480.

Gilden, D.H., Hayward, A.R., Krupp, J., Hunter-Laszio, M.,

Huff, J.C. and Vafai, A. (1987a) Varicella-zoster virus infection of human mononuclear cells. Virus Res., 7: 117–129.

Gilden, D.H., Rozemann, Y., Murray, R., Devlin, M. and Vafai, A. (1987b) Detection of varicella-zoster virus nucleic acid in neurons of normal human thoracic ganglia. Ann. Neurol., 22: 377–380.

Gilden, D.H., Devlin, M.E., Wellish, M., Mahalingam, R., Huff, C., Hayward, A. and Vafai, A. (1988) Persistence of varicella-zoster virus DNA in blood mononuclear cells of patients with varicella or zoster. Virus Genes, 2: 299–305.

Gilden, D.H., Kleinschmidt-DeMasters, B.K., Wellish, M., Hedley-Whyte, E.T., Rentier, B. and Mahalingam, R. (1996) Varicella zoster virus, a cause of waxing and waning vasculitis. NEJM case 5–1995 revisited. Neurology, 47: 1441–1446.

Gilden, D.H., Kleinschmidt-DeMasters, B.K., LaGuardia, J.J., Mahalingam, R. and Cohrs, R. (2000) Neurologic complications of the reactivation of varicella-zoster virus. N. Engl. J. Med., 342: 635–645.

Gold, E. (1966) Serologic and virus-isolation studies of patients with varicella or herpes-zoster infection. N. Engl. J. Med., 274: 181–185.

Hardy, I., Gershon, A.A., Steinberg, S.P., LaRussa, P. and the Varicella Vaccine Collaborative Study Group (1991) The incidence of zoster after immunization with live attenuated varicella vaccine. N. Engl. J. Med., 325: 1545–1550.

Hayakawa, Y. and Hyman, R.W. (1987) Isomerization of the UL region of varicella-zoster virus DNA. Virus Res., 8: 25–31.

Head, H. and Campbell, A.W. (1900) The pathology of herpes zoster and its bearing on sensory localization. Brain, 23: 353–523.

Hyman, R.W., Ecker, J.R. and Tenser, R.B. (1983) Varicella-zoster virus RNA in human trigeminal ganglia. Lancet, 2: 814–816.

Kennedy, P.G. and Steiner, I. (1994) A molecular and cellular model to explain the differences in reactivation from latency by herpes simplex and varicella-zoster viruses. Neuropathol. Appl. Neurobiol., 20: 368–374.

Kennedy, P.G., Grinfeld, E. and Gow, J.W. (1998) Latent varicella-zoster virus is located predominantly in neurons in human trigeminal ganglia. Proc. Natl. Acad. Sci. U.S.A., 95: 4658–4662.

Kennedy, P.G., Grinfeld, E. and Gow, J.W. (1999) Latent varicella-zoster virus in human dorsal root ganglia. Virology, 258: 451–454.

Kinchington, P.R. Reinhold, W.C., Casey T.A., Straus, S.E., Hay, J. and Ruyechan, W.T. (1985) Inversion and circularization of the varicella-zoster virus genome. J. Virol., 56: 194–200.

Koropchak, C.M., Solem, S.D., Diaz, P.S. and Arvin, A.M. (1989) Investigation of varicella-zoster virus infection of lymphocytes by in situ hybridization. J. Virol., 63: 2392–2395.

Krause, P.R. and Klinman, D.M. (2000) Varicella vaccination: Evidence for frequent reactivation of the vaccine strain in healthy children. Nat. Med., 6: 451–454.

Kutish, G., Mainprize, T. and Rock, D. (1990) Characterization of the latency-related transcriptionally active region of bovine herpesvirus 1 genome. J. Virol., 64: 5730–5737.

LaGuardia, J.J., Cohrs, R.J. and Gilden, D.H. (1999) Prevalence of varicella-zoster virus DNA in dissociated human trigeminal ganglia neurons and non-neuronal cells. J. Virol., 73: 8571–8577.

LaRussa, P., Steinberg, S.P., Shapiro, E., Vazquez, M. and Gershon, A.A. (2000) Viral strain identification in varicella vaccinees with disseminated rashes. Ped. Infect. Dis. J., 19: 1037–1039.

Lekstrom-Himes, J.A., Wang, K., Pesnicak, L., Krause, P.R. and Straus, S.E. (1998) The comparative biology of latent herpes simplex virus type 1 and type 2 infections: latency-associated transcript promoter activity and expression in vitro and in infected mice. J. Neurovirol., 4: 27–37.

Leventon-Kriss, S., Gotlieb-Stematsky, T., Vonsover, A. and Smetana, Z. (1979) Infection and persistence of varicella-zoster virus in lymphoblastoid Raji cell line. Med. Microbiol. Immunol., 167: 275–283.

Lungu, O., Annunziato, P.W., Gershon, A., Staugaitis, S.M., Josefson, D., LaRussa, P. and Silverstein, S.J. (1995) Reactivated and latent varicella-zoster virus in human dorsal root ganglia. Proc. Natl. Acad. Sci. U.S.A., 92: 10980–10984.

Lungu, O., Panagiotidis, C.A., Annunziato, P.W., Gershon, A.A. and Silverstein, S.J. (1998) Aberrant intracellular localization of varicella-zoster virus regulatory proteins during latency. Proc. Natl. Acad. Sci. U.S.A., 95: 7080–7085.

Mahalingam, R., Wellish, M., Wolf, W., Dueland, A.N., Cohrs, R., Vafai, A. and Gilden, D.H. (1990) Latent varicella-zoster viral DNA in human trigeminal and thoracic ganglia. N. Engl. J. Med., 323: 627–631.

Mahalingam, R., Wellish, M., Lederer, D., Forghani, B., Cohrs, R. and Gilden, D.H. (1993) Quantitation of latent varicella-zoster virus DNA in human trigeminal ganglia by polymerase chain reaction. J. Virol., 67: 2381–2384.

Mahalingam, R., Wellish, M., Cohrs, R., Debrus, S., Piette, J., Rentier, B. and Gilden, D.H. (1996) Expression of protein encoded by varicella-zoster virus open reading frame 63 in latently infected human ganglionic neurons. Proc. Natl. Acad. Sci. U.S.A., 93: 2122–2124.

Mainka, C., Fuss, B., Geiger, H., Hofelmayr, H. and Wolff, M.H. (1998) Characterization of viremia at different stages of varicella-zoster virus infection. J. Med. Virol., 56: 91–98.

Meier, J.L. and Straus, S.E. (1992) Comparative biology of latent varicella-zoster virus and herpes simplex virus infections. J. Infect. Dis., 166(Suppl. 1): 13–23.

Meier, J.L., Holman, R.P., Croen, K.D., Smialek, J.E. and Straus, S.E. (1993) Varicella-zoster virus transcription in human trigeminal ganglia. Virology, 193: 193–200.

Mitchell, W.J., Lirette, R.P. and Fraser, N.W. (1990) Mapping of low abundance latency-associated RNA in the trigeminal ganglia of mice latently infected with herpes simplex virus type 1. J. Gen. Virol., 71: 125–132.

Myers, M.G. (1979) Viremia caused by varicella-zoster virus:

Association with malignant progressive varicella. J. Infect. Dis., 140: 229–233.

Nagashima, K., Nakazawa, M. and Endo, H. (1975) Pathology of the human spinal ganglia in varicella-zoster virus infection. Acta Neuropathol., 33: 105–117.

Pevenstein, S.R., Williams, R.K., McChesney, D., Mont, E.K., Smialek, J.E. and Straus, S.E. (1999) Quantitation of latent varicella-zoster virus and herpes simplex virus genomes in human trigeminal ganglia. J. Virol., 73: 10514–10518.

Priola, S.A., Gustafson, D.P., Wagner, E.K. and Stevens, J.G. (1990) A major portion of the latent pseudorabies virus genome is transcribed in trigeminal ganglia of pigs. J. Virol., 64: 4755–4760.

Rand, K.H., Rasmussen, L.E., Pollard, R.B., Arvin, A. and Merigan, T. (1977) Cellular immunity and herpesvirus infections in cardiac transplant patients. N. Engl. J. Med., 296: 1372–1377.

Rock, D.L. and Fraser, N.W. (1983) Detection of HSV-1 genome in central nervous system of latently infected mice. Nature (London), 302: 523–525.

Rock, D.L. and Fraser, N.W. (1985) Latent herpes simplex virus type 1 DNA contains two copies of the virion DNA joint region. J. Virol., 55: 849–852.

Sawtell, N.M., Poon, D.K., Tansky, C.S. and Thompson, R.L. (1998) The latent herpes simplex virus type 1 genome copy number in individual neurons is virus strain specific and correlates with reactivation. J. Virol., 72: 5343–5350.

Sharrar, R.G., LaRussa, P., Galea, S., Steinberg, S., Sweet, A., Keatley, M., Wells, M., Stephenson, W. and Gershon, A. (2000) The postmarketing safety profile of varicella vaccine. Vaccine, 19: 916–923.

Shibuta, H., Ishikawa, T., Hondo, R., Aoyama, Y., Kurata, K. and Matumoto, M. (1974) Varicella virus isolation from spinal ganglion. Arch. Virusforsch., 45: 382–385.

Steiner, I. (1996) Human herpes viruses latent infection in the nervous system. Immunol. Rev., 152: 157–173.

Stevens, J.G., Wagner, E.K., Devi-Rao, G.B., Cook, M.L. and Feldman, L.T. (1987) RNA complementary to a herpesvirus gene mRNA is prominent in latently infected neurons. Science, 235: 1056–1059.

Straus, S.E., Owens, J., Ruyechan, W.T., Takiff, H.E., Casey, T.A., Vande Woude, G.F. and Hay, J. (1982) Molecular cloning and physical mapping of varicella-zoster virus DNA. Proc. Natl. Acad. Sci. U.S.A., 79: 993–997.

Twomey, J.J., Gyorkey, F. and Norris, S.M. (1974) The monocyte disorder with herpes zoster. J. Lab. Clin. Med., 83: 768–777.

Von Barensprung, F.G.F. (1863) Beitrage zur Kenntnis des Zoster. Ann. Chir. Krankenh., 11: 96–104.

Wagner, E.K. (1994) The herpes simplex type 1 virus latency gene. In: Y. Becker and G. Darai (Eds.), Frontiers of Virology, Vol. 3. Springer, Heidelberg, pp. 210–221.

Wilson, A., Sharp, M., Koropchak, C.M., Ting, S.F. and Arvin, A.M. (1992) Subclinical varicella-zoster virus viremia, herpes zoster, and T lymphocyte immunity to varicella-zoster viral antigens after bone marrow transplantation. J. Infect. Dis., 165: 119–126.

Zabolotny, J.M., Krummenacher, C. and Fraser, N.W. (1997) The herpes simplex virus type 1 2.0-kilobase latency-associated transcript is a stable intron which branches at a guanosine. J. Virol., 71: 4199–4208.

Zwaagstra, J., Ghiasi, H., Slanina, S.M., Nesburn, A.B., Wheatley, S.C., Lillycrop, K., Wood, J., Latchman, D.S., Patel, K. and Wechsler, S.L. (1990) Activity of herpes simplex virus type 1 latency associated transcript promoter in neuron-derived cells: evidence for neuron specificity and for a large LAT transcript. J. Virol., 64: 5019–5028.

Herpes Zoster and Postherpetic Neuralgia, 2nd Revised and Enlarged Edition
Pain Research and Clinical Management, Vol. 11
Edited by C.P.N. Watson and A.A. Gershon

CHAPTER 8

Neurological complications of herpes zoster

Maija Haanpää [*]

Peijas Hospital, Sairaalakatu 1, FIN-01400 Vantaa, Finland

1. Introduction

Varicella-zoster virus (VZV) is a human neurotropic herpesvirus that resides dormant in sensory ganglia along the whole neuraxis after the primary infection, varicella. The most typical clinical manifestation of the reactivation is herpes zoster (HZ), usually a painful dermatomal rash, which represents ganglionitis, peripheral neuritis and dermatitis caused by VZV. Somatosensory abnormalities, caused primarily by neural inflammation, are common in acute HZ (Haanpää et al., 1999a). About one-third of the patients have mechanical allodynia and one-fourth of patients have pinprick hypoaesthesia, and the presence of these abnormalities elevates the risk of postherpetic neuralgia (PHN) (Haanpää et al., 2000). In quantitative somatosensory testing, warm and cold thresholds are elevated in one-fifth and tactile thresholds are elevated in one-fourth of patients with HZ. All somatosensory abnormalities tend to normalise with time (Haanpää et al., 1999b), and most patients recover from zoster neuritis without any complications in some weeks.

Neurological complications other than PHN are rare in HZ (Table I). The risk is increased in patients who are immunocompromised or have a disseminated form of the disease. Central nervous system (CNS) complications include meningitis, encephalitis, myelitis, and cerebral angiitis. The most com-mon mechanism of viral spread seems to be the direct extension of the infection into cerebrospinal fluid (CSF) spaces from the infected ganglia via the meningeal ramus, leading to local meningitis (Ruppenthal, 1980; Schmidbauer et al., 1992). Because viraemia is not uncommon in HZ (Mainka et al., 1998), haematogenous spread to CNS can take place especially in immunocompromised patients (Schmidbauer et al., 1992). In trigeminal HZ, transaxonal spread from the infected ganglia into the brainstem and the cranial arteries can cause brainstem encephalitis and arteritis, respectively. In immunocompromised patients, a focal CNS infection can disseminate widely into the CNS parenchyma, and haematogenous infection of the subependymal microvasculature can lead to periventriculitis and ventriculitis with subsequent spread of the virus to distant parts of CNS (Schmidbauer et al., 1992; Kleinschmidt-DeMasters et al., 1996).

In addition to the CNS complications and peripheral sensory neuritis, lower motor neuron type (i.e. peripheral) paresis can occur in HZ. Motor weakness can also be a part of the symptoms of encephalitis, myelitis or a cerebrovascular event caused by angiitis. In these cases the paresis is of upper motor neuron type (i.e. central). The most common neurological complication of HZ, namely PHN, is discussed in Chapters 13–24. The course of HZ in immunosuppressed patients is presented in Chap-

---

* Correspondence to: Dr. Maija Haanpää, Peijas Hospital, Sairaalakatu 1, FIN-01400 Vantaa, Finland. E-mail: maija.haanpaa@hus.fi

TABLE I

Complications of herpes zoster in two population-based studies from Rochester, Minnesota

Complication	Galil et al. (1997) (%)	Ragozzino et al. (1982) (%)
Any complication	11.6	12.0
Postherpetic neuralgia[1]	7.9	9.3
Ocular complications	2.2	1.9
Motor deficit	0.9	1.0
Meningitis, encephalitis or CNS vasculitis	0.5	0.2
Herpes zoster oticus	0.2	0.2

[1]Defined as pain continuing after healing of rash.

ter 10. This chapter summarises neurological manifestations of reactivation of VZV with or without rash in immunocompetent patients.

2. Subclinical spread of inflammation into the central nervous system in herpes zoster

HZ has been regarded as a simple model of peripheral unilateral neuritis caused by VZV, but evidence from neuropathological reports suggests that viral invasion and inflammation may extend to the CNS as well. In addition to leptomeningitis, inflammatory changes in the anterior and posterior horn of the spinal cord and in the brainstem have been described (Reske-Nielsen et al., 1986; Watson et al., 1991; Schmidbauer et al., 1992; Denny-Brown et al., 1944; Fabian et al., 1997).

A recent study describes a series of 56 immunocompetent HZ patients without clinical symptoms of CNS infection (Haanpää et al., 1998). CSF were obtained from 46 patients on day 1 to 18 from the eruption of rash, and 16 consecutive patients with cranial or cervical HZ underwent magnetic resonance imaging (MRI) 1 to 5 weeks following rash. In 14/46 (35%) patients there was evidence of VZV in the CSF either in the form of a positive PCR or anti-VZV-IgG. Leucocytosis (range 5–1440/μl) was found in 21/46 (46%) patients. Zoster-related MRI changes were found in the brainstem in 9/16 (56%)

patients and in the cervical cord in 2. This suggests an inflammatory process in the CNS parenchyma. Three patients had enhancement of the trigeminal nerve in addition to the brainstem lesions. According to these results, the entrance of the VZV into the CSF space is common in HZ, and MRI changes can often be detected in patients with cranial or cervical HZ without any symptoms of a CNS infection.

An earlier report compares the EEG findings in 42 patients with HZ and 6 patients with HZ associated encephalitis (Peterslund and Hansen, 1989). Thirty-one percent of patients with HZ had EEG changes with reduced rhythm frequency ranging from 7 to 2 Hz activity. The location of HZ did not influence the frequency of EEG abnormalities. When compared to EEG in HZ associated encephalitis, the findings were qualitatively the same, but tended to be more severe in the encephalitis cases. The abnormal EEG findings suggest subclinical encephalitis in HZ patients, and the general symptoms such as prolonged fatigue after HZ may be explained by this.

3. Neurological complications due to reactivation of varicella-zoster virus without rash

It has been shown that VZV can reactivate subclinically (Gershorn et al., 1982; Devlin et al., 1992; Mainka et al., 1998) or without rash. Pain in a dermatomal distribution without rash due to reactivation of VZV is named 'zoster sine herpete' (Gilden et al., 1994). Three virologically confirmed cases with radicular pain in thoracic segments have been reported (Gilden et al., 1994; Amlie-Lefond et al., 1996). Cases of trigeminal 'zoster sine herpete' have also been published (Easton, 1970; Barrett et al., 1993). However, reactivation of VZV without rash encompasses a much broader syndrome complex than localised pain. In fact, VZV can affect all levels of the nervous system in the absence of skin lesions. It has been reported to cause multiple cranial neuropathies (Mayo and Booss, 1989; Golden et al., 1990; Izzat and Sharma, 1992; Osaki et al., 1995), polyneuritis (Mayo and Booss, 1989), meningitis (Echevarria et al., 1994), meningoencephalitis

(Powell et al., 1995), encephalitis (Mayo and Booss, 1989; Hokkanen et al., 1997), myelitis (Mayo and Booss, 1989) and cranial vasculitis (Nau et al., 1998) without rash in immunocompetent individuals. In a Spanish series, VZV was the most common cause of acute aseptic meningitis in adults (Echevarria et al., 1997).

4. Peripheral motor paresis

Motor involvement following HZ was first described in 1866 (Broadbent, 1866). According to population-based studies, the incidence of lower motor neuron-type paresis in HZ is about 1% (Ragozzino et al., 1982; Galil et al., 1997), whereas in a study of 1210 zoster patients at the Mayo Clinic, incidence of segmental paresis was 5% (Thomas and Howard, 1972). The low recorded incidence of motor deficit in thoracic HZ is probably related to the difficulty in diagnosing weakness of intercostal and abdominal muscles. In a small series, EMG revealed fibrillation in the paraspinal muscles in up to 70% of patients with HZ (Greenberg et al., 1992), which suggests that subclinical motor involvement is common in HZ. In our own series of 40 immunocompetent patients with HZ, EMG abnormalities were detected in 21/40 (53%) patients; subclinical in 13 and associated with motor paresis in 8 cases (Haanpää et al., 1997). EMG changes were confined to the myotomes suggested by rash in 9 patients and were more widespread in 12 patients. In 5 patients, the EMG changes became progressively more widespread in repeated examinations in spite of good clinical recovery. Although the rash was unilateral in all patients, 6 patients had bilateral EMG changes in their paraspinal muscles. These findings suggest that the virus spreads centrally from ganglia into the spinal cord and further to anterior roots to cause peripheral motor paresis.

EMG findings reported in HZ patients include (1) fibrillation and positive sharp wave potentials, compatible with Wallerian degeneration, (2) fasciculation potentials, compatible with axonal or anterior horn cell dysfunction, and (3) polyphasic potentials,

compatible with reinnervation (Gardner-Thorpe et al., 1976; Cioni et al., 1994; Haanpää et al., 1997). On MRI, contrast enhancement of the spinal nerve roots over several segments was observed in a patient with a rash in the groin and a weakness of the iliopsoas and quadriceps muscles, but on subsequent scanning the enhancement was found to be confined to the rash segment (Hanakawa et al., 1997). These findings suggest a more widespread virus-induced inflammation than would have clinically been expected.

The onset of motor weakness is usually rapid, reaching peak levels within hours or days. The interval between the eruption of rash and the onset of weakness ranges from one day to several weeks (Thomas and Howard, 1972). The prognosis of clinical paresis is good, with a complete or nearly complete recovery of function in 75% to 100% of patients (Thomas and Howard, 1972; Haanpää et al., 1997). The prognosis is independent of the initial degree of weakness.

Some uncommon motor manifestations associated with HZ have been described in the literature. Hemidiaphragmatic paresis associated with cervical zoster, even causing respiratory failure (Derveaux and Lacquet, 1982), and detrusor paralysis associated with sacral zoster and leading to urinary retention (Gardner-Thorpe et al., 1976; Jellinek and Tulloch, 1976) have been reported. Cases of the Guillain–Barré syndrome following shingles have also been described (Dayan et al., 1972; Ormerod and Cockerell, 1993; Mondelli et al., 1997).

5. Cranial polyneuritis

Cranial or cervical HZ may affect the cranial nerves, leading to the development of a characteristic catalogue of symptoms (Payten and Dawes, 1972; Aviel and Marshak, 1982; Rothschild et al., 1994). One of the best known is HZ oticus, also called the Ramsay–Hunt syndrome, which is characterised by a vesicular rash on the auricle and facial paralysis. However, the classic vesicular eruption of the pinna is not always present. If vesicles appear, they can appear before, during, or after the facial paralysis (Robillard et al., 1986). In HZ oticus, multiple cranial nerves are often involved, particularly the eight, producing hearing impairment and vertigo, but cranial nerves V, IX, X, XI and XII may also be affected (Aviel and Marshak, 1982; Adour, 1994; Rothschild et al., 1994). On MRI, enhancement of the VII and VIII cranial nerves and the labyrinth is typical of HZ oticus (Osumi and Tien, 1990; Kuo et al., 1995). Two cases of the Ramsay–Hunt syndrome with a pontine lesion, suggesting concomitant brainstem encephalitis, have been reported (Sartoretti-Schefer et al., 1999; Mizock et al., 2000). Using PCR, VZV has been detected in the facial nerve sheath, mucosa of the middle ear, posterior auricular muscles, temporal bone, and CSF (Wackym, 1997; Murakami et al., 1998). The prognosis of the facial paralysis in the Ramsay–Hunt syndrome is poorer than in Bell's palsy (i.e. idiopathic facial paralysis), but according to a retrospective analysis of 80 patients, early (<3 days) administration of acyclovir-prednisone treatment improved the prognosis significantly (Murakami et al., 1997).

6. The central nervous system complications of herpes zoster

6.1. Meningitis

VZV is a common cause of aseptic meningitis, which can present itself with or without rash. The rash may precede the meningeal symptoms or follow it. The course of the disease is benign; complete recovery may be expected in one to two weeks (Echevarria et al., 1997).

6.2. Encephalitis

Encephalitis occurs in up to 5% of the patients hospitalised because of HZ (Mazur and Dolin, 1978). In addition to symptoms and signs of meningeal irritation, patients show signs of cerebral involvement. They may be disoriented, confused, somnolent or agitated, but their mental state improves during the following weeks in most cases (Appelbaum et al., 1962; Jemsek et al., 1983; Hokkanen et al., 1997). Neuropsychological findings soon after HZ encephalitis include slowing of cognitive processes, memory impairment, and emotional and behavioural changes, which is typical of subcortical-type cognitive impairment (Hokkanen et al., 1997). In the acute phase, EEG shows a generalised disturbance of background activity, and SPECT reveals bilateral, mostly frontal, perfusion defects in many patients (Jemsek et al., 1983; Peterslund and Hansen, 1989; Hokkanen et al., 1997). In neuropathological examination, mononuclear leptomeningitis and localised or generalised alterations of the CNS parenchyma are seen (Ruppenthal, 1980). The tendency for lesions of encephalitis to occur at grey–white matter junctions is compatible with the neuroradiological and neuropsychological findings (Hokkanen et al., 1997). The presence of these lesions warrants the diagnosis of multifocal leucoencephalitis and is regarded to indicate viral invasion to small intraparenchymal arterioles causing small ischemic foci, and subsequent development necrosis and demyelination (Kleinschmidt-DeMasters et al., 1996). The proportion of necrosis and demyelination depends on the degree of additional oligodendrocyte infection by the virus (Devinsky et al., 1991). Although the prognosis of HZ encephalitis is good in most cases, cognitive impairment can remain permanent in some patients, and the disease may be even fatal in the immunocompromised.

6.3. Myelitis

Symptoms of myelitis appear usually from days to weeks after the appearance of cutaneous zoster ipsilaterally to the rash, with motor dysfunction predominating and evolving into paraplegia, followed by spinothalamic and to a lesser extent posterior column sensory deficit and sphincter disturbances (Devinsky et al., 1991; Echevarria et al., 1997). The outcome ranges from complete recovery to death, and the course of the disease may be acute, remitting-exacerbating, or chronic (Gilden et al., 1994). MRI of the spinal cord may show local swelling and hyperintense lesions in T2-weighted images (Hwang et al., 1991; Friedman, 1992; Tien et al., 1993). Gadolinium enhancement on T1-weighted images may be seen, suggesting severe inflammation leading to subsequent scarring (Esposito et al., 1993). Pathologically, the dorsal root entry zone and the posterior horn of the spinal cord segment corresponding to the affected dermatome are most severely involved. Spread of VZV into the spinal cord has been demonstrated in all patients in one series (Devinsky et al., 1991). Direct viral invasion into the cord is regarded as the major cause for the symptoms, but vasculitis with ischemic necrosis and immune-mediated demyelination have been proposed as additional pathogenetic mechanisms (Devinsky et al., 1991; Echevarria et al., 1997).

6.4. Cerebral angiitis and delayed hemiplegia

The neurological syndrome of thrombotic cerebral vasculopathy due to zoster-associated cerebral angiitis is a very rare disorder. There are approximately 60 cases in the literature (Sarazin et al., 1995). It appears from days to months after the onset of rash, usually after ophthalmic HZ (Martin et al., 1990). Cerebrovascular events after cervical (Fukumoto et al., 1986; Ross et al., 1991) or lingual (Geny et al., 1991) HZ have also been reported. Patients have clinical stroke-like symptoms, which usually suggest involvement of the territory of the ipsilateral carotid artery. The presentation of the neurological symptoms is usually monophasic, but recurrent ischemic episodes, either transient ischemic attacks or cerebral infarcts, can be seen (Sarazin et al., 1995). This syndrome has a mortality rate of at least 20%, with survivors experiencing major neurological morbidity (Sarazin et al., 1995).

Imaging studies reveal an infarction in the distribution of the involved vessels, and angiography or magnetic resonance angiography show the constriction or occlusion of the arteries, usually the anterior or middle cerebral artery (Kuroiwa and Furukawa, 1981; Doyle et al., 1983; Tien et al., 1993). Neuropathological evaluation reveals localised arteritis with thrombosis, infarcts and haemorrhagic lesions

in the brain, and VZV antigens or virus-like particles have been found in the wall of the affected vessels (Doyle et al., 1983; Martin et al., 1990). Direct spread of the virus from the ganglionic reactivation sites to the arterial wall by neural pathways is regarded as the main cause of the vascular changes (Kuroiwa and Furukawa, 1981; Martin et al., 1990; Sarazin et al., 1995).

6.5. Diagnosis and treatment of the central nervous system complications of herpes zoster

In cases with recent rash associated with neurological symptoms, there is a clinical suspicion of a zoster-associated neurological complication, but in patients without rash the diagnosis is more difficult. If the possibility of VZV as a causative agent comes into the clinician's mind, both VZV PCR and antibodies against VZV should be determined in the CSF. MRI and if necessary, magnetic resonance angiography, are the most appropriate imaging methods. Either positive PCR finding or evidence of the intrathecal antibody production against VZV suggest that VZV is the causative agent of the syndrome. In these cases, antiviral treatment with intravenous acyclovir (10 to 15 mg per kilogram of body weight three times daily for 7 to 10 days), and in cases of cerebrovascular angiitis or the Ramsay–Hunt syndrome, short-course prednisone treatment (1 mg kg^{-1} day^{-1}) are recommended (Murakami et al., 1997; Gilden et al., 2000).

7. Neurological complications of the fetus following maternal herpes zoster

Altogether five cases of congenital varicella syndrome following maternal HZ have been reported (Mustonen et al., 1998). It includes cutaneous scars, eye abnormalities, limb hypoplasia, brain abnormalities (i.e. cortical atrophy, mental retardation and seizures) and poor sphincter control. In a series of 201 neurologically symptomatic neonates, four (2%) of them had intrathecal production of antibodies to VZV (Mustonen et al., 1998). Chickenpox or HZ had not been observed in any of the mothers during pregnancy. The neonates with intrathecal VZV antibody production had seizures as their only neurological symptom. This finding suggests that intrauterine VZV infection with neurological complications of the fetus can be acquired without cutaneous symptoms in the mother. It also suggests that the clinical spectrum of congenital VZV infection seems to be broader than expected. The diagnosis is based on antibody measurements from serum and CSF. Antiviral treatment may prevent recurrent symptoms and progression of neurological injury.

8. Summary

According to studies on HZ patients without symptoms of neurological complications, entrance of VZV into the CSF space is common, and MRI changes in the brainstem can also be detected quite often in patients with cranial or cervical zoster. Subclinical lower motor neuron involvement, detected by EMG, is not uncommon in patients with HZ. Aseptic meningitis caused by VZV is common, but the other forms of the CNS complications, i.e. encephalitis, myelitis and cerebral vasculitis, are rare. Involvement of cranial nerves can cause cranial polyneuritis, of which the Ramsay–Hunt syndrome (vesicular rash on the auricle and facial paralysis) is the most well-known. All these complications are caused mainly by the direct spread of the virus from the infected ganglion into the spinal cord or brainstem. As the spread of VZV and development of neurological symptoms can occur also in the absence of skin lesion, one must bear in mind VZV as a possible causative agent of various neurological symptoms. An early search for VZV viral DNA by PCR or antibody in the CSF is essential for diagnosis. If either of these is found to be positive, antiviral treatment should be commenced without delay. The prognosis of neurological complications is usually good in immunocompetent patients, but neurological sequelae such as cognitive impairment after encephalitis, weakness of the lower limbs or sphincter disturbances after myelitis, or spastic hemiparesis or aphasia after cerebral infarction can remain in some patients. In the immunocompromised patients the neurological complications of HZ can be even fatal, but even in this group of patients early diagnosis and aggressive treatment may produce a favourable response.

References

Adour, K.K. (1994) Otological complications of herpes zoster. Ann. Neurol., 35: 62–64.

Amlie-Lefond, C., Mackin, G.A., Ferguson, M., Wright, R.R., Mahalingham, R. and Gilden, D.H. (1996) Another case of virologically confirmed zoster sine herpete, with electrophysiologic correlation. J. NeuroVirol., 2: 136–138.

Appelbaum, E., Kreps, S.I. and Sunshine, A. (1962) Herpes zoster encephalitis. Am. J. Med., 32: 25–31.

Aviel, A. and Marshak, G. (1982) Ramsay Hunt syndrome: a cranial polyneuropathy. Am. J. Otolaryngol., 3: 61–63.

Barrett, A.P., Katelaris, C.H., Morris, J.G.L. and Schifter, M. (1993) Zoster sine herpete of the trigeminal nerve. Oral Surg. Oral Med. Oral Pathol., 75: 173–175.

Broadbent, W.H. (1866) Case of herpetic eruption in the course of branches of the brachial plexus, followed by partial paralysis in corresponding motor nerves. BMJ, 2: 460.

Cioni, R., Giannini, F., Passero, C., Paradiso, C., Rossi, S., Fimiani, M. and Battistini, N. (1994) An electromyographic evaluation of motor complications in thoracic herpes zoster. Electromyogr. Clin. Neurophysiol., 34: 125–128.

Dayan, A.D., Ogul, E. and Graveson, G.S. (1972) Polyneuritis and herpes zoster. J. Neurol. Neurosurg. Psychiatry, 35: 170–175.

Denny-Brown, D., Adams, R.D. and Fitzgerald, P.J. (1944) Pathologic features of herpes zoster. A note on geniculate herpes. Arch. Neurol. Psychiatry, 51: 216–231.

Derveaux, L. and Lacquet, L.M. (1982) Hemidiaphragmatic paresis after herpes zoster. Thorax, 37: 870–871.

Devinsky, O., Cho, E.S., Petito, C.K. and Price, R.W. (1991) Herpes zoster myelitis. Brain, 114: 1181–1196.

Devlin, M.E., Gliden, D.H., Mahalingham, R., Dueland, A.N. and Cohrs, R. (1992) Peripheral blood mononuclear cells of the elderly contain varicella-zoster virus DNA. J. Infect. Dis., 165: 619–622.

Doyle, P.W., Gibson, G. and Dolman, C.L. (1983) Herpes zoster ophthalmicus with contralateral hemiplegia: identification of cause. Ann. Neurol., 14: 84–85.

Easton, H.G. (1970) Zoster sine herpete causing acute trigeminal neuralgia. Lancet, ii: 1065–1066.

Echevarria, J.M., Casas, I., Tenorio, A., de Ory, F. and Martinez-Martin, P. (1994) Detection of varicella-zoster virus-specific DNA sequences in cerebrospinal fluid from patients with acute aseptic meningitis and no cutaneous lesions. J. Med. Virol., 43: 331–335.

Echevarria, J.M., Casas, I., Martinez-Martin, P. (1997) Infections of the nervous system caused by varicella-zoster virus: a review. Intervirology, 40: 72–84.

Esposito, M.B., Arrington, J.A., Murtaugh, F.R., Coleman, J.M. and Sergay, S.M. (1993) MRI of the spinal cord in a patient with herpes zoster. AJNR, 14: 203–204.

Fabian, V.A., Wood, B., Crowley, B. and Kakulas, B.A. (1997) Herpes zoster brachial neuritis. Clin. Neuropathol., 16: 61–64.

Friedman, D.P. (1992) Herpes zoster myelitis: MR appearance. AJNR, 13: 1404–1406.

Fukumoto, S., Kinjo, M., Hokamura, K. and Tanaka, K. (1986) Subarachnoidal hemorrhage and granulomatous angiitis of the basilar artery: demonstration of the varicella-zoster-virus in the basilar artery lesions. Stroke, 17: 1024–1028.

Galil, K., Choo, P.W., Donahue, D.V.M. and Platt, R. (1997) The sequelae of herpes zoster. Arch. Intern. Med., 157: 1209–1213.

Gardner-Thorpe, C., Foster, J.B. and Barwick, D.D. (1976) Unusual manifestations of herpes zoster. J. Neurol. Sci., 28: 427–447.

Geny, C., Yulis, J., Azoulay, A., Brugiers, P., Saint-Val, C. and Degos, J.D. (1991) Thalamic infarctation following lingual herpes zoster. Neurology, 41: 1846.

Gershorn, A., Steinberg, S., Borkowsky, E., Lennette, D. and Lennette, E. (1982) IgM to varicella-zoster virus: demonstration in patients with and without clinical zoster. Ped. Infect. Dis., 1: 164–167.

Gilden, D.H., Wright, R.R., Schneck, S.A., Gwaltney, J.M. and Mahalingham, R. (1994) Zoster sine herpete, a clinical variant. Ann. Neurol., 35: 530–533.

Gilden, D.H., Kleinschmidt-DeMasters, B.K., LaGuardia, J.J., Mahalingham, R. and Cohrs, R.J. (2000) Neurologic complications of the reactivation of varicella-zoster virus. N. Engl. J. Med., 342: 635–645.

Golden, L.I., Deeb, Z.E. and deFries, H. (1990) Atypical findings in cephalic herpes zoster polyneuritis: case reports and radiographic findings. Laryngoscope, 100: 494–497.

Greenberg, M.K., McVey, A.L. and Hayes, T. (1992) Segmental motor involvement in herpes zoster: an EMG Study. Neurology, 42: 1122–1123.

Haanpää, M., Häkkinen, V. and Nurmikko, T. (1997) Motor involvement in acute herpes zoster. Muscle Nerve, 20: 1433–1438.

Haanpää, M., Dastidar, P., Weinberg, A., Levin, M., Miettinen, A., Lapinlampi, A., Laippala, P. and Nurmikko, T. (1998) Cerebrospinal fluid and magnetic resonance imaging findings in patients with acute herpes zoster. Neurology, 51: 1405–1411.

Haanpää, M., Laippala, P. and Nurmikko, T. (1999a) Pain and somatosensory dysfunction in acute herpes zoster. Clin. J. Pain, 15: 78–84.

Haanpää, M., Laippala, P. and Nurmikko, T. (1999b) Thermal

and tactile perception thresholds in patients with herpes zoster. Eur. J. Pain, 3: 375–386.

Haanpää, M., Laippala, P. and Nurmikko, T. (2000) Allodynia and pinprick hypoaesthesia in acute herpes zoster, and the development of postherpetic neuralgia. J. Pain Symptom. Manag., 20: 50–51.

Hanakawa, T., Hashimoto, S., Kawamura, J., Nakamura, M., Suenaga, T. and Matsuo, M. (1997) Magnetic resonance imaging in a patient with segmental zoster paresis. Neurology, 49: 631–632.

Hokkanen, L., Launes, J., Poutiainen, E., Valanne, L., Salonen, O., Sirén, J. and Iivanainen, M. (1997) Subcortical type cognitive impairment in herpes zoster encephalitis. J. Neurol., 244: 239–245.

Hwang, Y.M., Lee, B.I., Chung, J.W., Ahn, J.H., Kim, K.W. and Kim, D.I. (1991) A case of herpes zoster myelitis: positive magnetic resonance imaging finding. Eur. Neurol., 31: 164–167.

Izzat, M. and Sharma, P.D. (1992) Isolated bilateral paralysis of the soft palate in an adult. J. Laryngol. Otol., 106: 839–840.

Jellinek, E.H. and Tulloch, W.S. (1976) Herpes zoster with dysfunction of bladder and anus. Lancet, ii: 1219–1222.

Jemsek, J., Greenberg, S.B., Taber, L., Harvey, D., Gershorn, A. and Couch, R.B. (1983) Herpes zoster-associated encephalitis: clinicopathologic report of 12 cases and review of the literature. Medicine, 62: 81–97.

Kleinschmidt-DeMasters, B.K., Amlie-Lefond, C. and Gilden, D.H. (1996) The patterns of varicella zoster virus encephalitis. Hum. Pathol., 27: 927–938.

Kuo, M.J., Drago, P.C., Prooprs, D.W. and Chavda, S.V. (1995) Early diagnosis and treatment of Ramsay Hunt syndrome: the role of magnetic resonance imaging. J. Laryngol. Otol., 109: 777–780.

Kuroiwa, Y. and Furukawa, T. (1981) Hemispheric infarction after herpes zoster ophthalmicus: computed tomography and angiography. Neurology, 31: 1030–1032.

Mainka, C., Fuss, B., Harmut, G., Höfelmayr, H. and Wolff, M.H. (1998) Characterization of viremia at different stages of varicella-zoster virus infection. J. Med. Virol., 56: 91–98.

Martin, J.R., Mitchell, W.J. and Henken, D.B. (1990) Neurotropic herpesviruses, neural mechanism and arteritis. Brain Pathol., 1: 6–10.

Mayo, D.R. and Booss, J. (1989) Varicella zoster-associated neurologic disease without skin lesions. Arch. Neurol., 46: 313–315.

Mazur, D.H. and Dolin, R. (1978) Herpes zoster at the NIH: a 20 year experience. Am. J. Med., 65: 738–744.

Mizock, B.A., Bartt, R. and Agbemazdo (2000) Herpes zoster oticus with pontine lesion: segmental brain-stem encephalitis. Clin. Infect. Dis., 30: 229–231.

Mondelli, M., Scarpini, C., Malandrini, A. and Romano, C. (1997) Painful polyneuropathy after diffuse herpes zoster. Muscle Nerve, 20: 229–231.

Murakami, S., Hato, N., Horiuchi, J., Honda, N., Gyo, K. and

Yanagihara, N. (1997) Treatment of Ramsay Hunt syndrome with acyclovir-prednisone: significance of early diagnosis and treatment. Ann. Neurol., 41: 353–357.

Murakami, S., Nakashiro, Y., Mizobuchi, M., Hato, N., Honda, N. and Gyo, K. (1998) Varicella-zoster virus distribution in Ramsay Hunt syndrome revealed by polymerase chain reaction. Acta Otolaryngol. (Stockh.), 118: 145–149.

Mustonen, K., Mustakangas, P., Smeds, M., Mannonen, L., Uotila, L., Vaheri, A. and Koskiniemi, M. (1998) Antibodies to varicella zoster virus in the cerebrospinal fluid of neonates with seizures. Arch. Dis. Child Fetal Neonatal Ed., 78: 57–61.

Nau, R., Lantsch, M., Stiefel, M., Polak, T. and Reiber, H. (1998) Varicella zoster virus-associated focal vasculitis without herpes zoster: recovery after treatment with acyclovir. Neurology, 51: 914–915.

Ormerod, I.E.C. and Cockerell, O.C. (1993) Guillain–Barré syndrome after herpes zoster infection: a report of 2 cases. Eur. Neurol., 33: 156–158.

Osaki, Y., Matsubayashi, K., Okumiya, K., Wada, T. and Doi, Y. (1995) Polyneuritis cranialis due to varicella-zoster virus in the absence of rash. Neurology, 45: 2293.

Osumi, A. and Tien, R.D. (1990) MR findings in a patient with Ramsay Hunt syndrome. J. Comput. Assist Tomogr., 14: 901–903.

Payten, R.J. and Dawes, D.K. (1972) Herpes zoster of the head and neck. J. Laryngol. Otol., 86: 1031–1055.

Peterslund, N.A. and Hansen, J.A. (1989) Electroencephalographic changes in patients with herpes zoster. Acta Neurol. Scand., 79: 407–411.

Powell, K.F., Wilson, H.G., Croxson, M.C., Marshall, M.R., Wong, E.H., Anderson, N.E. and Thomas, M.G. (1995) Herpes zoster meningoencephalitis without rash: varicella zoster virus DNA in CSF. J. Neurol. Neurosurg. Psychiatry, 59: 198–199.

Ragozzino, M.W., Melton, L.J., Kurland, L.T., Chu, C.P. and Perry, H.O. (1982) Population-based study on herpes zoster and its sequelae. Medicine, 61: 310–316.

Reske-Nielsen, E., Oster, S. and Pedersen, B. (1986) Herpes zoster ophthalmicus and the mesencephalic nucleus. Acta Pathol. Microbiol. Immunol. Scand., 94: 263–269.

Robillard, R.B., Hilsinger, A.L. Jr. and Adour, K.K. (1986) Ramsay Hunt facial paralysis: clinical analysis of 185 patients. Otolaryngol. Head Neck Surg., 95: 292–297.

Ross, M.H., Abend, W.K., Schwartz, R.B. and Samuels, M.A. (1991) A case of C2 herpes zoster with delayed bilateral pontine infarction. Neurology, 41: 1685–1686.

Rothschild, M.A., Drake, W. III and Scherl, M. (1994) Cephalic zoster with laryngeal paralysis. ENT J., 73: 850–852.

Ruppenthal, M. (1980) Changes of the central nervous system in herpes zoster. Acta Neuropathol. (Berl.), 52: 59–68.

Sarazin, L., Duong, H., Bourgouin, P.M., Melanson, M., Chalk, C., Richardson, J. and Vézina, J.L. (1995) Herpes zoster vasculitis: demonstration by MR angiography. J. Comput. Assist Tomogr., 19: 624–627.

Sartoretti-Schefer, S., Kollias, S. and Valavanis, A. (1999) Ramsay Hunt syndrome associated with brain stem enhancement. Am. J. Neuroradiol., 20: 278–280.

Schmidbauer, M., Budka, H., Pilz, P., Kurata, T. and Hondo, R. (1992) Presence, distribution and spread of productive varicella zoster virus infection in nervous tissue. Brain, 115: 383–398.

Thomas, J.E. and Howard, F.M. (1972) Segmental zoster paresis — a disease profile. Neurology, 22: 459–466.

Tien, R.D., Felsberg, G.J. and Osumi, A.K. (1993) Herpesvirus infections of the CNS: MR findings. AJNR, 161: 167–176.

Wackym, P.A. (1997) Molecular temporal bone pathology: II. Ramsay Hunt syndrome (herpes zoster oticus). Laryngoscope, 107: 1165–1175.

Watson, C.P.N., Deck, H.J., Morshead, C., Van der Kooy, D. and Evans, R.J. (1991) Post-herpetic neuralgia: further postmortem studies of cases with and without pain. Pain, 44: 105–117.

Herpes Zoster and Postherpetic Neuralgia, 2nd Revised and Enlarged Edition
Pain Research and Clinical Management, Vol. 11
Edited by C.P.N. Watson and A.A. Gershon

CHAPTER 9

Dermatologic aspects of herpes zoster

Barry A.S. Lycka [1], Diane Williamson [2] and R. Gary Sibbald [3,*]

[1] *920 10665 Jasper Avenue, Edmonton, AB T5J 3S9, Canada,* [2] *Dermatology Day Care and Wound Healing Clinic, Sunnybrook and Women's College Health Sciences Centre, Toronto, ON M5G 2C4, Canada and* [3] *Department of Medicine, University of Toronto, Room BW4-658, 585 University Ave., Toronto, ON M5G 2C4, Canada*

1. Introduction

Herpes zoster, HZ, known as shingles, is a distinctive neurocutaneous entity that has been recognized for many centuries. In this chapter, the distinctive dermatologic features are outlined in terms of clinical presentation, histopathology and therapy.

The name herpes is derived from the Greek word meaning 'to creep' (Taylor-Robinson and Caunt, 1972). In its modern usage, this refers to the fact that the eruption consists of spreading vesicles. The term zoster is another Greek derivation, meaning 'girdle'. This describes the characteristic 'wrapped around' distribution which is commonly seen on the trunk. Similarly, the term shingles refers to a girdle-like distribution. Hence, the descriptive name clearly characterizes the disease: grouped vesicles on an inflamed base usually localized to one or two dermatomes without crossing the midline. This rash is often preceded, accompanied and followed by pain.

2. Clinical features

The first manifestation of zoster is usually pain, which can be severe. It may be sharply localized or diffuse and is often described as burning, aching or lancinating. Forty percent of patients experience pain more than 4 days prior to the skin eruption and 35% experience it less than 48 h prior to the skin condition (Wood et al., 1989). In some cases, the pain starts more than 100 days prior to the development of the distinctive skin rash. This is referred to as 'preherpetic neuralgia' (Gilden et al., 1991). Based on the distribution of the pain, it may mimic migraine, acute glaucoma, myocardial infarction, pleurisy, appendicitis or duodenal ulcer. Fever, malaise, myalgia, paraesthesia or pruritus may accompany the pain. The rash starts soon after as maculopapular, fixed erythematous areas that develop into fluid-filled vesicles within 12–24 h. Characteristically, it starts in a localized part of one, occasionally two, and rarely more contiguous dermatomes and spreads in a linear fashion over the next 3–5 days, stopping abruptly at the midline. Fixed urticarial erythema precedes closely grouped vesicles that tend to enlarge, umbilicate, and then become pustular as leukocytes invade them. As the haemorrhagic component of the vesicles develops, the surrounding urticarial erythema dissipates. This haemorrhagic blistering, often in grouped, grape-like clusters, is so distinctive that its presence in a lin-

---

* Correspondence to: R. Gary Sibbald, Department of Medicine, University of Toronto, Room BW4-658, 585 University Ave., Toronto, ON M5G 2C4, Canada. Phone: +1 (416) 978-4499; Fax: +1 (416) 978-4568.

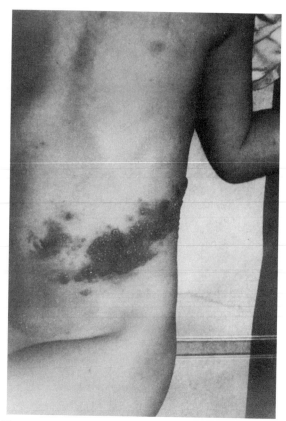

Fig. 1. Herpes zoster. Note prominent purpura. (Courtesy of Dr. Orest Talpash.)

ear distribution must be thought of as herpes zoster until proven otherwise (Fig. 1). Individual lesions may also become necrotic and ulcerate. The lymph nodes draining the affected area are often enlarged and tender.

Mild infections, which run a shorter course, can occur whereby macules and papules regress in 7–10 days without progressing to vesicles (Burgoon et al., 1957). In typical infections, crusting of the lesions occurs in 7–10 days, after which the patient is thought to be no longer contagious. Re-epithelialization then follows and is usually complete in 2–3 weeks in younger individuals (i.e. children and young adults) and in 3–4 weeks in older individuals. The eruption usually resolves with no residual rash, although occasionally post-inflammatory hyper- and hypopigmentation may be seen. If severe ulceration

occurs or healing is delayed, permanent scarring of the skin may result. This is most commonly seen in elderly, undernourished or immunocompromised patients (Ragozzino et al., 1982).

Any dermatome may be affected, but the dermatomes are not affected with equal frequency (Ragozzino et al., 1982). The distribution of the rash of HZ tends to mirror the areas most heavily affected by the primary VZV infection. As chicken pox tends to be centripetally distributed, thoracic dermatomes are most commonly affected, accounting for approximately half of all cases. This distribution may be due to contiguous spread from infected skin to the ganglia at the time of primary infection, or, alternatively, reactivation stimuli may be more common in this area. The second most commonly affected location is the first, or ophthalmic, branch of the trigeminal nerve. This occurs in 10–20% of affected individuals (Ragozzino et al., 1982), and has a particular propensity for elderly patients. Cervical and lumbosacral involvement account for the remainder of cases.

A common belief is that patients with involvement of the nasociliary branch of the trigeminal nerve are at greater risk of ocular complications. It is important to note, however, that any periocular involvement warrants careful monitoring (Duncan, 1991) as iritis, keratitis, conjunctivitis, acute retinal necrosis and the development of Argyll–Robertson pupillary abnormality may all occur (see Chapter 11).

Occasionally, HZ may be manifested by pain without skin involvement (Lewis, 1958; Easton, 1970). This is referred to as 'zoster sine herpete' and is presumably due to an abortive eruption. Some of these cases may represent a very prolonged interval between the onset of the preherpetic neuralgia and the characteristic rash of HZ (Gilden et al., 1991). However, in others the rash does not manifest. The diagnosis in this situation is very difficult, and is often made on a post hoc basis by finding rising antibody titres to the virus (i.e., a four-fold rise over 10 days).

HZ of the maxillary division of the trigeminal nerve produces vesicles of the uvula and tonsillar area. Involvement of the mandibular branch produces vesicles on the floor of the mouth, buccal mucous membrane and the anterior part of the tongue. Toothache may be the presenting sign.

The Ramsay–Hunt syndrome is characterized by the triad of pain in the ear, vesicles (affecting the tympanum, ear, tonsillar fauces, anterior pillar, pinna and the external auditory canal) and facial paralysis with loss of taste on the anterior two-thirds of the tongue. Suspected involvement of the geniculate ganglion has not yet been confirmed with pathological studies (see Chapter 15).

Visceral involvement may be responsible for abdominal pain and can mimic an acute surgical abdominal emergency such as acute appendicitis (Elliot and Mitchell Sams, 1990). Many a dermatologist has kept a surgeon at bay with the diagnosis of visceral HZ.

Although most cases of HZ are viewed as sharply localized to one or more dermatomes, careful observation will often reveal a few sparse papules and vesicles outside of the affected dermatome(s) (Huff, 1988). Tyring (1992) documented this finding in approximately 33% of immunocompetent patients. Resembling the lesions of varicella, these are considered to represent haematogenous spread and an inadequate host immune defence system to contain the lesions. The dissemination is thought to occur within circulating leukocytes, particularly monocytes.

Cutaneous dissemination, arbitrarily defined as more than 20 lesions outside the affected dermatome(s) (Ragozzino et al., 1982), is much rarer, occurring in only 2% of cases. The main risk factor is immunosuppression. Dissemination in immunocompromised patients occurs in up to 15–30% of cases (Sokol and Firat, 1965; Schimpf et al., 1972). Systemic involvement, resulting in pneumonia, hepatitis and encephalitis, is often associated with cutaneous dissemination and as a result can be fatal.

A particularly severe zoster in a young individual may be the presenting complaint of human immunodeficiency virus (HIV) infection. Tyring et al. (1995) reported that 15 of 419 patients presenting with herpes zoster entered into a study had HIV infection. When peripheral T_4 counts dip below 500, viral infections can present in unusual ways and may be the presenting complaint of HIV infection.

3. Complications

3.1. Pain

Almost all patients have pain associated with acute HZ. Distinct from this is the commonest and most intractable sequel of HZ, postherpetic neuralgia (PHN) (Huff, 1988). The true frequency of PHN depends on the definition used and the population studied. One definition is of pain persisting more than four weeks after the onset of the infection (Hope-Simpson, 1965). The reported incidence of PHN varies between 5% and 57%, according to different studies (Schmader and Studenski, 1989). More about PHN is detailed elsewhere in this book (see Chapters 14–24).

3.2. Cutaneous complications

3.2.1. Bacterial infection
Infection of cutaneous lesions was reported in 2.3% of cases in a 60-day follow-up study of complications of HZ (Galil et al., 1997). The most common infective complication is impetigo. Erysipelas and cellulitis can also occur.

3.2.2. Scarring
Individual lesions can scar as a sequel to necrotic zoster, dermal ulceration or infection. Sarcoid lesions (Bisaccia et al., 1983) and granuloma formation (Wright et al., 1989) have been reported within HZ scars.

3.2.3. Post-inflammatory hyperpigmentation
Significant thick crusts are often noted, particularly following secondary bacterial infection or ulceration. These crusts resolve, leaving local dusky erythematous macules that may then become pigmented.

3.2.4. Gangrene
Rarely, in association with a significant immunocompromised state, gangrenous skin lesions may result from deep necrosis and ulceration (Huff, 1988).

3.3. Ocular complications

Eye complications occur in approximately 2% of patients with HZ (Ragozzino et al., 1982; Galil et al., 1997) and in 67% of patients with ophthalmic nerve involvement. In short, HZ may complicate any aspect of the ophthalmic or peri-ophthalmic structures. For a more in-depth review of these complications the reader is referred to Chapter 11.

3.4. Motor complications

Although motor neuropathy is one of the least common complications of HZ, occurring in approximately 1% of cases (Ragozzino et al., 1982; Galil et al., 1997), its effects are often associated with significant morbidity. Degeneration of the anterior horn cells and motor fibres develops, similar to that seen in poliomyelitis (Chang et al., 1987). The motor weakness usually follows days to weeks after the rash, but it can on occasion precede both the pain and the rash of HZ. Facial weakness (Ramsay–Hunt syndrome), diaphragmatic paralysis, abdominal herniation due to T_{10} and T_{11} involvement (Landthaler and Heuser, 1979), loss of bowel and bladder function (Fugelso et al., 1973), and weakness of an arm or leg have all been reported. Ocular palsies are rare. Motor involvement tends to be more common in the elderly or when HZ is associated with underlying malignancy. The majority of patients either completely recover or they may show significant improvement with time.

3.5. Sensory complications

Sensory nerve involvement by HZ may result in damage to the 8th cranial nerve. Symptoms of this include tinnitus, deafness, vertigo and vomiting, making the differentiation from Menière's syndrome difficult.

3.6. Systemic complications

Another complication associated with immunosuppression is encephalitis (Dolin et al., 1978). This most

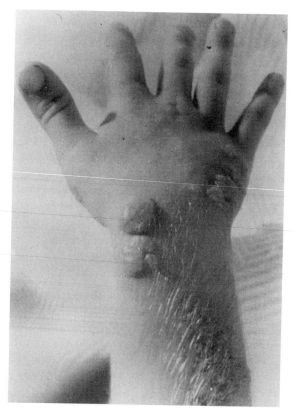

Fig. 2. Herpes zoster in a neonate. Note severe bullae. (Courtesy of Dr. Orest Talpash.)

commonly follows HZ affecting the head and neck (Jemseck et al., 1983). Onset follows skin lesions by 1 or 2 weeks, and may be manifested by seizures, delirium, hallucinations, confusion, coma and ataxia. Examination of the cerebrospinal fluid aids diagnosis by showing an increased number of white blood cells and elevated protein. If available, the cerebrospinal fluid can also be analysed using polymerase chain reaction (PCR) to detect VZV-DNA. Most patients recover without complications (Jemseck et al., 1983). Other rare complications of HZ include myelitis, pneumonia and hepatitis. All appear to be associated with widespread involvement.

3.7. HZ in pregnancy, infancy and childhood

The risk to the developing foetus is very small, probably because of the lack of significant viraemia

(Eyal et al., 1983; Enders, 1984). Most cases run a benign course, even if the eruption occurs early in pregnancy.

HZ in the neonate is usually an uncomplicated illness (Rogers and Tindall, 1972). It is thought to occur secondarily to in-utero exposure to the virus (Brunell and Kotchmar, 1981). Rarely, however, infants may be affected by severe bullous disease (Fig. 2).

4. Histopathology

The cutaneous lesions of HZ are histologically indistinguishable from varicella or herpes simplex infection. In all, the most common feature is an intraepidermal blister formed by 'ballooning degeneration' of infected epidermal cells in the lower to middle epidermis. This results in marked acantholysis (Fig. 3). Ballooning degeneration causes marked swelling of epidermal cells. Balloon cells have a homogeneous, eosinophilic cytoplasm. Eosinophilic inclusion bodies may also be present. These are separated by clear zones from the nuclear membrane and are known as Cowdry type A inclusions. Because balloon cells lose their intercellular bridges, acantholysis occurs, leading to dissolution of the lower epidermis.

Reticular degeneration may also occur. This is a process in which the epidermal cells become greatly distended by intracellular oedema, so that many of the cells burst. This occurs mainly at the upper portion and at the periphery of viral vesicles. Reticular degeneration is not specific for herpetic infections; it also occurs in all kinds of dermatitis, leading to dissolution of the lower epidermis.

Multinuclear giant cells are characteristic of herpetic lesions. These occur due to fusion of adjacent infected cells, in or near blisters. Smears taken from the floor of an early, freshly opened vesicle and

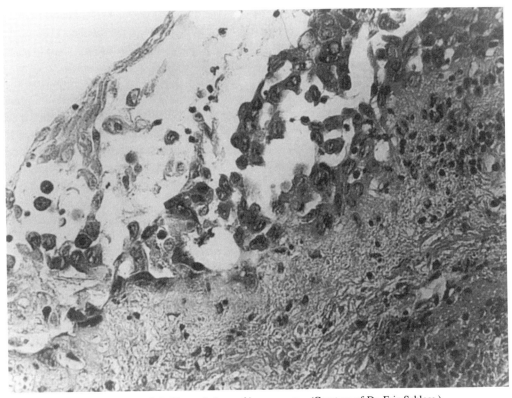

Fig. 3. Characteristic histopathology of herpes zoster. (Courtesy of Dr. Eric Schloss.)

stained with a Giemsa or toluidine blue stain (available in most hospital laboratories) show this characteristic feature. Such a preparation is known as a Tzank smear and gives a rapid method for identification of herpetic infection. Many hospital laboratories have replaced the Tzank smear with an immunofluorescent herpes antigen test. Viral fluid and cells from the base of the lesion are dried on a slide and stained using a specific immunofluorescent antigen–antibody sandwich technique. This procedure can be completed in less than one hour with inexpensive, commercially available kits. The presence of herpes simplex 1 or 2, herpes zoster or no detectable virus can help with therapeutic decisions in difficult cases.

The host inflammatory reaction promoted by HZ infection consists of an early response of lymphocytes and monocytes and the later appearance of neutrophils. This may progress to a leukocyclastic vasculitis with haemorrhage and purpura. In sensory ganglia, these histopathological features of inflammation, haemorrhage and necrosis are very pronounced.

The presence of HZ virus in the ganglia has been demonstrated by electron microscopy (Ghatak and Zimmerman, 1973) and by culture with monkey kidney cells (Bastian et al., 1975). Inflammatory and degenerative changes extend from the involved ganglion along the sensory nerves to the skin or proximally to the spinal cord, producing myelitis.

5. HZ and immunosuppression

HZ is thought to manifest itself in response to a decline in impaired cell-mediated immunity. It is particularly associated with lymphoproliferative malignancies, i.e. Hodgkin's disease and non-Hodgkin's lymphoma, and with HIV infection. In fact, 25% of HIV-positive individuals will have at least one episode of HZ at some point during the course of their disease (Friedman-Kien et al., 1986).

A frequently asked question is whether a patient presenting with HZ should be evaluated for systemic cancer or other underlying diseases which compromise the immune system. Such evaluations are not necessary or cost effective (Ragozzino et al., 1982) as the HZ usually presents late in the course of a cancer, or as a complication of radiation or chemotherapy. The exception to this is HIV infection, which can present as HZ. With this in mind, appropriate risk factors should be asked about, and a high index of suspicion together with a routine enquiry of the systems and a physical examination should suffice. If there is any doubt, more thorough laboratory investigations are indicated.

6. Diagnosis of HZ

In most cases, the diagnosis of HZ is obvious. However, because the pain may precede the development of vesicles by a few to, very rarely, more than 100 days (Gilden et al., 1991), HZ must be considered in the differential diagnosis of any unexplained localized acute pain syndrome.

Problems in diagnosis may arise early in the course of the disease. Localized dermatoses, such as crawling insect bites, allergic and irritant contact dermatitis and localized infections such as impetigo and folliculitis may at first mimic the disease. However, the progression of HZ to its characteristic painful, grouped lesions in a dermatomal distribution usually distinguishes these entities. A few subtle clinical pointers may, however, aid diagnosis. The distribution pattern may help, with zosteriform herpes simplex occurring most commonly in the maxillary distribution of the facial nerve and in the sacral areas. Recurrent lesions of the buttocks are almost always herpes simplex and *not* zoster. This site is the third most common for herpes simplex after the lips and genitals and is due to couples cuddling front to back ('cupping'). Pain is also more pronounced with HZ than with herpes simplex and zosteriform herpes simplex tends to recur whereas HZ usually occurs only once.

Despite this, the distinction between herpes simplex and HZ can still pose difficulties in some cases. In one randomized controlled study, 4.5% of clinically suspected cases of HZ were in fact herpes simplex virus on culture (Tyring et al., 1995). The presentation of the two conditions may at first seem identical and neither a Tzank smear nor electron microscopy of the vesicular fluid will differentiate the two entities. When specific immunofluorescent staining is available, the distinction between herpes simplex type 1 and 2 and herpes zoster can, however, be made in a short time. If this technique is unavailable, viral cultures can be taken, with herpes simplex taking 24–48 h to grow and herpes zoster often requiring 5–7 days. Prior to taking a culture, any crust should be lifted to expose the basal epidermal cells from which the culture is taken. Early pre-crusted lesions should be selected if present. Unfortunately, this method has a 50% false negative rate. More sophisticated methods of diagnosis, which may not be available in all centres, include VZV-DNA detection by PCR in a scraping from the base of a vesicle. Titration of complement-fixing antibody in acute and convalescent sera may be useful for atypical infections, where a four-fold increase in titre is required for diagnosis.

7. Therapy of HZ

Prior to the 1960s, a number of therapies were reported as efficacious but were never tested in a controlled fashion. These included injections of pituitary extract, vitamin B1 and B12, cobra venom, quinine, proteolytic enzymes, autohaemotherapy, sodium iodide and ergotamine (De Moragas and Kierland, 1957; Portenoy et al., 1986). Currently, therapy must be thought of as having three goals: to relieve the symptoms of acute pain, to decrease the duration, dissemination and infectivity of the skin rash and to prevent or shorten the duration of complications such as postherpetic neuralgia. Since the latter is covered extensively elsewhere in this book, comments will be confined to the treatment of acute HZ.

7.1. General measures

Since HZ is self-limited, most patients will recover completely without specific therapy. However, topical measures are justified for symptom relief. One useful measure is the use of wet dressings or compresses. These serve three functions. First, the application of fluid to the vesiculated, eroded or ulcerated skin restores a relatively physiological environment to the exposed nerve endings which are responsible for transmitting sensations such as pain and itching. Second, by softening and dissolving crusts, compresses remove solidified protein which would otherwise serve as a nidus for infection. Third, removal of the crusts and vesicles reduces the damaging effect of fluid entrapment and therefore reduces maceration. The fluids used for compressing can be normal saline, tap water, Burrow's solution (aluminum acetonide) and colloidal oatmeal (Aveeno™). These are usually applied for 10–15 min four times daily. If the skin lesions are impetiginized, a topical antibiotic ointment such as mupirocin or bacitracin (alone or in combinations) can be applied thereafter. Neomycin should be avoided alone or in combination products because of its allergic sensitising potential and cross-sensitivity with aminoglycosides. Since the patient is contagious by direct contact until the lesions have crusted, it is thought that this process may decrease the time of contagion. It may also hasten the healing process presumably by decreasing secondary bacterial infection.

Topical antipruritics or analgesic creams or lotions can be administered in the form of pramoxine or menthol, preferably without topical steroids. Storing these preparations in the refrigerator may provide an additive cooling, anti-itch effect.

Antipyretic agents may also be administered. Acetaminophen is preferable to acetylsalicylic acid in children because of the association of the latter with Reye's syndrome. Other analgesics are also important in HZ therapy. Controlling pain, especially at night so the patient can rest, is essential. Over-the-counter analgesics, nonsteroidal anti-inflammatory agents, tricyclic antidepressants, gabapentin and narcotic analgesics should all be considered, based on the severity of the pain.

Quality of life during the acute painful episode may be improved using tricyclic antidepressants. Second-generation agents high in noradrenaline may offer optimal clinical benefit (e.g. nortriptyline). The authors often start with 10–25 mg at night and gradually increase the dose, titrating therapeutic benefit and side effects.

Health care professionals who have not had an episode of chicken pox in the past and who come into contact with infected individuals should have a varicella zoster complement titre performed on a single blood specimen. If this is less than 1:8 or negative, immunization with the zoster (Oka) vaccine is strongly recommended.

7.2. Systemic antibacterial agents

The role of oral and parenteral antibacterial agents is controversial. Because of the intensity of the eruption, many physicians are tempted to prevent secondary bacterial infections. They assume the progressive cloudiness of the vesicular eruption, which becomes pustular, is bacterial infection. This is, however, uncommon and such therapy is usually not needed. The presence of frank purulence, honey-coloured crusting and deep ulceration do suggest superimposed impetiginization. Since the most common offending organisms is *Staphylococcus aureus*, a penicillinase-resistant semisynthetic penicillin, a cephalosporin or a broad-spectrum antibiotic aimed at this organism are the most appropriate. More specifically, cloxacillin, cephalexin, amoxicillin clavulanate, trimethoprim and sulfamethoxasole are all appropriate antibiotics.

7.3. Topical pain therapy

Topical agents are fully described in Chapter 21.

7.4. Glucocorticosteroids

One of the most controversial therapies for HZ is the use of glucocorticosteroid drugs. The indications cited are both for the relief of acute pain and the prevention of postherpetic neuralgia. Since the latter topic is addressed elsewhere in the book (Chapter 18), the former will be concentrated on. The use of systemic corticosteroid therapy has been suggested as a viable alternative since Nickel (1951) and

Sulzberger et al. (1951) used adrenocorticotrophic hormone (ACTH) in the treatment of HZ infections. A number of subsequent investigations followed in which corticosteroid derivatives were used in the management of HZ (Frank and Lysiak, 1953: Gelfand, 1954; Sauer, 1955; Appelman, 1955: Elliot, 1964; Sutton, 1984). However, these early investigations failed to utilise proper experimental methodology, making their conclusions suspect. A survey of 73 practising dermatologists, 56 of whom responded, showed that 81% routinely used corticosteroids in otherwise healthy patients older than age 60 who had HZ (Levinson and Shaw, 1985). Critics maintain an increased risk of herpes dissemination (Irons, 1964; Anderson and Janott, 1987) and avascular necrosis of the femoral head (Mills, 1986) as reasons against their use. More recently, a lack of efficacy has been claimed (Huff, 1988) and in view of recent studies (Wood et al., 1994; Whitley et al., 1996), together with the availability of effective antiviral therapies, these drugs now have little to recommend them.

7.5. Antiviral agents

Antiviral agents have been employed in the treatment of HZ for over 30 years. Although this is elaborated elsewhere in this book, a few points warrant mention. Idoxuridine, cytosine arabinoside, vidarabine and, more recently, acyclovir, valacyclovir and famciclovir have all been used in the acute management of HZ. Thymidine kinase inactivating anti-herpes drugs (acyclovir, valacyclovir, famciclovir) are generally conceded to promote faster resolution of vesicles and to decrease the amount of acute pain experienced (Wood et al., 1989). Their main benefit is to reduce the duration of postherpetic neuralgia (Wood et al., 1994; Tyring et al., 1995; Whitley et al., 1996). For maximal benefit, oral antivirals should be started within the first 24–72 h of onset of the skin rash. They are generally recommended for immunocompromised patients and in those patients at higher risk of developing postherpetic neuralgia (i.e., patients over 50 years of age, and those with a co-existing illness). In the Tyring study (Tyring et al., 1995), famciclovir 500 mg t.i.d. for 7 days decreased duration of postherpetic neuralgia for all patients by 60 days, and for patients over 50 years of age the duration was decreased by 100 days. Comparable benefits are probably obtained with valacyclovir 1000 mg t.i.d. for 7 days or acyclovir 800 mg 5 times daily, again for 7 days. There is no added benefit to using 10 days of oral antivirals over the standard 7-day course. The newer second-generation agents, valacyclovir (57%) and famciclovir (77%), have a higher oral absorption rate than acyclovir (12–20%), allowing a decrease in dosage frequency from 5 to 3 times daily. There was no increase in side effects with these agents when compared to placebo in the controlled studies.

8. Conclusion

Despite the fact that HZ has been described for hundreds of years, its treatment still presents a challenge, both in the immunocompetent host and even more so in the immunocompromised patient. The judicious use of pain relievers ameliorates the acute phase of the condition. In view of the higher risk of potentially life-threatening complications of HZ in immunocompromised patients and the high morbidity associated with postherpetic neuralgia, valacyclovir or famciclovir is recommended for both immunocompromised patients as well as those at high risk of developing PHN (individuals with ophthalmic zoster or over age of 50 years). The benefit of these newer generation antivirals in all patients has been documented and patients with new and evolving skin lesions should be given the choice to assess the benefits of therapy on an individual basis.

Pain with herpes zoster may be severe. Early consultation to a pain consultant is strongly recommended. In individuals over 70 years, the pain of postherpetic neuralgia is second to cancer-associated pain as the most common cause of pain-related suicide in the elderly.

Obviously, the ultimate goal is to prevent HZ. Vaccination against varicella virus is now universal in some Western countries. However, long-term studies to confirm the length of immunity conferred by the immunization are awaited. Should the vaccine not confer lifelong immunity, the worry is that primary varicella will become an adult disease, with its associated relatively high morbidity and mortality rate, rather than a benign childhood disease. The childhood Oka vaccine is currently being studied to boost immunity and decrease the risk of herpes zoster in individuals over 50 years that had varicella zoster infection (chicken pox) in childhood. At present, the best we can hope for is to palliate the acute situation, aim to decrease the risk of PHN and systemic complications with antiviral agents, where appropriate, and to observe for and treat complications.

References

Anderson, D.J. and Janott, E.N. (1987) Herpes zoster in a patient on methotrexate given prednisone to prevent postherpetic neuralgia. Ann. Intern. Med., 107: 783.

Appelman, D.H. (1955) Treatment of herpes zoster with ACTH. N. Engl. J. Med., 153: 693–695.

Bastian, F.O., Rabson, A.S., Yee, C.L., et al. (1975) Herpes virus varicellae. Arch. Pathol., 97: 331–333.

Bisaccia, E., Scarborough, D.A. and Carr, R.A. (1983) Cutaneous sarcoid granuloma formation in herpes zoster scars. Arch. Dermatol., 119: 788–789.

Brunell, P.A. and Kotchmar, G.S. (1981) Zoster in infancy: failure to maintain virus latency following intrauterine infection. J. Pediatr., 98: 71–76.

Burgoon, C.F., Burgoon, J.S., Baldridge, G.D. (1957) The natural history of herpes zoster. JAMA, 164: 265–269.

Chang, C.M., Woo, E., Yu, Y.L., et al. (1987) Herpes zoster and its neurological complications. Postgrad. Med. J., 63: 85–92.

De Moragas, J.M. and Kierland, R.R. (1957) The outcome of patients with herpes zoster. Arch. Dermatol., 75: 193–196.

Dolin, R., Reichman, R.C., Mazur, M.H., et al. (1978) Herpes zoster — varicella infections in immunosuppressed patients. Ann. Intern. Med., 89: 375–379.

Duncan, W.C. (1991) Skin and the eye. Dialog. Dermatol., 29(1).

Easton, H.G. (1970) Zoster sine Herpete causing acute trigeminal neuralgia. Lancet, 2: 1065.

Elliot, F.A. (1964) Treatment of herpes zoster with high doses of prednisone. Lancet, 2: 610–611.

Elliot, G.W. and Mitchell Sams, W. (1990) Viral vesicular diseases. In: W. Mitchell Sams and P.J. Lynch (Eds.), Principles and Practice of Dermatology. Churchill Livingstone, New York, pp. 103–105.

Enders, G. (1984) Varicella-zoster in children. Prog. Med. Virol., 29: 166–169.

Eyal, A., Friedman, M., Peretz, B.A., et al. (1983) Pregnancy complicated by herpes zoster. J. Reprod. Med., 28: 600–603.

Frank, L. and Lysiak, R. (1953) Herpetic and postherpetic pain treated with cortisone and ACTH. N.Y. J. Med., 53: 2379.

Friedman-Kien, A.E., Lafleur, F.L., Gendler E., et al. (1986) Herpes zoster: a positive early clinical sign for development of AIDS in high-risk individuals. J. Am. Acad. Dermatol., 14: 1023–1028.

Fugelso, P.D., Reed, W.B., Newman, S.B., et al. (1973) Herpes zoster of the anogenital area affecting urination and defaecation. Br. J. Dermatol., 89: 285.

Galil, K., Choo, P.W., Donahue, J.G., et al. (1997) The sequelae of herpes zoster. Arch. Intern. Med., 157: 1209–1213.

Gelfand, M.L. (1954) Treatment of herpes zoster with cortisone. JAMA, 154: 911–912.

Ghatak, N.R. and Zimmerman, H.M. (1973) Spinal ganglion in herpes zoster. A light and electron microscopic study. Arch. Pathol., 95: 411–415.

Gilden, D.H., Dueland, A.N., Cohrs, R., et al. (1991) Preherpetic neuralgia. Neurology, 41: 1215–1218.

Hope-Simpson, R.E. (1965) The nature of herpes zoster: a long term study and a new hypothesis. Proc. R. Soc. Med., 58: 9–20.

Huff, J.C. (1988) Herpes zoster. Curr. Probl. Dermatol., 1: 1–40.

Irons, G.V. (1964) Steroids and herpes zoster. JAMA, 189: 649.

Jemseck, J., Greenberg, S.B., Taber, I., et al. (1983) Herpes zoster associated encephalitis — clinicopathologic report of 12 cases and review of the literature. Medicine (Baltimore), 62: 81–96.

Landthaler, M. and Heuser, M. (1979) Paralytische Bauchwandherni bei Zoster. Hautarzt, 30: 432–433.

Levinson, J.C., Shaw, J.C. (1985) Treatment of herpes zoster with corticosteroids: fact or fiction. West. J. Med., 142: 117–118.

Lewis, G.W. (1958) Zoster sine herpete. Br. Med. J., 2: 418–419.

Mills, K. (1986) Herpes zoster and corticosteroid therapy. Med. J. Aust., 145: 60.

Nickel, W.R. (1951) Herpes zoster treated with ACTH. Arch. Dermatol., 64: 372.

Portenoy, R.K., Duma, C. and Foley, K.M. (1986) Acute herpetic and postherpetic neuralgia: clinical review and current management. Ann. Neurol., 20: 651–664.

Ragozzino, M.W., Melton, L.J., Kurland, L.T., et al. (1982) Population based study of herpes zoster and its sequelae. Medicine (Baltimore), 61: 310–316.

Rogers, R.S. and Tindall, J.P. (1972) Herpes zoster in children. Arch. Dermatol., 106: 204–207.

Sauer, G.C. (1955) Herpes zoster: treatment of post-herpetic neuralgia with cortisone corticotropin and placebo. Arch. Dermatol., 77: 488–489.

Schimpf, S., Serpick, A., Stoler, B., et al. (1972) Varicella zoster in patients with cancer. Ann. Intern. Med., 76: 241–245.

Schmader, K.E. and Studenski, S. (1989) Are current therapies useful for the prevention of postherpetic neuralgia? A critical analysis of the literature. J. Gen. Intern. Med., 4: 83–89.

Sokol, H. and Firat, D. (1965) Varicella zoster in Hodgkin's disease. Am. J. Med., 39: 452–455.

Sulzberger, M.B., Sauer, G.C., Herman, F., et al. (1951) Effects of ACTH and cortisone on certain diseases and physiological functions of the skin. I. Effects of ACTH. J. Invest. Dermatol., 16: 323–337.

Sutton, G. (1984) Steroid therapy in the treatment of herpes zoster. Br. J. Clin. Pract., 38: 21–24.

Taylor-Robinson, D. and Caunt, A.E. (1972) Varicella Virus. Springer, New York, pp. 1–78.

Tyring, S.K. (1992) The natural history of varicella zoster virus. Semin. Dermatol., 11: 211–217.

Tyring, S., Barbarash, R.A., Nahlik, J.E., et al. (1995) Famciclovir for the treatment of acute herpes zoster: effects on acute disease and postherpetic neuralgia. A randomized double-blind placebo-controlled trial. Collaborative Famciclovir Herpes Zoster Study Group. Ann. Intern. Med., 123: 89–96.

Whitley, R.J., Weiss, H., Gnann, J.W., et al. (1996) Acyclovir with and without prednisone for the treatment of herpes zoster, a randomized placebo-controlled trial. Ann. Intern. Med., 125: 376–383.

Wood, M.J., Ogan, P.H., McKendrick, M.W., Care, C.D., et al. (1989) Efficacy of oral acyclovir treatment of acute herpes zoster. Am. J. Med., 85 (Suppl. 2A): 79–83.

Wood, M.J., Johnson, R.W. and McKendrick, M.W. (1994) A randomized trial of acyclovir for 7 days or 21 days with and without prednisolone for treatment of acute herpes zoster. N. Engl. J. Med., 330: 896–900.

Wright, A.L., Cotton, D.W.K., Winfield, D.A., et al. (1989) Granuloma formation in herpes zoster scars. Dermatologica, 179: 45–46.

Herpes Zoster and Postherpetic Neuralgia, 2nd Revised and Enlarged Edition
Pain Research and Clinical Management, Vol. 11
Edited by C.P.N. Watson and A.A. Gershon

CHAPTER 10

Zoster in immunosuppressed patients

Anne A. Gershon [*]

Department of Pediatrics, Columbia University College of Physicians and Surgeons, New York, NY 10032, USA

1. Introduction

It was recognized for almost 100 years ago that vari-cella-zoster virus (VZV) causes both varicella and zoster, and it was proposed that zoster resulted from reactivation of latent infection with the virus about 50 years ago (Garland, 1943). Experiments using both polymerase chain reaction (PCR) and in situ hy-bridization have now demonstrated that latent VZV is harbored in human sensory ganglia (Croen et al., 1988; Mahalingham et al., 1990, 1993, 1996; Lungu et al., 1995, 1998; Kennedy et al., 1999), and the hypothesis that zoster is caused by viral reactivation has been proven (Hayakawa et al., 1984; Straus et al., 1984; Williams et al., 1985). How and why VZV remains latent, and the factors and mechanisms by which it reactivates, nevertheless, are still unknown. One clue to the mechanism however, is the increased incidence of zoster in immunosuppressed patients, suggesting that immunity plays a significant role in reactivation of latent VZV. Hope-Simpson postulated that as immunity to VZV wanes with time after the primary infection (chickenpox), reactivation of the virus occurs; he proposed that zoster develops when the immune response to VZV fell below a "criti-cal level" with time in the elderly (Hope-Simpson, 1965).

2. Humoral immunity to VZV

Studies of humoral immunity indicated that specific antibodies play little or no role in the pathogen-esis of reactivation of VZV (Brunell et al., 1975; Hardy et al., 1991a,b). Antibodies to the virus that develop after chickenpox are detectable by a variety of methods including immunofluorescence, ELISA, and latex agglutination (Gershon et al., 1992). It is far simpler to measure humoral immunity to VZV than CMI responses, which may account for early attempts to determine whether antibodies might play a role in development of zoster.

It was appreciated for years by pediatricians that children with agammaglobulinemia are not at in-creased risk to either develop severe varicella nor do they have an increased risk of zoster compared to healthy children. Zoster was observed to develop in patients despite pre-existing positive VZV antibody titers (Brunell et al., 1975), and there is also a brisk antibody response early in zoster, with high spe-cific antibody titers usually present in disseminated zoster (Uduman et al., 1975). Therefore treatment of zoster with high-titered immune globulin would not be likely to cure the illness Subsequently, passive immunization was shown not to prevent develop-ment of zoster or to have any therapeutic value in

---

[*] Correspondence to: Dr. A.A. Gershon, Department of Pediatrics, Columbia University College of Physicians and Surgeons, 650 W. 168th Street, New York, NY 10032, USA. Phone: +1 (212) 305-9445; Fax: +1 (212) 342-5218; E-mail: aag1@columbia.edu

the illness (Merigan and Stevens, 1978; Stevens and Merigan, 1980). Increased rather than decreased antibody titers were found in the aged, also suggesting that low antibody titers did not predispose to zoster (Gershon and Steinberg, 1981). Thus it was proposed that cellular immunity (CMI) to VZV probably plays a more significant role in host defense.

3. Cellular immunity

It became possible to measure CMI to VZV in 1974. The first assay to be developed was proliferation of lymphocytes due to exposure to VZV antigens (Jordan and Merigan, 1974). Partially purified lymphocytes from patients before and after varicella were studied in vitro. A comparison was made between the response of lymphocytes that were stimulated with VZV and control antigen, measuring incorporation of radioactive thymidine into cells, and a ratio was calculated. After varicella, there was at least 3 times as much DNA synthesis in lymphocytes stimulated with VZV antigen compared to control antigen. Using this assay, low (i.e. less than 3×) proliferative responses specific to VZV were found in heart transplant patients during the time when they are at high risk to develop zoster (Rand et al., 1977), and in patients prior to being treated for lymphoma, who were also at high risk to develop zoster (Arvin et al., 1978). Prospective longitudinal studies on lymphoma patients revealed loss of positive lymphocyte transformation responses to VZV in 13 of 13 patients who developed zoster, but not in 13 matched controls who had high levels of VZV CMI. Despite low VZV CMI in 21 other patients, however, zoster did not occur. Thus low CMI to VZV was a necessary, but not sufficient requirement for reactivation of VZV. Antibody levels, in contrast, were not lower in zoster patients than in matched controls (Arvin et al., 1980). Subsequent prospective studies on leukemic children who were immunized with live attenuated varicella vaccine also revealed that vaccinated children with low CMI to VZV were at risk to develop zoster while those with normal or high CMI levels were not. As anticipated, antibody titers in vaccinated leukemic

children who developed zoster and those who did not were similar before zoster developed (Hardy et al., 1991a,b). Elderly individuals are thought to be predisposed to develop zoster because their CMI response to VZV diminishes with age (Miller, 1980; Berger et al., 1981; Burke et al., 1982). Low CMI to VZV, alone, however does not guarantee that zoster will develop; most individuals with low CMI to VZV do not develop the illness. Yet to be explained, moreover, is why, on occasion, otherwise healthy children and young adults may develop zoster.

4. Can subclinical zoster occur?

In longitudinal studies in renal transplant patients who experienced chickenpox in the past, it was observed that significant fluctuations of VZV antibody titers occurred in the absence of symptoms of VZV infection (Luby et al., 1977). These observations suggested the possibility of subclinical reactivation of VZV. Meyers et al. detected a return from negative to positive lymphocyte transformation to VZV in 89% of 18 bone marrow transplant (BMT) patients following clinical zoster, and also in 52% of 29 patients who did not have symptoms of zoster. They proposed that after BMT, the silent shift of CMI to VZV from low to normal positive levels might be due to subclinical reactivation of VZV (Meyers et al., 1980). Moreover, it was known that IgM was detectable not only after chickenpox, but also after zoster, and the observation that positive IgM titers developed in some asymptomatic patients also suggested subclinical reactivation of VZV (Gershon et al., 1982). In both of these studies, however, boosting of immunity following an exposure to the virus could not be ruled out. Such boosting was observed in healthy and immunocompromised patients after exposure to VZV (Brunell et al., 1975; Arvin et al., 1983; Gershon et al., 1984).

Ljungman and colleagues followed 102 patients before and after BMT; the incidence of clinical zoster and apparent subclinical reactivation of VZV were similar, 36 and 26%, respectively. In the patients with proposed subclinical reactivation, the diagnosis was based upon a four-fold or greater rise in titer of antibodies to VZV, or an increase of lymphocyte transformation response from 'susceptible' to 'immune' levels without symptoms. While silent reinfection with VZV could not be ruled out, these patients were expressly asked to avoid exposure to individuals with varicella or zoster. Moreover, they were isolated from others when hospitalized (Ljungman et al., 1986). Wilson et al. found, using PCR, that viremia with VZV was demonstrable in 19% of 37 BMT patients who had no symptoms of zoster (Wilson et al., 1992). It seems most likely that these observations are indicative of subclinical reactivation of VZV, but reinfection with a viremia is not completely ruled out.

It is now recognized that decreased levels of CMI to VZV predispose to development of zoster, which may be either clinically apparent or subclinical. Following reactivation of VZV, positive CMI responses to the virus usually persist, and second attacks of clinical zoster are uncommon, even in immunocompromised patients. The return to positive VZV CMI levels not only occurs in BMT patients, but has also been observed in the elderly after zoster (Hayward et al., 1991). It is also of interest that poor CMI to VZV in susceptible adults who have been immunized with live attenuated varicella vaccine does not seem to predispose to zoster. This observation suggests there may be little or no latent VZV infection since the majority have never experienced viremia or harbored VZV on the skin which is believed to be the mechanism by which latent infection occurs (Hardy et al., 1991a,b).

5. Clinical zoster in immunocompromised patients

Following either allogeneic and autologous BMT, various studies have found that 20–40% and more recently as many as 60–70% of patients develop clinical zoster, almost entirely during the first or second year after transplantation, but usually following the first 100 days after transplantation (Locksley et al., 1985; Schuchter et al., 1989; Han et al., 1994; Koc

et al., 2000; Leung et al., 2000). Of BMT patients, those transplanted for lymphoma have the highest reported rates of zoster. Patients with malignancies, particularly lymphoma and leukemia, also experience a high rate of reactivation of VZV and clinical zoster. In one study in the 5 years after diagnosis of malignancy, the incidence of zoster was 5 times higher than in the general adult population (Raggozino et al., 1982). There are some data to suggest that the sites of the primary tumor and/or local radiotherapy predispose to development of zoster in that particular location (Rusthoven et al., 1988).

In a retrospective study of 231 patients who underwent BMT between 1969 and 1982, the probability of developing zoster was 30% (Locksley et al., 1985). There were 23 deaths associated with VZV infection, although many of these cases of zoster occurred before acyclovir therapy became available. Patients with acute graft-versus-host disease were more likely to develop dissemination and death from zoster. Cranial nerve zoster was particularly severe and painful. Abdominal zoster could present with protracted pain and fever prior to onset of rash, making diagnosis difficult. Two patients in this study died with generalized visceral VZV infection with no skin lesions (Locksley et al., 1985).

In another retrospective study of 153 patients who underwent autologous BMT, 28% developed zoster (at a median of 5 months later); 77% had localized zoster and 23% had generalized lesions (Schuchter et al., 1989). Some of these latter cases may have been second attacks of varicella. Most of these patients were treated with intravenous acyclovir, and there were no VZV-associated deaths. Morbidity, however, in 25%, included alopecia, postherpetic neuralgia, and neurologic dysfunction. Patients with systemic lupus erythematosis also have an increased incidence of zoster, due to immunologic impairment secondary to immunosuppressive therapy they have received (Nagasawa et al., 1990).

Although zoster is generally considered to be rare in children, children with malignancy and/or who have undergone BMT are also at increased risk to develop zoster, and the magnitude of their risk approaches that of adult cancer patients. Of

1132 children with malignant disease followed at St. Jude Children's Hospital in Memphis, TN (1962–1972), 101 developed zoster (Feldman et al., 1973). The incidence was highest, 22%, in children with Hodgkin's disease; the overall incidence was 9%. The following complications were noted: pneumonia, meningoencephalitis, thrombocytopenia, iritis, keratitis, and prolonged cutaneous zoster. In a smaller, more recent study of 199 children (1975–1985), 25% of leukemic children with prior varicella developed zoster; the overall rate was 16.5% (Novelli et al., 1988). A study of 236 children aged 2–18.5 years, who underwent autologous BMT in France, reported a 25% incidence of zoster, with no cases of visceral dissemination (Wacker et al., 1989).

Not only are immunocompromised patients more likely to develop zoster than immunocompetent individuals, but also they are at greater risk for development of both cutaneous and visceral dissemination of virus. Their incidence of post-herpetic neuralgia does not seem to be increased (Balfour, 1988), but acute pain may be severe (Rusthoven et al., 1988). The risk of dissemination appears to be related to the degree of immunocompromise.

Visceral zoster presenting with abdominal complaints such as pain, nausea, and vomiting, and hepatic involvement has been described, even in the absence of skin lesions (Stemmer et al., 1993; Rogers et al., 1995; David et al., 1998).

6. Zoster in HIV-infected patients

These patients are at increased risk to develop both classic zoster and a chronic, indolent form of the illness. Zoster, especially in a young adult, may be the presenting sign of HIV infection (Colebunders et al., 1988; Friedman-Kien et al., 1988). While most of these patients recover completely from zoster, some may develop a chronic skin infection due to VZV. These skin lesions are generalized, sparse, and may last for weeks. Some of these patients respond to administration of acyclovir, but VZV resistant to acyclovir has also been isolated from some of these patients (Pahwa et al., 1988; Hoppenjans et al., 1990; Linnemann et al., 1990). It is of particular interest and not fully explained, that while zoster is common in HIV-infected children and adults, it rarely causes visceral dissemination. The incidence of zoster increases as CMI and CD4 levels decrease as HIV infection progresses (Veenstra et al., 1995).

Pahwa and her colleagues reported a bizarre case of VZV infection that lasted 14 months in a severely immunodeficient HIV-infected child (Pahwa et al., 1988). When this 4-year-old girl was exposed to varicella, varicella-zoster immune globulin (VZIG) was given for passive immunization. Acyclovir was also administered after varicella developed, and the child recovered. Six weeks later, she developed localized thoracic zoster, for which she was again given acyclovir. Four weeks after the acyclovir was discontinued, she developed a few chronic disseminated VZV skin lesions. There were usually 1–2 vesicles at one time and never more than 10. Many lesions became hyperkeratotic and wart-like in appearance. It was possible to stop or control lesions with high doses of intravenous acyclovir, but they recurred when the drug was stopped. Antigens of VZV were demonstrated in lesions by immunofluorescence, but a viral culture was positive on only one occasion. This isolate was highly resistant to acyclovir, although it is unknown if resistance actually developed on treatment. Eventually, the girl developed a vasculitis, clinically attributed to VZV, that involved her central nervous system, leading to her death.

HIV-infected children who develop varicella in the setting of severe immunodeficiency are at an extraordinary high risk to develop zoster. In prospective studies of HIV-infected children, those who had less than 15% CD4 lymphocytes when they developed varicella had a 70% chance of developing zoster within a few years after varicella (Gershon et al., 1997). A comparison of the incidence of zoster in various types of patients is shown in Table I. Thus not only is a low CMI response prior to onset of zoster, but the CMI response at the time of the primary infection appears to be related, as well. It is possible that a strong CMI response to primary infection plays a role in controlling the degree of latent

TABLE I

Incidence of zoster per 1000 person-years of observation

Number	Group of patients	Incidence
548	Vaccinated children with leukemia	8
96	Children with leukemia, following natural varicella	25
331	Adults with HIV (varicella before HIV infection)	51 [2]
30	Children with HIV (varicella after HIV infection)	163 [2]
	With > 20% CD4 levels at varicella ($n = 20$)	30
	With < 20% CD4 levels at varicella ($n = 10$) [1]	467 [2]

Modified from Gershon et al. (1997). Adult data from Veenstra et al. (1995).

[1] 70% developed zoster.

[2] Incidence in HIV-infected children (including those with < 20% CD4 levels at varicella) and adults significantly different ($P =< 0.05$) by log-rank and Wilcoxon tests.

infection that occurs after varicella. Possibly those with low CMI develop a higher burden of latent infection than those with more intact CMI.

Unusual forms of zoster have also been described in HIV-infected patients. These include encephalitis, which may be difficult to diagnose if it occurs without any skin manifestations (Silliman et al., 1993; Burke et al., 1997; Iten et al., 1999). In addition, VZV may cause retinitis in HIV-infected patients (Moorthy et al., 1997). The prognosis for these patients may be improved with institution of antiviral therapy.

7. Diagnosis

The best method to diagnose VZV infections is either to demonstrate viral antigens or infectious virus in skin lesions. This will differentiate skin rashes caused by VZV from rashes caused by herpes simplex virus with which they may clinically be confused (Kalman and Laskin, 1986). Viral antigens may be demonstrated by scraping the base of a vesicular lesion, making a smear on a microscope slide, fixing the specimen, and staining it with commercially prepared fluorescein labeled monoclonal antibodies to VZV and HSV (Gershon and Forghani, 1995). This is a practical diagnostic test since it is widely available and yields an answer within about 1 h. Fluid may also be aspirated from vesicles and placed in viral transport medium for culture of VZV, which usually takes several days.

The diagnosis of VZV infection may also be made by antibody determinations although this method is somewhat inaccurate. The presence of specific IgM on one serum sample obtained during the acute illness is diagnostic. A four-fold or greater increase in antibody titers to VZV in sera obtained at onset of illness and again 2 weeks later is usually significant although, there are shared antigens between VZV and HSV that may on occasion lead to an erroneous identification (Gershon and Forghani, 1995). There are a variety of antibody tests for VZV with differing availability and sensitivity, so the physician is encouraged to consult the local laboratory when planning to obtain antibody titers for diagnostic purposes.

PCR is particularly useful to diagnose VZV infections. It is more sensitive than culture and can be performed on blood, CSF, vesicular fluid, and possibly other body fluids as well (LaRussa et al., 1993, 1994; Rogers et al., 1995; Burke et al., 1997; Iten et al., 1999).

8. Antiviral therapy and prophylaxis

Given the relative ease of administration of acyclovir, its low rate of toxicity, and its clear efficacy in speeding the healing of VZV infections, it is recommended that immunocompromised patients with zoster be promptly treated with this medication. Therapy is given not only as a life-saving measure, but also to decrease morbidity. High doses of intravenous acyclovir (1500 mg/m^2/day for children, and 30 mg/kg/day for adults, divided into three doses) are recommended (Whitley, 1992; Whitley and Gnann, 1992; Whitley and Straus, 1993). Treatment is usually given for 1–2 weeks, depending on the clinical course of the patient.

Since zoster is not always severe in immunocompromised patients, the oral form of acyclovir at high dosage may be considered in selected patients who are minimally immunosuppressed and whose zoster is mild and very localized. The oral formulation of acyclovir has been found to hasten the healing of zoster in elderly patients; a dose of 800 mg 5 times a day is given (Huff et al., 1993). There are no firm data on which to select a dose of oral acyclovir for HIV-infected children. Based on the author's experience, a dose of 900 mg/m^2 q.i.d. for 7–10 days or until 3 days after no new lesions have occurred could be tried. In deciding upon a dose of acyclovir for children, it is preferable to calculate the dosage on the basis of surface area rather than on weight. Patients who do not appear to be responding to oral acyclovir should be hospitalized and treated promptly with intravenous acyclovir.

Long-term oral therapy with acyclovir has been used to try to prevent recrudescence of chronic VZV infection in HIV-infected patients. Reactivation of VZV has occurred in some patients while they were receiving acyclovir (ACV) however, and double-blind placebo-controlled studies have not been done. Nevertheless, there is some anecdotal information suggesting efficacy (Pahwa et al., 1988; Hoppenjans et al., 1990; Linnemann et al., 1990). The decision whether to use long-term acyclovir must be individualized for every patient. There have been a number of recorded instances in which VZV resistant to acyclovir have developed after long-term oral therapy (Pahwa et al., 1988; Hoppenjans et al., 1990; Linnemann et al., 1990). Prompt development of zoster upon cessation of prophylactic acyclovir has also been a serious clinical problem (Selby et al., 1989; Sempere et al., 1992; Steer et al., 2000). Moreover, because of the increasing problem of viral drug resistance, long-term use of ACV should be avoided wherever possible.

Newer antiviral drugs for oral administration, famciclovir and valacyclovir, have the advantage of pharmacokinetic profiles that result in higher levels of active drug in the serum and therefore allow less frequent oral dosing. The adult dose of famciclovir is 500 mg orally three times a day, and that of valacyclovir is 1000 mg orally three times a day. Because higher serum levels of these drugs are attained following oral dosing, they are preferred over acyclovir for the treatment of zoster in adolescents and adults if oral therapy is to be used. There is little experience with these drugs in immunocompromised patients, however, and they should generally be used with caution and only in patients thought not to be significantly immunocompromised.

For zoster that is suspected or proven to be caused by VZV resistant to acyclovir, foscarnet may be employed. The usual intravenous dose of foscarnet is 180 mg/kg/day in two divided doses, adjusted according to renal function. Foscarnet has been found to be effective for acyclovir-resistant VZV in HIV-infected patients (Breton et al., 1988; Balfour et al., 1994). Foscarnet is significantly less well tolerated than acyclovir, often leading to renal toxicity and disturbance of electrolyte balance, and thus patients given this drug should be monitored closely.

9. Zoster in immunocompromised children vaccinated against chickenpox

Live attenuated varicella vaccine was developed in Japan by Takahashi and his colleagues in 1974 (Takahashi et al., 1974). This vaccine is highly protective against varicella in healthy and certain immunocompromised children, such as those with underlying leukemia (Gershon et al., 1999). It has been tested in three general groups, healthy children, healthy adults, and leukemic children. A summary of the efficacy and safety of varicella vaccine in these groups is shown on Table II. It will be noted from this table that although protection is the rule, some vaccinees may manifest a mild breakthrough case of chickenpox following exposure to VZV. A major reason for the development of this vaccine was

TABLE II

Summary of estimated safety and efficacy of varicella vaccine in various groups

Group	Seroconversion rate		Rate of vaccine-associated rash	Protective efficacy
	After 1 dose	After 2 doses		
Healthy children	95%	Not given	5%	90%
Healthy adults	85%	95%	5–10%	90%
Leukemic children	85%	95%	50%	90%

Based on data from Gershon et al. (1999).

to prevent severe or fatal varicella in children with leukemia.

Because it was known that children with leukemia had a high incidence of zoster, there was great interest in determining whether vaccination would be associated with a decreased incidence of this disease. Two studies reported from Japan, found zoster in 8/52 (15%) vaccinated children and in 11/63 (18%) controls, and 4/44 (9%) of vaccinees and 8/37 (22%) controls (Takahashi et al., 1974). Studies from the United States have indicated more clearly that the incidence of zoster after vaccination of leukemic children is lower than after natural infection. In a small study, none of 34 vaccinated leukemics, but 15 of 73 (21%) unmatched controls developed zoster ($P = 0.017$) (Brunell et al., 1986).

In the American Collaborative Vaccine Study, the rate of zoster was 2% in vaccinees and 15% in controls (Hardy et al., 1991a,b). Ninety-six leukemic vaccinees were prospectively matched, according to chemotherapeutic protocol, age, and sex, to 96 leukemic children who had experienced natural varicella. A life-table analysis revealed that the probability of developing zoster was greater in controls than in the vaccinees. Thus immunization offered a protective effect not only against varicella, but also against zoster in leukemic children. There are several possibilities as to why zoster may be less common after vaccination than after natural infection. The virus is attenuated, and it may not have access to sensory nerves if the skin is not infected, as is frequently the case after vaccination.

It was observed in Japan and in American studies that zoster occurs far more frequently in children who had experienced a VZV-associated rash than in those who never had a VZV-associated rash after immunization (Takahashi et al., 1974). In the American Collaborative Study, of 13 vaccinated leukemic children who developed zoster, 11 (85%) had a prior history of a VZV-related rash, either vaccine-associated (eight children) or breakthrough varicella (three children) (Hardy et al., 1991a). Both children with no history of rash developed zoster at the injection site of the vaccine. In the 268 vaccinees who had any type of previous VZV-related rash, the relative risk of subsequent development of zoster was 5.75, compared to the 280 vaccinees who had no VZV-associated rash. In this study, two cases of zoster were due to vaccine-type virus and two were caused by wild-type VZV. Those children with zoster caused by the wild-type virus had experienced mild breakthrough varicella after exposure to VZV. Bone marrow transplantation was also associated with an increased risk of zoster in the leukemic children who had been immunized (relative risk 7.5). These data support the concept that skin infection with VZV leads to latent neuronal infection.

Now that all children in the United States and Canada are being vaccinated routinely, similar benefits should accrue to those who go on to become immunocompromised in later life. One would predict that they should have less of a problem with zoster than immunocompromised patients seen in the late 1980s and 1990s.

10. Prevention

In a study of immunization of BMT patients with an inactivated varicella vaccine to boost their CMI response to VZV, the severity of varicella was decreased in comparison to control patients who were given placebo. The number of skin lesions that vaccinees manifested was about 10 times less than seen in controls, and none of the vaccinees had severe pain (Redman et al., 1997). Although the number of patients studied was small and the incidence of zoster was not affected by vaccination, these studies seem important to be confirmed and extended. There are no controlled data to support use of live varicella vaccine to boost immunity in immunocompromised patients and prevent zoster. A double-blind controlled study, however, is currently underway in elderly individuals, using a special formulation of VZV vaccine that is significantly more potent than the one licensed for prevention of varicella. Results from this study are expected to be available in several years.

11. The future

Our knowledge about the pathogenesis of zoster and how it can be prevented and treated has increased tremendously during the past 30 years. Predictably, even more progress will be made. The pathogenesis of zoster will certainly be clarified, and the mechanism by which CMI prevents its development will be discovered. It will probably be determined whether certain aspects of CMI, in particular cytotoxic T-cells, antibody-dependent cellular toxicity (ADCC), and natural killer (NK) cells are important in controlling latent virus. The specific antigens of VZV that are important in the CMI response to the virus need to be identified. In addition, hopefully the molecular mechanisms of pathogenesis, establishment, and control of latency will be determined. Studies are already underway to determine whether a live varicella vaccine can be used to boost immunity to VZV in the elderly and in HIV-infected children who have had natural varicella, to prevent or modify zoster. Early studies, indicating that vaccine can boost CMI to VZV, suggest that this approach might be effective (Berger et al., 1984; Gershon et al., 1996; Levin et al., 1998). Eventually, if the

population at large is vaccinated during childhood, the overall incidence of zoster may be predicted to decline, even in immunocompromised patients.

References

Arvin, A., Koropchak, C.M. and Wittek, A.E. (1983) Immunologic evidence of reinfection with varicella-zoster virus. J. Infect. Dis., 148: 200–205.

Arvin, A.M., Pollard, R.B., Rasmussen, L. and Merigan, T. (1978) Selective impairment in lymphocyte reactivity to varicella-zoster antigen among untreated lymphoma patients. J. Infect. Dis., 137: 531–540.

Arvin, A.M., Pollard, R.B., Rasmussen, L. and Merigan, T. (1980) Cellular and humoral immunity in the pathogenesis of recurrent herpes viral infections in patients with lymphoma. J. Clin. Invest., 65: 869–878.

Balfour, H.H. (1988) Varicella zoster virus infections in immunocompromised hosts. A review of the natural history and management. Am. J. Med., 85(2A): 68–73.

Balfour, H.H., Benson, C., Braun, J., Cassnes, B., Erice, A., Friedman-Kien, A., Klein, T., Polsky, B. and Safrin, S. (1994) Management of acyclovir-resistant herpes simplex and varicella-zoster infections. J. Acquired Immune Defic. Syndr., 7: 254–260.

Berger, R., Florent, G. and Just, M. (1981) Decrease of the lympho-proliferative response to varicella-zoster virus antigen in the aged. Infect. Immun., 32: 24–27.

Berger, R., Luescher, D. and Just, M. (1984) Enhancement of varicella-zoster-specific immune responses in the elderly by boosting with varicella vaccine. J. Infect. Dis., 149: 647.

Breton, G., Fillet, A.-M., Katlama, C., Bricaire, F. and Caumes, E. (1988) Acyclovir-resistant herpes zoster in human immunodeficiency virus-infected patients: results of foscarnet therapy. Clin. Infect. Dis., 27: 1525–1527.

Brunell, P., Gershon, A.A., Uduman, S.A. and Steinberg, S. (1975) Varicella-zoster immunoglobulins during varicella, latency, and zoster. J. Infect. Dis., 132: 49–54.

Brunell, P.A., Taylor-Wiedeman, J., Geiser, C.F., Frierson, L. and Lydick, E. (1986) Risk of herpes zoster in children with leukemia: varicella vaccine compared with history of chickenpox. Pediatrics, 77: 53–56.

Burke, B.L., Steele, R.W., Beard, O.W., Wood, J.S., Cain, T.D. and Marmer, D.J. (1982) Immune responses to varicella-zoster in the aged. Arch. Intern. Med., 142: 291–293.

Burke, D.G., Kalayjian, R.C., Vann, V.R., Madreperla, S.A., Shick, H.E. and Leonard, D.G.B. (1997) Polymerase chain reaction detection and clinical significance of varicella-zoster virus in cerebrospinal fluid from human immunodeficiency virus-infected patients. J. Infect. Dis., 176: 1080–1084.

Colebunders, R., Mann, J., Francis, H., Bila, K.L.I., Ilwaya, M., Kakonde, N., Quinn, T.J.C. and Piot, P. (1988) Herpes zoster in African patients: a clinical predictor of human immunodeficiency virus infection. J. Infect. Dis., 157: 314–319.

Croen, K.D., Ostrove, J.M., Dragovic, L.Y. and Straus, S.E. (1988) Patterns of gene expression and sites of latency in human ganglia are different for varicella-zoster and herpes simplex viruses. Proc. Soc. Natl. Acad. Sci. USA, 85: 9773–9777.

David, D.S., Tegtmeier, B.R., O'Donnel, M.R., Paz, I.B. and McCartty, T.M. (1998) Visceral varicella-zoster after bone marrow transplantation: report of a case series and review of the literature. Am. J. Gasteroenterol., 93: 810–813.

Feldman, S., Hughes, W.T. and Kim, H.Y. (1973) Herpes zoster in children with cancer. Am. J. Dis. Child., 126: 178–184.

Friedman-Kien, A., Lafleur, F., Gendler, F., Hennessey, N., Montagna, R., Halbert, S., Rubenstein, S., Krasinski, K., Zang, E. and Poiesz, B.A. (1988) Herpes zoster: a possible early clinical sign for development of acquired immunodeficiency syndrome in high-risk individuals. J. Am. Acad. Dermatol., 14: 1023–1028.

Garland, J. (1943) Varicella following exposure to herpes zoster. New Engl. J. Med., 228: 336–337.

Gershon, A. and Forghani, B. (1995) Varicella-Zoster Virus. In: E. Lennette (Ed.), Diagnostic Procedures for Viral, Rickettsial, and Chlamydial Infections. American Public Health Association, Washington, DC, pp. 601–613.

Gershon, A., LaRussa, P., Steinberg, S., Lo, S.H., Mervish, N. and Meier, P. (1996) The protective effect of immunologic boosting against zoster: an analysis in leukemic children who were vaccinated against chickenpox. J. Infect. Dis., 173: 450–453.

Gershon, A., Mervish, N., LaRussa, P., Steinberg, S., Lo, S.-H., Hodes, D., Fikrig, S., Bonagura, V. and Bakshi, S. (1997) Varicella-zoster virus infection in children with underlying HIV infection. J. Infect. Dis., 176: 1496–1500.

Gershon, A. and Steinberg, S. (1981) Antibody responses to varicella-zoster virus and the role of antibody in host defense. Am. J. Med. Sci., 282: 12–17.

Gershon, A., Steinberg, S., Borkowsky, W., Lennette, D. and Lennette, E. (1982) IgM to varicella-zoster virus: demonstration in patients with and without clinical zoster. Pediatr. Infect. Dis., 1: 164–167.

Gershon, A., Steinberg, S. and LaRussa, P. (1992) Varicella-Zoster Virus. In: E.H. Lennette (Ed.), Laboratory Diagnosis of Viral Infections. Marcel Dekker, New York, pp. 749–765.

Gershon, A., Takahashi, M. and White, C.J. (1999) Live attenuated varicella vaccine. In: S. Plotkin and W. Orenstein (Eds.), Vaccines, 3rd edn., WB Saunders, pp. 475–507.

Gershon, A.A., Steinberg, S. and Gelb, L., NIAID-Collaborative-Varicella-Vaccine-Study-Group. (1984) Clinical reinfection with varicella-zoster virus. J. Infect. Dis., 149: 137–142.

Han, C.S., Miller, W., Haake, R. and Weisdorf, D. (1994) Varicella zoster infection after bone marrow transplantation: incidence, risk factors and complications. Bone Marrow Transplant., 13: 277–283.

Hardy, I.B., Gershon, A., Steinberg, S., LaRussa, P. et al. (1991a) Incidence of zoster after live attenuated varicella vaccine. In: International Conference on Antimicrobial Agents and Chemotherapy, Chicago, IL.

Hardy, I.B., Gershon, A., Steinberg, S., LaRussa, P., et al. (1991b) The incidence of zoster after immunization with live attenuated varicella vaccine. A study in children with leukemia. New Engl. J. Med., 325: 1545–1550.

Hayakawa, Y., Torigoe, S., Shiraki, K., Yamanishi, K. and Takahashi, M. (1984) Biologic and biophysical markers of a live varicella vaccine strain (Oka): identification of clinical isolates from vaccine recipients. J. Infect. Dis., 149: 956–963.

Hayward, A., Levin, M., Wolf, W., Angelova, G., Gilden, D. (1991) Varicella-zoster virus-specific immunity after herpes zoster. J. Infect. Dis., 163: 873–875.

Hope-Simpson, R.E. (1965) The nature of herpes zoster: a long term study and a new hypothesis. Proc. R. Soc. Med., 58: 9–20.

Hoppenjans, W.B., Bibler, M.R., Orme, R.L. and Solinger, A.S. (1990) Prolonged cutaneous herpes zoster in acquired immunodeficiency syndrome. Arch. Dermatol., 126: 1048–1050.

Huff, J.C., Drucker, J.L., Clemmer, A., Laskin, O., Connor, J.D., Bryson, Y.J. and Balfour, H.H. (1993) Effect of oral acyclovir on pain resolution in herpes zoster: a reanalysis. J. Med. Virol., Suppl. 1: 93–96.

Iten, A. et al. (1999) Impact of CSF PCR on the management of HIV-infected patients with VZV infection of the CNS. J. Neurovirol., 5: 172–180.

Jordan, G.W. and Merigan, T.C. (1974) Cell-mediated immunity to varicella-zoster virus; in vitro lymphocyte responses. J. Infect. Dis., 130: 495–501.

Kalman, C.M. and Laskin, O.L. (1986) Herpes zoster and zosteriform herpes simplex virus infections in immunocompetent adults. Am. J. Med., 81: 775–778.

Kennedy, P.G., Grinfeld, E. and Gow, J.W. (1999) Latent VZV in human dorsal root ganglia. Virology, 258: 451–454.

Koc, Y., Miller, K.B., Schenkein, D.P., Griffith, J., Akhtar, M., DesJardin, J. and Snydman, D.R. (2000) Varicella zoster virus infections following allogeneic bone marrow transplantation: frequency, risk factors, and clinical outcome. Biol. Blood Marrow Transpl., 6: 44–49.

LaRussa, P., Hughes, P., Pearce, J., Lepow, M., Steinberg, S., Lipsitz, S. and Gershon, A. (1993) Use of polymerase chain reaction (PCR) assay to identify and type varicella zoster virus. In: Society for Pediatric Research Annual Meeting, Washington, DC, Abstract 1026.

LaRussa, P., Steinberg, S. and Gershon, A. (1994) Diagnosis and typing of varicella-zoster virus (VZV) in clinical specimens by polymerase chain reaction (PCR). In: 34th ICAAC, Orlando, FL.

Leung, T.F., Chik, K.W., Li, C.K., Shing, M.M., Chan, P.K. and Yuen, P.M. (2000) Incidence, risk factors and outcome of varicella-zoster infection in children after hematopoetic stem cell transplantation. Bone Marrow Transplant., 25: 167–172.

Levin, M., Barber, D., Goldblatt, E., Jones, M., LaFleur, B., Chan, C., Stinson, D., Zerbe, G.O. and Hayward, A. (1998) Use of a live attenuated varicella vaccine to boost varicella-specific immune responses in seropositive people 55 years of age and older: duration of booster effect. J. Infect. Dis., 178: S109–112.

Linnemann, C.C., Biron, K.K., Hoppenjans, W.G. and Solinger, A.M. (1990) Emergence of acyclovir-resistant varicella zoster virus in an AIDS patient on prolonged acyclovir therapy. AIDS, 4: 577–579.

Ljungman, P., Lonnqvist, B., Gahrton, G., Ringden, O., Sundqvist, V.-A. and Wahren, B. (1986) Clinical and subclinical reactivations of varicella-zoster virus in immunocompromised patients. J. Infect. Dis., 153: 840–847.

Locksley, R.M., Flournoy, N., Sullivan, K.M. and Meyers, J. (1985) Infection with varicella-zoster virus after marrow transplantation. J. Infect. Dis., 152: 1172–1181.

Luby, J., Ramirez-Ronda, C., Rinner, S., Hull, A. and Vergne-Marini, P. (1977) A longitudinal study of varicella zoster virus infections in renal transplant recipients. J. Infect. Dis., 135: 659–663.

Lungu, O., Annunziato, P., Gershon, A., Stegatis, S., Josefson, D., LaRussa, P. and Silverstein, S. (1995) Reactivated and latent varicella-zoster virus in human dorsal root ganglia. Proc. Natl. Acad. Sci. USA, 92: 10980 10984.

Lungu, O., Panagiotidis, C., Annunziato, P., Gershon, A. and Silverstein, S. (1998) Aberrant intracellular localization of varicella-zoster virus regulatory proteins during latency. Proc. Natl. Acad. Sci. USA, 95: 780–785.

Mahalingham, R., Wellish, M., Cohrs, R., Debrus, S., Piette, J., Rentier, B. and Gilden, D.H. (1996) Expression of protein encoded by varicella-zoster virus open reading frame 63 in latently infected human ganglionic neurons. Proc. Natl. Acad. Sci. USA, 93: 2122–2124.

Mahalingham, R., Wellish, M., Lederer, D., Forghani, B., Cohrs, R. and Gilden, D. (1993) Quantitation of latent varicella-zoster virus DNA in human trigeminal ganglia by polymerase chain reaction (PCR). J. Virol., 67: 2381–2384.

Mahalingham, R., Wellish, M., Wolf, W., Dueland, A.N., Cohrs, R., Vafai, A. and Gilden, D. (1990) Latent varicella-zoster viral DNA in human trigeminal and thoracic ganglia. New Engl. J. Med., 323: 627–631.

Merigan, T.C. and Stevens, D.A. (1978) The use of zoster immune globulin in the prevention of varicella and treatment of zoster. In: Fifteenth Congress of the International Blood Transfusion Society, Paris, France.

Meyers, J.D., Flurnoy, N. and Thomas, E.D. (1980) Cell-mediated immunity to varicella-zoster virus after allogeneic bone marrow transplantation. J. Infect. Dis., 141: 479–487.

Miller, A.E. (1980) Selective decline in cellular immune response to varicella-zoster in the elderly. Neurology, 30: 582–587.

Moorthy, R.S., Weinberg, D.V., Teich, S.A., Berger, B.B., Minturn, J.T., Kumar, S., Rao, N.A., Fowell, S.M., Loose, I.A. and Jampol, L.M. (1997) Management of varicella zoster virus retinitis in AIDS. Br. J. Ophthalmol., 81: 189–194.

Nagasawa, K., Yamauchi, Y., Tada, Y., Kusaba, T., Niho, Y. and Yoshikawa, H. (1990) High incidence of herpes zoster in patients with systemic lupus erythematosus: an immunological analysis. Ann. Rheum. Dis., 49: 630–633.

Novelli, V.M., Brunell, P.A., Geiser, C.F., Narkewicz, S. and Frierson, L. (1988) Herpes zoster in children with acute lymphocytic leukemia. Am. J. Dis. Child., 142: 71–72.

Pahwa, S., Biron, K., Lim, W., Swenson, P., Kaplan, M., Sadick, N. and Pahwa, R. (1988) Continuous varicella-zoster infection associated with acyclovir resistance in a child with AIDS. J. Am. Med. Assoc., 260: 2879–2882.

Raggozino, M., Melton, J., Kurland, L., Chu, C. and Perry, H. (1982) Risk of cancer after herpes zoster. New Engl. J. Med., 307: 393–397.

Rand, K.H., Rasmussen, L.E., Pollard, R.B., Arvin, A. and Merigan, T. (1977) Cellular immunity and herpesvirus infections in cardiac transplant patients. New Engl. J. Med., 296: 1372–1377.

Redman, R., Nader, S., Zerboni, L., Liu, C., Wong, R.M., Brown, B.W. and Arvin, A.M. (1997) Early reconstitution of immunity and decreased severity of herpes zoster in bone marrow transplant recipients immunized with inactivated varicella vaccine. J. Infect. Dis., 176: 578–585.

Rogers, S.Y., Irving, W. and Russell, N.H. (1995) Visceral varicella zoster infection after bone marrow transplantation without skin involvement and the use of PCR for diagnosis. Bone Marrow Transplant., 15: 805–807.

Rusthoven, J.J., Ahlgren, P., Elhakin, T., Pinfold, P., Reid, J., Stewart, L. and Feld, R. (1988) Varicella-zoster infection in adult cancer patients: a population study. Archiv. Int. Med., 148: 1561–1566.

Schuchter, L.M., Wingard, J.R., Piantadosi, S., Burns, W.H., Santos, G.W. and Saral, R. (1989) Herpes zoster infection after autologous bone marrow transplantation. Blood, 74: 1424–1427.

Selby, P.J., Powles, R.L., Easton, D., Perren, T.J., Stolle, K. Jameson, B., Fiddian, A.P., Tryhorn, Y. and Stern, H. (1989) The prophylactic role of intravenous and long-term oral acyclovir after allogenic bone marrow transplantation. Br. J. Cancer, 59: 434–438.

Sempere, A., Sanz, G.F., Senet, L., de al Rubia, I., Jarque, F., Lopez, M.J., Arilla, M., Guinot, M., Martin, G., Martinez, J., Marty, M.L. and Sanz, M.A. (1992) Long-term acyclovir prophylaxis for prevention of varicella-zoster virus infection after autologous bone stem cell transplantation in patients with acute leukemia. Bone Marrow Transplant., 10: 495–498.

Silliman, C.C., Tedder, D., Ogle, J.W., Simon, J., Kleinschmidt-DeMasters, B.K., Manco-Johnson, M. and Levin, M.J. (1993) Unsuspected varicella-zoster virus encephalitis in a child with acquired immunodeficiency syndrome. J. Pediatr., 123: 418–422.

Steer, C.B., Szer, J., Sasadeusz, J., Matthews, J.P., Beresford,

J.A. and Grigg, A. (2000) Varicella-zoster infection after allogeneic bone marrow transplantation: incidence, risk factors and prevention with low-dose aciclovir and ganciclovir. Bone Marrow Transplant., 25: 657–664.

Stemmer, S.M., Kinsman, K., Tellchow, S. and Jones, R.B. (1993) Fatal noncutaneous visceral infection with varicella-zoster virus in a patient with lymphoma after autologous bone marrow transplantation. Clin. Infect. Dis., 16: 497–499.

Stevens, D. and Merigan, T. (1980) Zoster immune globulin prophylaxis of disseminated zoster in compromised hosts. Arch. Int. Med., 140: 52–54.

Straus, S.E., Reinhold, W., Smith, H.A., Ruyechan, W., Henderson, D., Blaese, R.M. and Hay, J. (1984) Endonuclease analysis of viral DNA from varicella and subsequent zoster infections in the same patient. New Engl. J. Med., 311: 1362–1364.

Takahashi, M., Otsuka, T., Okuno, Y., Asano, Y., Yazaki, T. and Isomura, S. (1974) Live vaccine used to prevent the spread of varicella in children in hospital. Lancet, 2: 1288–1290.

Uduman, S.A., Gershon, A.A. and Brunell, P.A. (1975) Should patients with zoster receive zoster immune globulin. J. Am. Med. Assoc., 234: 1049.

Veenstra, J., Krol, A., van Praag, R., Frissen, P., Schellekens, P., Lange, J., Coutinho, R. and van der Meer, J. (1995) Herpes zoster, immunological deterioration and disease progression in HIV-1 infection. AIDS, 9: 1153–1158.

Wacker, P., Hartmann, O., Benhamou, E., Salloum, E. and Lemerle, J. (1989) Varicella-zoster virus infections after autologous bone marrow transplantation in children. Bone Marrow Transplant., 4: 191–194.

Whitley, R. (1992) Therapeutic approaches to varicella-zoster virus infections. J. Infect. Dis., 166: S51–57.

Whitley, R.J. and Gnann, J.W. (1992) Acyclovir: a decade later. New Engl. J. Med., 327: 782–789.

Whitley, R.J. and Straus, S. (1993) Therapy for varicella-zoster virus infections: where do we stand. Infect. Dis. Clin. Pract., 2: 100–108.

Williams, D.L., Gershon, A., Gelb, L.D., Spraker, M.K., Steinberg, S. and Ragab, A.H. (1985) Herpes zoster following varicella vaccine in a child with acute lymphocytic leukemia. J. Pediatr., 106: 259–261.

Wilson, A., Sharp, M., Koropchak, C., Ting, S. and Arvin, A. (1992) Subclinical varicella-zoster virus viremia, herpes zoster, and T lymphocyte immunity to varicella-zoster viral antigens after bone marrow transplantation. J. Infect. Dis., 165: 119–126.

Herpes Zoster and Postherpetic Neuralgia, 2nd Revised and Enlarged Edition
Pain Research and Clinical Management, Vol. 11
Edited by C.P.N. Watson and A.A. Gershon

CHAPTER 11

Ophthalmic zoster

Deborah Pavan-Langston [*]

Department of Ophthalmology, Harvard Medical School, and Massachusetts Eye and Ear Infirmary, Clinical Virology, 243
Charles St., Boston, MA 02114, USA

1. Epidemiology

The steadily rising incidence of herpes zoster is a function of increased disturbance of cell-mediated immunity in a population that is aging, more often treated with immunosuppressive agents, and in the midst of an HIV epidemic. Ophthalmic zoster, or HZO, is second only to thoracic in frequency with up to 250,000 cases annually in the United States. Of these, 50–70% suffer visual morbidity (Hope-Simpson, 1965; Ragozzino et al., 1982; Harding et al., 1987; Donahue et al., 1995; Weller, 1995; Pavan-Langston and Dunkel, 1996; Pepose, 1997; Gilden et al., 2000). Studies have shown that the trigeminal sensory ganglion is the most frequent site of latency for varicella virus (VZV). It reactivates in 10–25% of the population, travels back down the first division of the Vth cranial nerve, and erupts in that dermatome to cause often devastating disease (Mahalingam et al., 1990, 1993). Demography is variable in reporting sexual predominance, but it is consistent in showing a steady increase in incidence and severity with age, particularly in the 5th–8th decade of life.

2. Clinical disease

Initial symptoms are usually fever, malaise, and chills, often with severe neuralgia over the distribution of V-1. Combing the hair or wearing a hat may be unbearably painful. The wide variety of ocular findings are listed in Table I. Ninety-three percent of patients suffer acute pain with persistence in about one-third of cases at 6 months time; the incidence is >70% in those over 80 years of age (Liesegang, 1984; Harding, 1993; Pavan-Langston, 2000).

Dermatitis develops in 90% of patients within 3 days of pain onset appearing in multiple crops of infectious watery vesicles on an erythematous, possibly hemorrhagic base (Fig. 1A,B). These form escars and frequently leave tell-tale scarring over the dermatomal map after a 2–4-week healing period. Rarely, *zoster sine herpete* occurs with ocular findings, but no dermatitis. Virus has been isolated from the aqueous in some of these cases (Yamamoto et al., 1995). Zoster dermatitis is generally not a recurring phenomenon.

Inflammation of the 'white' of the eye takes the form of conjunctivitis, episcleritis and scleritis. These often occur acutely and may recur months to years later. Conjunctivitis tends to be diffuse while the underlying episclera and sclera are focal

---
[*] Correspondence to: Dr. D. Pavan-Langston, Massachusetts Eye and Ear Infirmary, Clinical Virology, 243 Charles St., Boston, MA 02114, USA. Phone: +1 (617) 573-4041; Fax: +1 (617) 573-4369; E-mail: dpl@vision.eri.harvard.edu

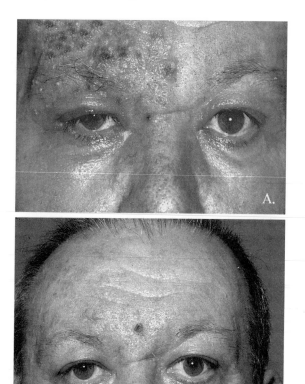

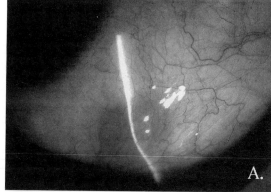

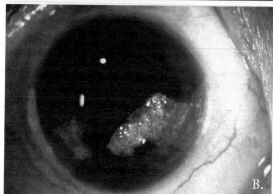

Fig. 1. (A) Acute zoster ophthalmicus involving the 1st division of the trigeminal nerve with crops of vesicles in various stages of maturity. (B) Same patient 1 month later with residual tell-tale scarring of forehead as dermatitis resolves.

Fig. 2. (A) Acute zoster nodular episcleritis which resolved slowly over several months with mild topical steroid and oral non-steroidal antiinflammatory agents. (B) Calcium deposition in subepithelial space to form band keratopathy in chronic ocular zoster.

inflammatory responses and may be flat or nodular (Fig. 2A). There may be residual scleral thinning.

Corneal involvement occurs in about 65% of cases and is a keratitis which assumes three general forms, all of which may occur separately or together. These are: (1) infectious epithelial pseudodendrites; (2) trophic mechanical ulcers; and (3) stromal immune reaction. With chronic ocular inflammation calcium often precipitates out of the tear film to deposit beneath the corneal epithelium (Fig. 2B).

The dendritiform lesions occur both acutely and in delayed recurrent disease in which case they may be called 'delayed mucous plaques'. They may be confused with herpes simplex dendritic lesions (Fig. 3A,B). Early and late VZV lesions may be PCR$^+$ for viral DNA and virus cultures have been

positive during acute disease (Piebenga and Laibson, 1973; Pavan-Langston and McCulley, 1973; Forrest and Kaufman, 1976; Marsh, 1976; Marsh and Cooper, 1987; Liesegang, 1985; Pavan-Langston et al., 1995; Yamamoto et al., 1995). Zoster dendrites may be differentiated from those caused by herpes simplex virus in that the former are raised, superficial lesions with tapered endings while the latter tend to cause frank epithelial defects with bulbous endings.

Mechanical (trophic) epithelial ulcers occur in more than 25% of patients at some point and are due to poor healing in the face of corneal anesthesia and aqueous tear deficiency secondary to the destructive ganglionitis with loss of the nasolacrimal reflex. This condition may be further aggravated by poor lid

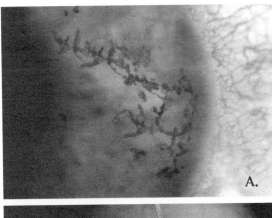

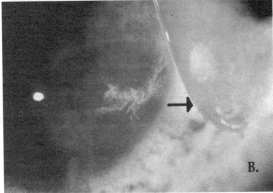

Fig. 3. (A) Acute pseudodendritic (branching) infectious varicella/zoster keratitis appearing on day 4 after onset of rash. (B) Late pseudodendritic zoster keratitis developing silently 1 year after acute disease and discovered incidentally upon moving therapeutic contact lens (arrow). Lesion was positive for VZV antigen by PCR.

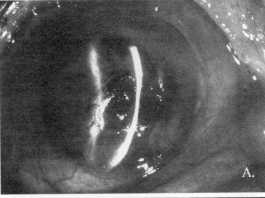

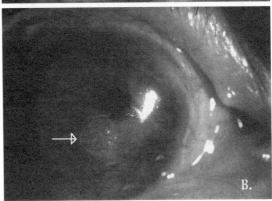

Fig. 4. (A) Thinning corneal ulcer (note narrowing of light beam) in anesthetic cornea. Perforation is threatened. (B) Same eye immediately after sterile tissue adhesive (cyanoacrylate glue) has been applied to seal ulcer (arrow). Plano T therapeutic lens was then placed over adhesive.

function (Liesegang, 1985; Pavan-Langston, 2000). The corneal surface is dull with a course punctate keratitis preceding actual breakdown of the epithelium. Persistence of the defect may result in collagenolytic enzyme release from keratocytes, corneal melting and perforation (Fig. 4A,B).

Stromal keratitis is essentially an immune reaction to viral antigen deposited during the acute attack and possibly during late subclinical migration of virus from the ganglion. Assay for VZV DNA has been positive in some reported cases (Wenkel et al., 1993; Yu et al., 1993; Pavan-Langston et al., 1995). A non-necrotic translucent disciform keratitis representing inflammatory edema may occur any time after the acute event, most commonly at 3–4 months time. Clusters of lymphocytes may be clinging to the

endothelium as keratic precipitates (KPs) (Marsh, 1976; Reijo et al., 1983). Another form of VZV immune reaction is a necrotic interstitial keratitis (IK) characterized by a dense white infiltrate often with new vessel growth into the cornea (Fig. 5A,B). Both of these forms of keratitis are similar to that seen in HSV disease and may be confused with it in the absence of a clear history of HZO. The resulting band keratopathy is opaque, may cause ulceration, and may be removed with EDTA chelation.

Iritis or iridocyclitis affects about 40% of HZO patients acutely and may recur years later (Womack and Liesegang, 1983). It is felt to be an immune reaction to invasion of the uveal structure by infectious VZV or to antigen deposited by the virus. VZV DNA has been detected in the aqueous (Liesegang,

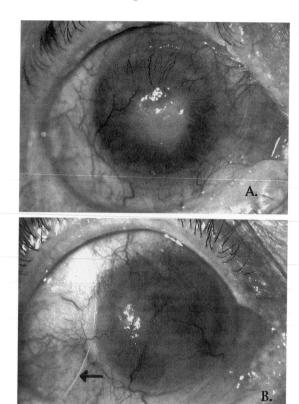

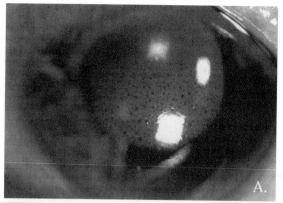

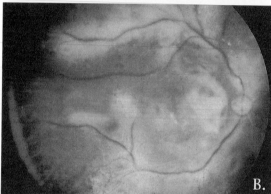

Fig. 5. (A) Chronic neurotrophic ulcerative keratitis over chronic stromal immune keratitis post HZO. Neovascular pannus is moving in 360° in cornea's attempt at tissue repair. (B) Same eye 6 months later after ulcer has healed under therapeutic contact lens (arrow) leaving immune stromal scarring under pannus.

Fig. 6. (A) Acute and chronic iritis with fresh lymphocytic keratic precipitates (KPs) coating back of cornea pupil irregularity due to iris sphincter atrophy secondary to repeated attacks of iritis. (B) Acute retinal necrosis (ARN) of retina due appearing 1 month after acute ocular zoster in immunocompetent patient. Note exudates follow pattern of vascular arcades.

1984; Yamamoto et al., 1995; Wilson, 1996). Clinical findings may include deep aching, cirumcorneal hyperemia, lymphocytic precipitates on the corneal endothelium (KPs), cells and protein flare in the aqueous, iris scarring to the lens, sectoral iris pigment atrophy, and sphincter damage (Fig. 6A). Secondary cataract formation from the combined insult of inflammation and the topical steroids necessary to treat it is common.

Glaucoma may be secondary to white blood cell blockage of the trabecular drainage system in the angle of the anterior chamber, or to inflammatory scarring of the iris to the corneal periphery thus sealing off the angle. Intraocular pressure may initially be low or normal due to inflammatory inhibition of normal aqueous production. As this production returns to normal with recovery secondary glaucoma may make itself known as the intraocular pressure steadily goes up (Naumann et al., 1968; Womack and Liesegang, 1983; Liesegang, 1984).

Extraocular muscle palsies may involve the 3rd, 4th, and/or 6th cranial nerves to produce marked restriction of eye movement, lid droop, and disturbing diplopia. Even the most severe of these, will, however, largely resolve over weeks leaving some residual ptosis in most patients.

The retinitis of HZO is not common, but may result in optic neuritis, major vascular occlusions, necrotizing retinitis with hemorrhaging and exudates (Culbertson et al., 1986; Browning et al., 1987;

Engstrom et al., 1994; Culbertson and Dix, 1996; Ganatra et al., 2000). Acute retinal necrosis (ARN) occurs in immunocompetent and suppressed patients involves the posterior pole with infiltrates, blotchy hemorrhages, arteriolitis and phlebitis (Fig. 6B). Vision drops rapidly as this progresses. The differential diagnosis includes HSV, cytomegalovirus, toxoplasma, syphilis, large cell lymphoma and Behçet's disease. Immunocompromised patients may also develop progressive outer retinal necrosis (PORN) which begins insidiously in the retinal periphery spreading with little overt inflammation to cause gradual constriction of the peripheral vision and lastly loss of central sight from retinal necrosis.

Neuralgia, both acute and late (post-herpetic, PHN), is more common in ophthalmic than other forms of zoster. They vary in incidence with increasing age (Ragozzino et al., 1982; Cobo et al., 1985, 1986, 1987; Donahue et al., 1995). Acute neuralgia is seen in less than 15% of patients under age 20 years, about 40% in patients between 30 and 50 years and only 20% in patients over this age. In contrast, chronic pain, or PHN lasting more than 1 year, is seen in less than 4% of patients under 20 years, 10% in those up to age 50 years, and 50% or higher in those in the 5th–8th decades of life (DeMoragas and Kierland, 1957). PHN is variably described as constant boring pain, sudden transient lancinating pain, pain elicited by usually non-painful stimuli, e.g. wind, severe itching. Maximum recovery is achieved by 2 years with little change in status after that time.

The HIV epidemic has played a major role in the increasing incidence of VZV disease, and consequently, HZO, especially in the young adult population. In the immunocompromised patient the dermatitis, and ocular inflammatory disease are more prolonged and often need intravenous antiviral therapy to induce resolution. In one study of HZO in HIV[+] patients, one-third had no ocular involvement (just dermatitis), one-third a keratitis, and half had iritis (Margolis et al., 1998). Only 4% had PHN which may reflect the relatively young age of the affected population. The dendritiform epithelial keratitis may occur acutely or as long as 6 years after the acute illness and assume a painful, chronic, drug-resistant form (Chern et al., 1998). Response to antiviral therapy is variable with a variety of drugs often tried before response is seen: topical trifluridine or vidarabine, oral acyclovir or famciclovir, i.v. foscarnet or cidofovir.

3. Prevention of HZO

The advent of the varicella vaccine may hold promise for dramatically reducing the overall incidence of zoster, and, therefore, HZO, in the foreseeable future. Limited data indicates that the incidence of zoster is notably lower in vaccinated healthy children and adults compared to those who suffered a natural infection (Gershon, 1995). Furthermore, the marked drop in zoster cell-mediated immunity by age 50 years and the excellent immune response to vaccine in the older population suggests that vaccinating even those patients who have had chicken pox in childhood may be highly effective in reducing the incidence of zoster in patients over 50 years of age (Levin et al., 1998).

4. Management of HZO (Table I)

The therapy of acute zoster is currently defined by use of systemic antivirals, and tricyclic antidepressants (TCAs) to inhibit acute and chronic pain.

4.1. Antivirals

Antiviral therapy is significantly more effective if begun within 72 h of rash onset. Compared to placebo acyclovir (Zostrix™) therapy, 800 mg p.o. 5×/day for 7–10 days, induces a prompt resolution of skin rash, cessation of pain, more rapid healing, reduced duration of viral shedding, and reduced duration of new lesion formation. There is also a significant reduction in the incidence and severity of acute dendritiform keratopathy, scleritis, episcleritis, iritis, the incidence (but not the severity if it occurred) of corneal stromal immune keratitis, and the incidence of late-onset ocular inflammatory disease (Cobo et

TABLE I

Guidelines to therapy of herpes zoster ophthalmicus

Acute disease

Antivirals: Treat for 7 days, preferably starting within 72 h of onset of rash.

a. Famciclovir (Famvir™) 500 mg p.o. t.i.d. (immunocompetent or compromised) <u>or</u>
b. Valaciclovir (Valtrex™) 1 g p.o. t.i.d. (immunocompetent), <u>or</u>
c. Acyclovir (Zovirax™) 800 mg p.o. 5 i.d.
d. Immunocompromised patients: i.v. ACV for 10 days. 10 mg/kg q. 8 h in adults and 500 mg/m^2 q. 8 h for children under 12 years of age.

Pain prevention/management

a. TCA antidepressants, e.g. nortriptyline, desipramine 10–100 mg p.o. q.h.s. or divided dose ×3 m (or longer PRN) starting lowest dose as early as possible after acute disease onset, titrating up PRN. Use with caution in patients with cardiac disease.
b. Non-narcotic or short-term narcotic analgesics, e.g. oxycodone, codeine, propoxyphene.

Skin therapy

a. Cool to tepid wet compresses (if tolerated) to keep involved skin clean.

Ocular anterior segment

a. Poor lid closure (exposure): topical antibiotic ophthalmic ointment t.i.d.
b. Corneal dendritiform keratopathy: therapy ×2–3 weeks (variably effective).
   1. 3% vidarabine ointment, or
   2. 1% trifluridine 5 i.d., or
   3. oral antivirals (see above).
c. Corneal immune disease, episcleritis, scleritis or iritis:
   1. Topical steroids (1.0–0.125% prednisolone or 0.1% dexamethasone q, 2 h → q.i.d. PRN disease severity. Slow taper over weeks to months. Antibiotic gtt/ointment prophylaxis.
   2. Oral NSAIDs, e.g. ibuprofen 400 mg p.o. t.i.d.
   3. Antivirals unnecessary.
   4. Mydriatic/cycloplegia for iritis (scopolamine q.d.).
d. Glaucoma:
   1. Topical β-blockers e.g. timolol or carteolol b.i.d.
   2. May add other agents, such as latanaprost q.d., brinzolamide or dorzolamide b.i.d.
   3. <u>No</u> miotics, e.g. pilocarpine.
   4. Topical steroids if glaucoma due to inflammatory trabeculitis.

---

al., 1985, 1986; Borruat et al., 1991; Harding and Porter, 1991; Hoang-Xuan et al., 1992). Effect on PHN is variable with some reports showing no efficacy, and others significant decrease in severity and incidence (Cobo et al., 1986; Harding and Porter, 1991; Hoang-Xuan et al., 1992; Aylward et al., 1994; McGill and White, 1994; Pepose, 1997).

Famciclovir (Famvir™) 500 mg p.o. t.i.d. for 1 week was significantly better than placebo or acyclovir in significantly decreasing the duration and incidence of acute pain, viral shedding, and lesion duration, and in reducing the duration of PHN in non-ocular zoster (DeGreef, 1995; Tyring et al.,

1995; Tyring, 1996). There are, as yet, no published reports on famciclovir and HZO, but a recent masked, multicenter study comparing the efficacy of FCV with ACV indicates that it is comparable in all ophthalmic parameters going out to 6 months of follow up (Tyring et al., 2000) PHN was not addressed.

Valaciclovir (Valtrex™) 1 g p.o. t.i.d. for 1 week appears to be as effective or better than ACV in non-ocular and ocular zoster. In one study comparing VCV with ACV in 1141 immunocompetent patients with zoster of a variety of dermatomes (35 with HZO), VCV was comparable to ACV in the duration

TABLE I

(continued)

Chronic/late disease

a. Corneal immune disease, episcleritis, scleritis, iritis, or dendritiform keratopathy.
   1. As under Acute HZO above.
b. Unhealthy epithelium in anesthetic cornea.
   1. Early lateral tarsorrhaphy and lubrication with artificial tears and tear ointments.
   2. Allow vascularization to progress to aid in healing any ulcer.
   3. Topical steroids with caution and only at low doses to minimize any inflammation.
c. Exposure keratopathy (poor lid closure) or corneal ulceration or thinning
   1. Lateral tarsorrhaphy.
   2. Therapeutic soft contact lens, e.g. Permalens™ or Kontur™ lenses.
   3. Tissue adhesive, e.g. Dermabond™, if progressive thinning.
   4. Conjunctival flap, or transplant. See Surgical procedures.
d. Glaucoma: As under Acute HZO above.
e. Post-herpetic neuralgia (PHN). All drugs below may be used additively.
   1. TCA antidepressants, e.g. nortriptyline, desipramine, or other TCAs): 10 mg titrated up to 100 mg q.h.s. PRN. Use caution if patient has cardiac disease.
   2. Gabapentin (Neurontin™): 300 mg p.o. q.d. starting dose. Efficacy may not be reached until 600 mg b.i.d.–t.i.d. Some may not respond at all.
   3. Slow-release opioids added if TCAs +/or gabapentin insufficiently effective: Oxycontin-SR™ 10–40 mg p.o. q. 12 h.
   4. Capsaicin cream one to three times daily to skin as tolerated.
   5. Sympathetic blockade or invasive pain management techniques, e.g. trigeminal ganglion ablation, rarely warranted as very rarely successful.
f. Acute retinal necrosis (ARN) p.o. or i.v. antivirals.
   1. Acyclovir, famciclovir, or valaciclovir. Doses per text.
g. Peripheral outer retinal necrosis (PORN) poor responsive to therapy.
   1. Combined intravitreal injections of ganciclovir and i.v. foscarnet variably effective.

of skin lesions but significantly better than ACV in acute pain resolution and reduced duration of PHN up to 1 year of follow up. The only ocular study compared ACV with VCV in 121 immunocompetent patients with acute HZO, and reported an incidence of keratitis, uveitis, and episcleritis that was similar in both groups (Colin et al., 2000). Neither group had any incidence of neurotrophic keratitis or scleritis, and acute pain was noted in about two-thirds of each group. It was concluded that VCV was a valid alternative to ACV in treatment of HZO. There are no studies comparing VCV with FCV or on the incidence of PHN after HZO treated with VCV.

4.2. Pain management

This is discussed elsewhere in this book in greater detail, but the principles do not differ greatly in HZO. In acute disease, tricyclic antidepressants, such as desipramine or nortriptyline 25–100 mg p.o. q.h.s. or in divided doses should be started along with antiviral therapy and continued for 2–3 months or longer as tolerated. This will both reduce acute pain and inhibit development of PHN. A cardiac history should be taken as TCAs may put a patient at risk of arrhythmia. Narcotic and non-narcotic analgesics should also be given acutely as needed (Galen, 1995; Bowsher, 1997; Dworkin et al., 1998).

The anticonvulsant gabapentin (Neurontin™) 300–600 mg p.o. t.i.d. is often effective at controlling PHN and may be given for months to years in doses as tolerated or needed (Galen, 1995; Bowsher, 1997; Dworkin et al., 1998). Periodic tapering should be attempted.

If the combination of gabapentin and TCAs is not totally effective or if one or both drugs are not tolerated in treatment of PHN, slow-release opioids, such as oxycodone-SR (Oxycontin-SR™) 10–20 mg p.o.

q.d.–b.i.d. may give relief. Because of slow-release, there is no 'high' and, therefore, little chance of addiction. Again, periodic tapering should be attempted as PHN may decrease spontaneously over time.

Topical therapy may also be useful in HZO PHN. Capsaicin cream q.d.–t.i.d. over many weeks will reduce substance P, a pain mediator, from the nerve endings. This will not only reduce PHN, but is one of the few substance that may relieve itching. Unfortunately, the cream may be locally irritating leading to patient intolerance. It should not be applied too close to the eyes. Lidoderm™ skin patches may also be used effectively in application over the forehead and scalp as needed.

4.3. Anti-inflammatory or other non-antiviral treatment of anterior segment disease

Episcleritis or scleritis is slowly responsive to mild topical steroid, such as 1/8% prednisolone b.i.d.–q.i.d. for several weeks to months in combination with oral non-steroidal anti-inflammatory agents (NSAIDs), such as ibuprofen 400 mg p.o. t.i.d. As steroids are tapered, oral NSAIDs are continued.

Acute zoster pseudodendritic keratitis often resolves with the systemic antivirals alone. Late lesions may not need treatment but if persistent, painful, or coming in repeated crops, vidarabine 3% ointment 5×/day for 2–3 weeks often suffices (Pavan-Langston et al., 1995). Response may be variable, however, necessitating trying other topical antivirals, such as trifluridine 1.0% 8×/day or systemic antivirals in full zoster dose (Chern et al., 1998; Margolis et al., 1998). Topical steroids will not exacerbate pseudodendrites and may be used to treat the acute inflammatory conjunctivitis, episcleritis, or an iritis with relative impunity.

Trophic sterile ulcerations in the anesthetic zoster cornea are treated with topical antibiotic drops, lubricating artificial tears, lateral tarsorrhaphy to narrow the lid opening, and, if healing does not ensue within a week or two, a constant-wear, therapeutic contact lens (Permalens™, Kontur™). If the cornea begins to thin in the open ulcer, tissue adhesive may be used to seal the ulcer and a Plano-T™ soft lens applied. The

majority of neurotrophic ulcers will heal with such treatment and the adhesive dislodge spontaneously. Topical steroids may be used more safely and in higher doses when the ulcer is sealed than when it is still open.

Stromal disease, being essentially immune in nature, is generally responsive to topical steroid therapy. Depending on the severity of reaction, starting doses may range from 1% prednisolone or 0.1 dexamethasone every 2 h, while awake to just b.i.d.–t.i.d. Tapering the dose begins as the immune disease begins to lessen going down in 50% steps over several weeks to months. The lower the dose, the longer it is maintained to prevent steroid rebound. The patient may ultimately be switched to 1/8% prednisolone q.i.d. from 1% q.d. and then carried through further taper. If the patient develops steroid glaucoma steroids such as Vexol™ or Lotemax™ may be substituted as they are less likely to cause pressure rise and are about half the equivalent strength of 1% prednisolone. Intraocular pressure (IOP) should be checked at each exam because of the risk of glaucoma both from HZO and from steroids. Topical antibiotics such as Polytrim™ drops q.i.d. or Polysporin™ ointment b.i.d. should be used in conjunction with steroids given more than once daily.

Iritis is treated in essentially the same manner as stromal immune keratitis. Dosage starts at a level compatible with the severity of the anterior chamber inflammation. Occasionally the IOP is low due to decreased aqueous production in the face of iritis. As the iritis responds to treatment and aqueous production recovers, the pressure may go up and reach glaucomatous levels.

Glaucoma is elevated IOP (generally 22–24 mm Hg or higher) of whatever cause. Because these eyes tend to be inflamed, it is best not to use miotics, such as pilocarpine, or the pupil may scar down. Drops such as β-blockers, e.g. timoptic, betoxalol, levobunalol, or α-adrenergics, e.g. brimonidine, or carbonic anhydrase inhibitors, e.g. brinzolamide, dorzoalamide, or prostaglandin inhibitors, e.g. latanaprost, may be used once or twice daily alone or in combination with other drug groups just named.

4.4. Therapy of retinitis

The retinitis of HZO is difficult to treat. Doses of systemic antivirals are given above in the discussion of retinitis. There is a significant reduction in the incidence of involvement of the fellow eye in treated versus untreated patients (13 vs. 70%) (Blumenkranz et al., 1986). Oral famciclovir or valaciclovir have been successful as adjictive therapy with i.v. ACV or foscarnet (Figueroa et al., 1997; Miller et al., 1997). Steroids, oral or i.v., have been used along with anticoagulants in efforts to reduce intraocular inflammation, vasculopathy and neuropathy with neither adverse affect nor objective proof that this treatment is effective. Regression of ARN begins within 5 days in acyclovir-treated patients but takes 3 weeks in untreated patients. The atrophic retina has a salt and pepper appearance, the optic nerve is pale, vision may be good to poor, and retinal detachment occurs within 8 weeks in 75% of the most severely involved eyes. The prognosis with PORN is much worse with prognosis very guarded in these usually HIV[+] patients. Combinations of acyclovir and ganciclovir do not really stop the relentless clinical course, but intravitreal ganciclovir and i.v. foscarnet coupled with laser photo-coagulation have been successful (Engstrom et al., 1994; Perez-Blazquez et al., 1997). There is a high incidence of retinal detachment in both ARN and PORN groups.

4.5. Surgical approaches in HZO

The most common procedures are lateral tarsorrhaphy or closure of the outer third of the lids to protect the anesthetic cornea, and lid reconstruction of badly scarred dysfunctional lids (Fig. 7). Corneal transplantation (penetrating keratoplasty, PK) has a limited role in HZO. As the majority of these eyes are anesthetic, transplanted eyes heal poorly with increased chance or wound dehiscence (Makensen et al., 1984). A scarred cornea that has retained a reasonable amount of sensation may be a candidate for such a surgical procedure in an effort to restore vision. If done, however, a lateral tarsorrhaphy should be placed at the same time to protect the new graft

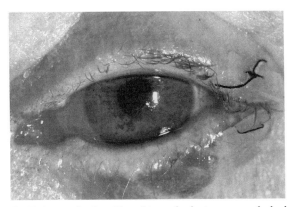

Fig. 7. A recently placed lateral tarsorrhaphy to narrow palpebral fissure thus reducing corneal exposure. Note zoster pseudodendrites on cornea.

(Reed et al., 1989). A newer procedure, keratoprosthesis, holds great promise for success in these cases, however (Yaghouti and Dohlman, 1999).

5. Summary

The eye and its adnexa are second only to thoracic involvement as the site of recurrent VZV in the form of zoster. The incidence is increasing steadily due to the relative immunosuppression seen in our aging population and in increased numbers of patients truly immunosuppressed by a variety of systemic clinical conditions. Because of the very real threat to vision and risk of long-term incapacitation, we are fortunate to have a variety of systemic antivirals and neurogenic agents to alleviate, in large part, many of the sequellae of this disease. There is still a significant amount of work to be done, however, toward the goal of eliminating this ocular pariah altogether.

References

Aylward, G., Claoue, C., Marsh, R. and Yasseem, N. (1994) Influence of oral acyclovir on ocular complications of herpes zoster ophthalmicus. Eye, 8: 70–74.

Blumenkranz, M., Culbertson, W. et al. (1986) Treatment of the acute retinal necrosis syndrome with intravenous acyclovir. Ophthalmology, 93: 296–300.

Borruat, F., Borruat, F., Buechi, E., Piguet, F., Fitting, P., Zografros, L. and Herbort, C. (1991) Prevention of ocular complications of herpes zoster ophthalmicus by adequate treatment with acyclovir. Klin. Monatsbl. Augenheilkd., 198(5): 358–360.

Bowsher, D. (1997) The effects of preemptive treatment of postherpetic neuralgia with amitriptyline: a randomized, double-blind, placebo-controlled trial. J. Pain Sympt. Manage., 13(6): 327–331.

Browning, D., Blumenkranz, M., Culbertson, W., et al. (1987) Association of varicella zoster dermatitis with acute retinal necrosis syndrome. Ophthalmology, 94: 602–606.

Chern, K., Conrad, D., Holland, G., Holsclaw, D., Schwartz, L. and Margolis, T. (1998) Chronic infectious varicella zoster virus epithelial keratitis in patients with Acquired Immune Deficiency Syndrome. Arch. Ophthalmol., 116: 1011–1017.

Cobo, L., Foulks, G., Liesegang, T., Lass, J., Sutphin, J., Wilhelmus, K. and Jones, D. (1985) Oral acyclovir in the therapy of acute Herpes zoster ophthalmicus: an interim report. Ophthalmology, 92: 1574.

Cobo, L., Foulks, G., Liesegang, T., Lass, J., Sutphin, J., Wilhelmus, K.G. and Jones, D. (1986) Oral acyclovir in the treatment of acute Herpes zoster ophthalmicus. Ophthalmology, 93: 763.

Cobo, M., Foulks, G., Liesegang, T., Lass, J., Sutphin, J., Wilhelmus, K. and Jones, D. (1987) Observations on the natural history of herpes zoster ophthalmicus. Curr. Eye Res., 6: 195–199.

Colin, J., Prisant, O., Cochener, B., Lescale, O., Rolland, B. and Hoang-Xuan, T. (2000) Comparison of the efficacy and safety of valaciclovir and acyclovir for the treatment of Herpes zoster ophthalmicus. Ophthalmology, 107: 1507–1512.

Culbertson, W., Blumenkranz, M., Pepose, J., Stewart, J., Curtin, V. et al. (1986) Varicella-zoster. Am. J. Ophthalmol., 93: 559–569.

Culbertson, W. and Dix, R. (1996) Varicella-zoster virus diseases: posterior segment of the eye. In: Ocular Infection and Immunity. Mosby, St. Louis, pp. 1131–1153.

DeGreef, H. (1995) Famciclovir, a new oral antiviral drug: its efficacy and safety in the treatment of uncomplicated herpes zoster in immunocompetent patients. Int. J. Antimicrob. Agents, 4: 241–246.

DeMoragas, J. and Kierland, R. (1957) The outcome of patients with Herpes zoster. Arch. Dermatol., 75: 193.

Donahue, J., Choo, P., Manson, J. and Platt, R. (1995) The incidence of herpes zoster. Arch. Int. Med., 155: 1605–1609.

Dworkin, R., Boon, R., Griffin, R. and De Phung (1998) Postherpetic neuralgia: impact of famciclovir, age, rash, severity, and acute pain in Herpes zoster patients. J. Infect. Dis., 178 (Suppl): S76–S80.

Engstrom, R., Holland, G., Margolis, T., Muccioli, C., Lindley, J. and Belfort, R. (1994) The progressive outer retinal necrosis syndrome. A variant of necrotizing herpetic retinopathy in patients with AIDS. Ophthalmology, 101: 1488–1502.

Figueroa, M., Garabito, I., Gutierrez, C. and Fortun, J. (1997)

Famciclovir for the treatment of acute retinal necrosis (ARN) syndrome. Am. J. Ophthalmol., 123: 255–257.

Forrest, W. and Kaufman, H. (1976) Zosteriform Herpes simplex. Am. J. Ophthalmol., 81: 86.

Galen, B. (1995) Neuropathic pain of peripheral origin: advances in pharmacologic treatment. Neurology, 45 (Suppl. 9): S17–S25.

Ganatra, J., Chandler, D., Santos, C., Kuppermann, B. and Margolis, T. (2000) Viral causes of the acute retinal necrosis syndrome. Am. J. Ophthalmol., 129: 166–172.

Gershon, A. (1995) Varicella-zoster virus: prospects for control. Adv. Pediatr. Infect. Dis., 10: 93–124.

Gilden, D., Kleinschmidt-DeMasters, B. et al. (2000) Neurologic complications of the reactivation of varicella-zoster virus. New Engl. J. Med., 342(9): 635–645.

Harding, S. (1993) Management of ophthalmic zoster. J. Med. Virol., Suppl. 1: 97–101.

Harding, S. and Porter, S. (1991) Oral acyclovir in herpes zoster ophthalmicus. Curr. Eye Res., 10 (Suppl)): 177–182.

Harding, S., Lipton, J. and Wells, J. (1987) Natural history of herpes zoster ophthalmicus: predictors of post herpetic neuralgia and ocular involvement. Br. J. Ophthalmol., 71: 353–358.

Hoang-Xuan, T., Buchi, E.R., Herbort, C.P., Denis, J., Frot, P., Thenault, S. and Pouliquen, Y. (1992) Oral acyclovir for herpes zoster ophthalmicus. Ophthalmology, 99: 1062–1071.

Hope-Simpson, R. (1965) The nature of herpes zoster: a long-term study and a new hypothesis. Proc. Soc. Med., 58: 9.

Levin, M., Barber, D., Goldblatt, E., Jones, M., LaFleur, B., Chan, C., Stinson, D., Zerbe, G. and Hayward, A. (1998) Use of a live, attenuated varicella vaccine to boost varicella-specific immune responses in seropositive people 55 years of age and older: duration of booster effect. J. Infect. Dis., 178 (Suppl. 1): S109–S112.

Liesegang, T. (1984) Varicella-zoster virus: systemic and ocular features. J. Am. Acad. Dermatol., 11: 165.

Liesegang, T. (1985) Corneal complications from Herpes zoster ophthalmicus. Ophthalmology, 92: 316.

Mahalingam, R., Wellish, M., Lederer, D., Forghani, B., Cohrs, R. and Gilden, D. (1993) Quantitation of latent varicella-zoster virus DNA in human trigeminal ganglia by polymerase chain reaction. J. Virol., 67(4): 2381–2384.

Mahalingam, R., Wellish, M., Wolfe, W., Dueland, A., Cohrs, R., Vafai, A. and Gildin, D. (1990) Latent varicella-zoster viral DNA in human trigeminal and thoracic ganglia. New Engl. J. Med., 323: 627–631.

Makensen, G., Sundmacher, R. and Witschel, D. (1984) Late wound complications after circular keratotomy for zoster keratitis. Cornea, 3: 95.

Margolis, T., Milner, M., Shama, A., Hodge, W. and Seiff, S. (1998) Herpes zoster ophthalmicus in patients with human immunodeficiency virus infection. Am. J. Ophthalmol., 125: 285–291.

Marsh, R. (1976) Ophthalmic herpes zoster. Br. J. Hosp. Med., 15: 609–618.

Marsh, R. and Cooper, M. (1987) Ophthalmic zoster: mucous plaque keratitis. Br. J. Ophthalmol., 71: 725–728.

McGill, J. and White, J. (1994) Acyclovir and post-herpetic neuralgia and ocular involvement. Br. Med J., 309: 1124–1128.

Miller, R., Brink, N., Cartledge, J., Sharvell, Y., Frith, P. (1997) Necrotising retinopathy in patients with advanced HIV disease. Genitourin. Med., 73(6): 462–466.

Naumann, G., Gass, J. and Font, R. (1968) Histopathology of Herpes zoster ophthalmicus. Am. J. Ophthalmol., 65: 533.

Pavan-Langston, D. (2000) Viral disease of the cornea and external eye. In: D. Albert and F. Jakobiec (Eds.), Principles and Practice of Ophthalmology, 2nd edn. W.B. Saunders, Philadelphia, PA, pp. 846–893.

Pavan-Langston, D. and Dunkel, E. (1996) Varicella-zoster of the anterior segment. In: Ocular Infection and Immunity, 1st edn., Mosby, Philadelphia, PA, pp. 946–985.

Pavan-Langston, D. and McCulley, J. (1973) Herpes zoster dendritic keratitis. Arch. Ophthalmol., 89: 25.

Pavan-Langston, D., Yamamoto, S. and Dunkel, E. (1995) Delayed herpes zoster pseudodendrites. Arch. Ophthalmol., 113: 1381–1385.

Pepose, J. (1997) The potential impact of varicella vaccine and new antivirals on ocular disease related to varicella-zoster virus. Am. J. Ophthalmol., 123: 243–249.

Perez-Blazquez, E., Traspas, R., Marin, I. and Montero, M. (1997) Intravitreal ganciclovir treatment in progressive outer retinal necrosis. Am. J. Ophthalmol., 124: 418–421.

Piebenga, L. and Laibson, P. (1973) Dendritic lesions in Herpes zoster ophthalmicus. Arch. Ophthalmol., 90: 268.

Ragozzino, M., Melton, M. and Kurland, L. (1982) Population based study of Herpes zoster and its sequellae. Medicine, 61: 310.

Reed, J., Joyner, S. and Knauer, W. III (1989) Penetrating keratoplasty for Herpes zoster keratopathy. Am. J. Ophthalmol., 107: 257.

Reijo, A., Antti, V. and Jukka, M. (1983) Endothelial cell loss in Herpes zoster keratouveitis. Br. J. Ophthalmol., 67: 751.

Tyring, S. (1996) Efficacy of famciclovir in the treatment of herpes zoster. Semin. Dermatol., 15(2) (Suppl. 1): 27–31.

Tyring, S., Barbarash, R., Nahlik, J., Cunningham, A., Marley, J. and Heng, M. (1995) Famciclovir for the treatment of acute herpes zoster: effects on acute disease and post-herpetic neuralgia. Ann. Int. Med., 123: 89–96.

Tyring, S., Engst, R., Corriveau, C., Robillard, N., Trottier, S., Van Slydken, S., Crann, R., Locke, L., Saltzman, R., Palestine, A. and the Collaborative Famciclovir Ophthalmic Zoster Research Group, Arch. Ophthalmol., in press.

Weller, T. (1995) Varicella-zoster virus. History, perspective, and evolving concerns. Neurology, 45 (Suppl. 8): S9–S10.

Wenkel, H., Rummelt, C., Rummelt, V., John, G., Fleckenstein, B. and Naumann, G. (1993) Detection of Varicella Zoster Virus DNA and Viral Antigen in Human Cornea After Herpes Zoster Ophthalmicus. Cornea, 12(2): 131–137.

Wilson, F.I. (1996) Varicella and Herpes zoster ophthalmicus. In: K. Tabbara and R. Hyndiuk (Eds.), Infections of the Eye. Little, Brown, Boston, MA, pp. 387–400.

Womack, L. and Liesegang, T. (1983) Complications of Herpes zoster ophthalmicus. Arch. Ophthalmol., 101: 42.

Yaghouti, F. and Dohlman, C.H. (1999), Innovations in keratoprosthesis: proved and unproved. In: F. Jakobiec and M. Krystolik (Eds.), Surgical Advances in Ophthalmology. International Ophthalmol Clinics, Lippencott, Williams, Wilkins, Philadelphia, PA, 39(1): 27–36.

Yamamoto, S., Shimomura, Y., Pavan-Langston, D., Dunkel, E. and Tano, Y. (1995) Detecting varicella-zoster virus DNA in iridocyclitis using polymerase chain reaction: a case of zoster sine herpete. Arch. Ophthalmol., 113: 1358–1359.

Yu, D., Lemp, M., Mathers, W., Espy, M., White, T. (1993) Detection of varicella-zoster virus DNA in disciform keratitis using polymerase chain reaction. Arch. Ophthalmol., 111: 167–168.

Herpes Zoster and Postherpetic Neuralgia, 2nd Revised and Enlarged Edition
Pain Research and Clinical Management, Vol. 11
Edited by C.P.N. Watson and A.A. Gershon

CHAPTER 12

Vaccination against zoster

Myron J. Levin [*]

University of Colorado School of Medicine, Pediatric Infectious Diseases, 4200 East Ninth Avenue, C-227,
Denver, CO 80262, USA

1. Introduction

Herpes zoster (HZ) is caused by reactivation of vari-cella-zoster virus (VZV) latent in sensory ganglia, subsequent retrograde spread of VZV down the cuta-neous nerve exiting that ganglion, and further repli-cation of VZV in the associated dermatome (Gilden et al., 2000). The prodromal pain and early acute pain of HZ results from the early ganglionitis. Late post-herpetic neuralgia probably represents changes in ganglia subsequent to the ganglionitis (Chapters 15 and 17).

Clinical observations made early in the past century established the close relationship between the virus causing chickenpox and that causing HZ (Bruusgaard, 1932). The isolation of VZV from both diseases made it possible to prove that these isolates were identical in growth characteristics, antigenic properties and genetic organization (Weller and Wit-ton, 1958). Ultimate proof came when VZV was iso-lated from a varicella lesion and subsequently from HZ in the same individual. Both isolates were identi-cal (Straus et al., 1984). Similarly, some individuals who have received the live attenuated varicella vac-cine have developed HZ with virus identical to the vaccine strain (Gelb et al., 1987).

2. What is known about latency of VZV?

The VZV genome is thought to be present in neurons (possibly also in some non-neuronal cells) in a circu-lar episome (Hyman et al., 1983; Croen et al., 1988; Clarke et al., 1995; Lungu et al., 1995; Meier et al., 1993; LaGuardia et al., 1999; see Chapter 7). At least five genes are active and some of their gene products have been detected in ganglia removed at autopsy (Croen et al., 1988; Meier et al., 1993; Cohrs et al., 1995, 1996; Mahalingam et al., 1996; Debrus et al., 1995; Kennedy et al., 1998, 1999; LaGuardia et al., 1999). VZV DNA and proteins are demonstrable in 75–85% of trigeminal and thoracic ganglia, and in other cranial nerve ganglia (Furuta et al., 1992, 1997; Mahalingam et al., 1990, 1992; Liedtke et al., 1993).

3. What is the relationship between VZV-specific immunity and HZ?

It has long been known that HZ is more frequent and more severe in patients who are immunodeficient (Feldman et al., 1973; Dolin et al., 1978; Colebun-ders et al., 1988; Wilson et al., 1992; Kawasaki et al., 1996; Derryck et al., 1998; Ljungman et al., 1986; see Chapter 10). Although this could be explained

* Correspondence to: Dr. M.J. Levin, University of Colorado School of Medicine, Pediatric Infectious Diseases, 4200 East Ninth Avenue, C-227, Denver, CO 80262, USA. Phone: +1 (303) 315-4620; Fax: +1 (303) 315-7909; E-mail: myron.levin@uchsc.edu

by the loss of a direct effect of VZV-specific immunity in maintaining latency, it is more likely that VZV reactivates sporadically (due either to random or specific physiological or environmental events), but is efficiently contained by VZV-specific immunity. This is supported by serological evidence for contained reactivation and instances of inapparent viremia (Gershon et al., 1982; Ljungman et al., 1986; Wilson et al., 1992). Consequently, in immunosuppressed patients the reactivating VZV is more likely to propagate in the sensory ganglion and is poorly contained after spread to the periphery. The occurrence of neuropathic syndromes in normal hosts without cutaneous manifestations of VZV suggests a partial breakdown in this process (Barrett et al., 1993; Gilden et al., 1994, 2000). The proposed mechanism of contained reactivation may be a factor in maintaining resistance to VZV infection long after varicella occurs in childhood.

This relationship appears not to involve humoral immunity, since children with isolated γ-globulin deficiency and adults with common variable immune deficiency do not suffer more frequent or severe VZV infections. Similarly, adults with isolated defects in antibody synthesis, such as those with multiple myeloma or chronic lymphocytic leukemia, in the phase before they receive chemotherapy, do not develop severe HZ. Conversely, children with severe combined immune deficiency, or bone marrow transplant recipients who receive replacement γ-globulin, develop severe VZV infections, indicating the primacy of VZV-specific T-cell mediated immunity (CMI) for recovery from VZV infection (Ljungman et al., 1986; Wilson et al., 1992).

4. Why is HZ more common and more severe with increasing age?

Aging is associated with a decline in VZV-specific CMI. This can be demonstrated by skin testing with VZV antigen or measuring lymphoproliferative responses by simple lymphoproliferative assays (LPA) of peripheral blood mononuclear cells exposed to VZV antigen in vitro (Miller, 1980; Berger et al.,

1981; Burke et al., 1982). More complex responder cell frequency (RCF) assays enumerate circulating CD4 memory cells that respond to VZV antigen (Hayward et al., 1994b). These responses appear to decline noticeably about age 40 and become progressively lower with aging (A.R. Hayward and M.J. Levin, unpublished; Hayward et al., 1991). Levels of VZV antibodies in older people remain at 80–90% of that of younger cohorts, although this has not been studied with respect to subclass, type, or affinity of antibody (Berger et al., 1981; Gershon and Steinberg, 1981; Levin and Hayward, 1996). These observations support the hypothesis that the burden of HZ in the elderly is explained by their inability to limit reactivation of VZV, either in situ in ganglia or after axonal spread. That is, aging results in immunological compromise with respect to VZV infection. At present, it is not known if the assays used to measure immunity in the elderly to date include critical components of the immune response against VZV, or if they even serve as surrogates for essential responses.

5. Hypothesis for prevention of HZ

It will be possible with a VZV vaccine to boost VZV-specific CMI in elderly individuals such that they will experience a decrease in the frequency or severity or HZ.

6. Will live VZV vaccines be safe in elderly people?

In view of the decline in VZV-specific CMI described above, there was some concern that these vaccines might be reactogenic. However, the proposed vaccines are based on the attenuated Oka strain and there are also reassuring observations that older people who come in contact with children with varicella do not become clinically reinfected. Moreover, older individuals with HZ are able to contain the infection within 7–10 days, although there is some evidence that viremia can occur, based on the frequency of distant extradermatomal lesion in

TABLE I

VZV vaccination of older individuals

Author/reference	n	Age (years)	Vaccine (PFU × 10³)	Antigen U/ml	Immune test	Duration (years)
Berger et al. (1984)	33	55–65	2.7[4]	NA[8]	LPA[9]	<0.16
Berger et al. (1985a)	29	50–65	6–12[4,5]	NA	LPA	<0.10
Starr et al. (1987)	25	50–74	4.4[6]	6.0	LPA	<0.33
Sperber et al. (1992)	95	18–49	0.28–2.8–28[6]	0.08–8.4	Antibody	1
Takahashi[1]	37	>50	3.0[5]	4.0	Skin test	1
Trannoy et al. (2000)	200	55–88	3.2–8.5–41.7[7]	0	LPA/RCF[10]	1
Levin et al. (1998)	202	60–82	3–6–12[6]	4.0–12.0	RCF/CK[11]/Antibody	6–8
Levin et al. (2000)	167	55–79	4.0 vs. nil[6]	5.2	RCF/CK/Antibody	3
Oxman[2]	28,000[3]	60→75	>20.0[6]	NA	RCF/Elispot	–[12]

[1] M. Takahashi and K. Yamanishi, personal communication.
[2] Personal communication for the VA Study CSP 403 Study Group.
[3] As of 1/15/01.
[4] Manufacturer = RIT.
[5] Received VZV skin test prior to vaccination.
[6] Manufacturer = Merck Research Laboratories.
[7] Manufacturer = Pasteur Merieux Connaught.
[8] NA = not available.
[9] Lymphocyte proliferation assay.
[10] Responder cell frequency assay.
[11] Induced cytokine assay.
[12] Planned for 3-year follow-up.

these patients (Balfour, 1988). Additional potential risks of proposed vaccines are difficult to evaluate, such as those due to their administration subcutaneously, which is not the normal route for acquiring VZV infection, and the maximal dose that might be tolerated.

Live attenuated varicella vaccines have been given to people age 55 and over in nine trials (Table I). At least 23,000 older subjects have now received doses varying from 3000 to >40,000 PFU; of these more than 28,000 have received at least 20,000 PFU. The vaccine was well tolerated in all trials. The occurrence of local pain, erythema, and induration is similar to that seen with other vaccines, such as for influenza. Similarly, systemic reactions, such as fever and malaise are rare. In an early trial with doses of 3000 to 12,000 PFU, 6 of 200 vaccinees had a possible VZV lesion within or distant from the injection site (Levin et al., 1998). These subjects were not ill. In another trial of 200 subjects, 50 who received >40,000 PFU had less local and systemic reactions than a control group receiving pneumococcal polysaccharide vaccine (Trannoy et al., 2000). One percent of the VZV vaccine recipients developed a rash at the injection site (Levin

et al., 1998; Trannoy et al., 2000). In an ongoing placebo-controlled trial of >20,000 PFU there has been no excess of local or systemic reactions in the vaccine recipients (M.N. Oxman and the CSP403 Study Group, personal communication). Nevertheless, it is important to be cautious, since there is limited experience in giving live varicella vaccine to older people, especially in the high titer proposed for HZ prevention. Furthermore, there is a potential risk if an individual is vaccinated who has an undiagnosed immunosuppressive illness, such as lymphoma.

7. Will live VZV vaccines be immunogenic in older people? (see Table I)

Evaluation of VZV-specific CMI, either as skin test (Hata, 1980), LPA (Berger et al., 1985b), or RCF (Hayward et al., 1991) in patients with HZ demonstrates that these response are boosted by 'natural' immunization with the antigenic load of the outbreak. Presumably it is this boost that permits or hastens recovery. Furthermore, the rarity of second cases of HZ suggests that this endogenous boosting is significant and long-lasting (Hope-Simpson, 1965). Conversely, the vaccines designed for prevention could fail to replicate as well as reactivated wild-type VZV and thereby fail to mimic natural boosting.

In the early 1980s Swiss investigators immunized 62 older volunteers with 2700 to 12,000 PFU of a VZV vaccine (Berger et al., 1984, 1985a). All had a negative LPA or VZV skin test prior to immunization. More than 50% developed a positive LPA 2–3 weeks later. In subjects who were skin tested, both vaccinees and placebo recipients developed positive skin test responses. This indicated that skin testing might be a useful immunogen. Moreover, some vaccinees were skin test positive and LPA negative, indicating that skin testing might have been more sensitive than the LPA in use for these experiments. The vaccine used for these experiments is no longer available for study.

Experiments in the USA began in 1987 with 25 older subjects receiving 4400 PFU of VZV vaccine (Starr et al., 1987). Most subjects less than age 60 years converted their LPA responses, whereas only 20% of those older than age 70 years did so. This was the first suggestion that age of vaccination might limit this preventative strategy. All of the early experiments had a limited follow-up period.

The first large trial of VZV vaccines for seropositive subjects was undertaken in 1992 with 95 adults (Sperber et al., 1992). Their mean age was only 32 years (the oldest was 49 years). Doses as high as 28,000 PFU were compared to similar amounts of vaccine that had been heat inactivated. Although only antibody responses were measured, these were stimulated equally by both types of vaccine. This suggested that the VZV antigen, in addition to replicating virions in live vaccines, is immunogenic and probably an important component of live vaccines. This had previously been considered when Bergen et al. found that reducing the VZV antigen content of a live VZV vaccine formulation resulted in a decrease in antibody and CMI at 1 year after primary vaccination of children (Bergen et al., 1990).

There are two completed and one on-going large study of a live VZV vaccine for elderly subjects. The trial of Trannoy et al. consisted of 200 subjects age 55–88 years (mean age, 65 years) (Trannoy et al., 2000). These were divided into cohorts of 50 that received either pneumococcal polysaccharide vaccine as placebo, 3200, 8500, or 41,650 PFU of live vaccine. The inclusion of the control group provided unequivocal information that the VZV vaccine is well tolerated in this age group. Specific CMI responses were measured by LPA and RCF using either a single VZV gene product, purified VZV glycoproteins, or a crude infected culture lysate. VZV-specific CMI was boosted 2–3-fold by 6 weeks after vaccination. RCF was superior to LPA, and responses with either method were best measured using crude antigen. An antibody increment of 30–40% was also noted. As in other studies, the magnitude of the antibody response did not correlate with that of the CMI response. In spite of the log difference in inoculum, no dose effect was observed for CMI or antibody.

Although there has been a considerable number of older subjects vaccinated with a live VZV vaccine, and these have been reassuring with respect to safety, the earlier studies shared one or more of the following deficiencies: (1) most were very small; (2) some had low-risk subjects less than 60 years of age; (3) some did not adequately evaluate CMI; (4) where skin testing was used to derive baseline information, it is likely that this altered the immune response independently of vaccination; (5) none investigated the essential issue of the persistence of the booster responses stimulated by vaccination.

The sole long-term trial was begun before the study of Trannoy et al. Four cohorts with at least 40 subjects of age 60–87 years received 3000, 6000, 12,000 PFU or 3000 PFU given twice with a 3-month interval (Levin et al., 1998). There was an early boost in antibody, but this measure returned to baseline within 1 year. There was also a transient boost in γ-interferon produced by mononuclear cells stimulated by VZV antigen in vitro. The lasting response was that of RCF, which was boosted 2-fold by immunization (Fig. 1, curve C). This booster effect persisted with a half-life of 56 months. Furthermore, although there was no dose effect observed 2 years after booster immunization, such an effect could be

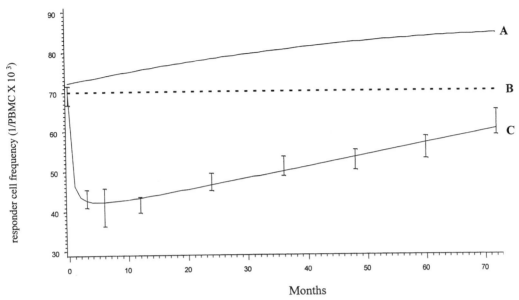

Fig. 1. Mean (±S.E.) of VZV responder cell frequency (RCF) in peripheral blood mononuclear cells (PBMC) from elderly recipients of live attenuated varicella vaccine compared with the expected RCF of a cohort of the same age who had not been vaccinated. Curve A represents expected RCF if the subjects had not been vaccinated. This was calculated from the distribution of RCF values of vaccinees at baseline, using the formula: RCF = −311.38 + 9.80 (age) − 0.06 (age)^2. Curve B represents the mean baseline RCF of all vaccinees. Curve C represents the RCF of vaccinees at times after vaccination. Frequency at time 0 was significantly less ($P < 0.05$) than at all other times. Number of observations: 0 months, 188; 3 months, 190; 12 months, 186; 24 months, 177; 36 months, 166; 48 months, 160; 60 months, 153; 72 months, 124.

observed thereafter between the highest and lowest doses administered (Fig. 2). The potential value of booster immunization is not appreciated by comparing the residual booster effect (Fig. 1; curve C) with the baseline measurements at the time of immunization (Fig. 1; curve B). Rather, it is necessary to correct for the ongoing natural decline of VZV-specific CMI that accompanies aging. This decline can be calculated from the distribution of RCF in various age groups at baseline before they were vaccinated (Fig. 1, Curve A). Thus, there is a continuing booster effect apparent as the difference between curve A and C in Fig. 1 at all points throughout the 6 years of follow-up.

8. What is known about the nature of boost in CMI following vaccination of older subjects?

The RCF assay utilized for the trials described above measures CD4$^+$ memory T-cells that express

the CD45R0 phenotype (Hayward et al., 1994a). Responding cells include those with MHC class II-restricted cytotoxicity for VZV antigen-bearing targets (Hayward et al., 1996). These cells make either γ-interferon or IL-4 (Zhang et al., 1994). Vaccinees also develop an increase in HLA class I-restricted mononuclear cells that lyse autologous Epstein–Barr virus transformed lymphoblasts transfected with plasmids coding for VZV antigens. Natural killer activity was also increased at 3 months after vaccination (Hayward et al., 1996).

In a companion experiment, a subset of vaccinees were immunized with tetanus toxoid 3 months before receiving their VZV vaccine, and RCF to both VZV and tetanus toxoid subsequently determined. There was only a weak correlation between responses to the two antigens. Half of the VZV-non-responders developed a tetanus-specific response, arguing against a global defect in failure of secondary immunization (Hayward et al., 1994a). The RCF

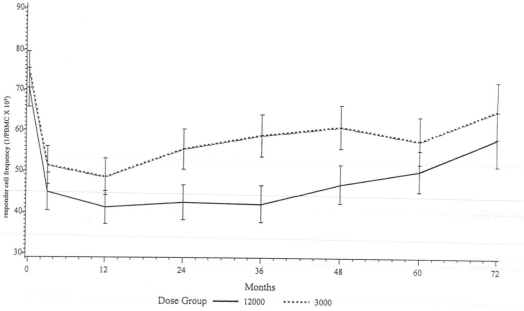

Fig. 2. Mean (±SE) of VZV responder cell frequency (RCF) in peripheral blood mononuclear cells (PBMC) from elderly recipients of two different doses of live attenuated varicella vaccine. A longitudinal analysis of their time response curves indicated that RCF at the 12,000 PFU dose is significantly greater ($P < 0.05$) through 48 months than at each corresponding point at the 3000 PFU dose. Number of observations: 3000 PFU/12,000 PFU = 0 months, 52/48; 3 months, 52/49; 12 months, 52/46; 24 months, 46/46; 36 months, 41/40; 48 months, 40/38; 60 months, 41/38; 72 months, 28/32.

responses at baseline or after boosting did not correlate with the presence of $CD3^+$, $CD4^+$, $CD8^+$, or $CD3CD45R0^+$ markers at baseline, suggesting that variation in memory cell phenotype did not explain variable response to VZV antigens.

9. How efficient are live vaccines in boosting CMI in older subjects?

Approximately 40% of vaccinees in the larger trials had no detectable response in the RCF assay prior to immunization (Levin et al., 1998; Trannoy et al., 2000; M. Takahashi and K. Yaminishi, personal communication). Following booster vaccination the percentage of nonresponders was 10–12%. Subsequently, the nonresponding proportion increased toward the baseline value. These observations could be partly explained by limitations in formatting the RCF assay such that at maximum sensitivity the assay can detect only ≥ 1 VZV-responding cell per 100,000 circulating mononuclear cells. Nevertheless, the existence of a large nonresponder group in any population of elderly individuals, and the presence of a residual fraction that does not boost after receiving VZV vaccine, could define those individuals who are especially likely to develop HZ. Similarly, the loss of responding cells observed in a significant proportion of vaccinees may be an indicator of the duration of the protective effect and the need for additional booster vaccinations.

10. Will an inactivated vaccine boost CMI in older subjects?

An inactivated vaccine has potential advantages for older subjects in terms of safety, especially for those who (unknowingly) have not had prior varicella or who have an unrecognized immunosuppressive illness or therapy. An early indication that an inactivated vaccine might be effective was the ability

VZV skin test antigen to enhance VZV-specific CMI. Moreover, trials of varicella vaccine in children using formulations with different ratios of PFU to VZV antigen indicated that the antigen content influenced antibody response (Bergen et al., 1990).

An inactivated VZV vaccine has been studied in bone marrow transplant recipients (Redman et al., 1997). Thirty-eight subjects were immunized with 4.5 U (equivalent to 2900 PFU of commercially available live vaccine) of VZV antigen. A single dose given to 14 patients 1 month after transplantation significantly increased the VZV-specific LPA at 3 months post-transplantation compared to a randomly assigned control group, but there was no protective effect. However, three doses given monthly, starting a month post-transplantation, was both immunogenic and protective. Although the incidence of HZ was the same as that of the control group, there was strong attenuation in terms of lesion number, initial pain, and post-herpetic neuralgia. The addition of a dose prior to bone marrow transplantation further enhanced LPA. Efficacy data on this four-dose schedule is not yet available (A. Arvin, personal communication). This experiment raises the possibility that a vaccine to prevent HZ might be more effective in attenuating the outbreaks (especially with respect to post-herpetic pain) than in preventing all cases. This outcome of 'breakthrough' HZ would be akin to the breakthrough varicella seen in children vaccinated with the varicella vaccine.

Since the bone marrow transplant recipients were severely immunosuppressed, it is even more likely that elderly subjects might respond to an inactivated vaccine. A trial comparing live attenuated and inactivated vaccine was undertaken in subjects with a mean age of 65 years (minimum age was 55 years) (Levin et al., 2000). Approximately 165 subjects received either 4000 PFU of a live VZV vaccine or an equal volume that had been heat inactivated. The inactivated vaccine had an immunoelectrophoresis profile similar to vaccine not exposed to heat. At 1 and 3 years post-vaccination, there was no difference in boost of RCF or half-life of the booster response. Cytotoxic T-cell activity was stimulated by both the live and the inactivated vaccine, but the live vaccine

stimulated a greater response (Hayward et al., 1996). The duration of the cytotoxic response has not been reported.

11. What is known about the efficacy of vaccines to present HZ?

To date, experiments with vaccines to prevent HZ have not been powered to determine efficacy. Passive surveillance for >1200 subject-years in vaccinees has suggested that the incidence of HZ may not have been reduced, but that the manifestations of the outbreak may have been greatly attenuated (Levin et al., 1998, 2000). This is consistent with the results of immunizing bone marrow transplant recipients. However, no conclusions are possible on this issue, since there are problems with: (a) sample size: (b) the nature of the surveillance; (c) the diagnostic methods available at the beginning of the studies to fully evaluate 'atypical' or 'breakthrough' HZ (e.g. no PCR).

12. What research is currently being undertaken?

An appropriately powered efficacy trial is underway. Because the long-term study of Levin et al. demonstrated a dose effect on the persistence of the booster response, the pivotal efficacy trial was preceded in 1997–1998 by several dose-finding experiments. Furthermore, the observations that inactivated VZV vaccine is immunogenic dictated that the candidate vaccines for these penultimate trials contain various combinations of live virus and VZV antigen. A multicenter trial evaluated six formulations (varying from 2000 to 67,000 PFU) of candidate vaccines to prevent HZ in 515 vaccinees ≥60 years of age (143 were age ≥76 years). Based on this preliminary dose-finding trial, an additional 357 subjects at three separate sites were given 34,000 or 50,000 PFU, including 20% who had stable chronic obstructive pulmonary disease or diabetes mellitus (M.N. Oxman et al., unpublished). A vaccine was chosen based on an endpoint boost in RCF at 3 months post-vaccination. This final study vaccine contains 10–20 times more virus and antigen than administered in the previous long-term studies.

The definitive test of concept began in December, 1998 as a double-blind efficacy trial that will encompass 37,800 vaccinees, two-thirds 60–69 years old and the remainder ≥70 years old. This study (M.N. Oxman and the CSP403 Study Group, personal communication) is utilizing 16 sites within the Veterans Administration Collaborative Trials system and six sites supported by the National Institute of Allergy and Infectious Diseases. Given the possibility that some cases of HZ might be attenuated by booster vaccination, rather than prevented, several types of endpoints have been chosen. These include not only cases of HZ and of post-herpetic neuralgia, but as the primary endpoint measures of 'burden of illness'. This is a parameter that integrates pain severity and duration over an extended observation period. For this purpose, the Zoster Brief Pain Inventory was prepared by modifying the published Brief Pain Inventory (Cleeland, 1990). It was validated in a separate study of more than 100 patients with acute HZ as a reliable measure of zoster pain (P. Coplan, K. Schmader et al., manuscript in preparation). Numerous other pain, quality of life, and medication use instruments are utilized to quantitate clinical endpoints. Assuming >3 cases of HZ per 1000 vaccinees per year, and given the composition of the study group, it will require approximately 4.5 years of follow-up (total study duration of 5.5 years) to determine a 60% efficacy. Case ascertainment is being achieved through an automated telephone response system that contacts all participants monthly to inquire about interval episodes. Putative cases are being documented by fluorescent antibody and PCR analysis of lesion scrapings, aided by acute and convalescent immunological assays.

Some consideration has been given to the possibility that the vaccine could be effective for a limited period, with subsequent decline in the protective effect, as suggested by the published long-term studies (Levin et al., 1998). Therefore, an experiment is underway in which remaining vaccinees from the original long-term study are receiving an additional booster dose of the current vaccine. This will evaluate the magnitude and duration of a second dose (M.J. Levin, J. Smith et al; unpublished).

13. Is there a surrogate marker for protection against herpes zoster?

There is no known marker that predicts protection against HZ. The suggestion of disease attenuation observed in the long-term trial correlates with boosting in RCF (Levin et al., 1998). However, this falls far short of validation, especially since it was noted early in that trial that some episodes of confirmed HZ occurred in subjects who had an excellent RCF profile (Levin et al., 1994). The difficulties with developing a surrogate are two-fold. First, the RCF assay is not optimal with respect to variability and requires large study populations to evaluate significance (Hayward et al., 1994b). Secondly, variability is increased when fresh cells are studied at many points over many years. Alternate methods are under study. Those that measure secretion of cytokines into the media of VZV-stimulated mononuclear cells do not offer an advantage over RCF (Hayward et al., 1998). The evaluation of assays of induced intracellular cytokines is ongoing (M.N. Oxman and CSP 403 Study Group, unpublished). An assay that is likely to be more promising is the enumeration of VZV-specific memory cells by Elispot assay. This assay was compared to RCF in 175 subjects who received booster doses of VZV vaccine. Elispot appears to be preferable because it has less variability, measures predominantly TH1 responses, has a wider dynamic range, and is more sensitive than proliferative assays (J. Smith, M. Caulfield et al., personal communication). Elispot is formatted to use frozen cells; thus, sequential time points can be evaluated in the same assay.

A surrogate marker would be valuable for rapid evaluation of candidate vaccines, and would be required if future changes are made in an established vaccine. Toward this end, CMI (RCF; induced cytokine assays; Elispot) will be measured in the efficacy trial in a substudy of 1200 vaccine/placebo recipients before and after booster vaccination. These assays will also be performed at onset of HZ and at regular intervals from all cases of HZ occurring in the full 37,800 subjects. One possibility, although unlikely, is that enough cases of HZ will occur in the 1200 subject subset to validate a marker. A second approach to validation would be to compare measures of specific CMI early after onset of HZ in the full study cohort with data obtained in the immunology substudy. If these measurements after acute HZ are significantly lower than values seen at pre- or post-immunization in age-matched subjects in the immunology substudy, then this would begin to relate such measurements to outcome. A third possibility is that some measure of CMI during attacks of HZ will correlate with the severity of these attacks (measured as burden of illness or post-herpetic neuralgia) in the two study arms. Finally, it will be important to determine if the vaccine-induced responses are of the same magnitude reached by patients who develop HZ. This would indicate that the vaccine can mimic natural boosting from HZ, which we believe is sufficient to prevent second attacks in most older individuals.

14. Are there epidemiological factors that might impact reactivation of VZV in the future?

The impact of varicella vaccine on future potential cases of HZ is unclear. Varicella vaccine is recommended for all normal children after 1 year of age, and catch-up vaccination is recommended for all other susceptible children and adults. Preliminary evidence indicates that sufficient numbers of at-risk individuals are being immunized to alter the normal epidemiological curve for varicella in the United States (J. Seward, personal communication). This limitation in the circulation of wild-type VZV will remove the environmental boost that probably contributes to the level of VZV-specific immunity in adults (Arvin et al., 1993; Asano et al., 1994; Gershon et al., 1990; Krause and Klinman, 1995). Natural boosting may be important for delaying, pre-

venting, or attenuating HZ in seropositive individuals, whether they are immune because of varicella or vaccination (Garnett and Grenfell, 1992). Environmental boosting could also impact the efficacy of a shingles vaccine, but is likely to have less of an effect because of more limited exposure in older people. Conversely, people who remain susceptible, and are not vaccinated, may benefit from a paucity of environmental VZV, since they will be more likely to avoid infection and thereby not develop HZ. Less clear is whether the development of varicella later in childhood or adulthood, which tends to result in more severe disease, will serve to delay VZV reactivation.

Approximately 1–3% of children in the USA receive nucleoside analogues (usually acyclovir) for treatment of varicella (Lieu et al., 1994; Yawn et al., 1997). This is more common in adolescents. This might reduce the number of skin lesions in children and adults, and thereby decrease the amount of latent VZV in ganglia. Conversely, very early therapy of varicella could decrease the level of VZV-specific immunity, and thereby increase the likelihood of HZ or reduce the response to a shingles vaccine. A comparison of VZV-specific RCF in acyclovir-treated and untreated children demonstrated no difference at 3 years after varicella (Rotbart et al., 1993).

The vaccine virus (Oka strain) becomes latent in ganglia. However, viremia and skin lesions appear to be minimal following vaccination, suggesting that the quantity of latent genome in ganglia will be less than after varicella. Moreover, Oka strain VZV is temperature sensitive and replicates 7-fold less readily in cultured human neurons than does the parent strain (Hayakawa et al., 1984; Somekh and Levin, 1993). HZ caused by Oka strain has been documented in immunocompromised and normal vaccinees (Gelb et al., 1987; Merck Research Laboratories, personal communication). The age-specific incidence of HZ in vaccinees is not known, and there are no experiments underway to determine this. The passive collection system maintained by the manufacturer suggests a lower incidence in vaccinees compared to historical controls, but this conclusion suffers from the probability of underreporting and the relatively short period of latency for vaccinees, compared with naturally infected individuals. An optimistic view of the preventative effect of vaccination could be drawn from the data of Hardy et al. (1991). They compared well-matched groups of leukemic children who had either prior varicella or Oka vaccine. The vaccinated group had an approximately 3-fold lower incidence of HZ than naturally infected patients, and vaccinees receiving two doses of vaccine had a lower incidence of HZ than those receiving a single dose (Gershon et al., 1996).

15. Conclusions

Developing an immunization strategy to prevent HZ in aging individuals is hampered by limited information concerning the age-related VZV-specific immune defects that are the basis of this disease. There is ample evidence that several measures of VZV-specific CMI can be boosted in older vaccinees by either a live attenuated or a heat-inactivated varicella vaccine. A carefully designed, appropriately powered efficacy trial is underway to evaluate a 'shingles' vaccine. Presumably this trial will also help us address certain lingering issues, such as: (1) the safety of large amounts of live varicella virus in a large cohort of elderly vaccinees; (2) the persistence of VZV-specific immune responses stimulated by this vaccine, and implications for additional doses if immunity wanes; and (3) the search for a surrogate marker associated with protection against HZ. The study may fail to clarify: (1) the significance, in terms of HZ risk, of those vaccinees who fail to boost after vaccination; (2) the relative importance of the live and inactive components of the vaccine. Furthermore, several community-based epidemiological factors, such as universal varicella vaccination, may influence the final interpretation of this trial.

References

Arvin, A.A., Koropchak, C.M. and Wittek, A.E. (1993) Immunologic evidence of reinfection with varicella-zoster virus. J. Infect. Dis., 148: 200–205.

Asano, Y., Suga, S. and Yoshikawa, T. et al. (1994) Experience and reason: twenty-year follow-up of protective immunity of the Oka strain live varicella vaccine. Pediatrics, 94: 524–526.

Balfour Jr., H.H. (1988) Varicella zoster virus infections in immunocompromised hosts. Am. J. Med., 85 (Suppl. 2A): 68–73.

Barrett, A.P., Katelaris, C.H. and Morris, J.G.L. et al. (1993) Zoster sine herpete of the trigeminal nerve. Oral Surg. Oral Med. Oral Pathol., 75: 17–75.

Berger, R., Amstutz, I. and Just, M. et al. (1985a) Booster vaccination of healthy adults with VZV antibody but without a VZV-specific cell-mediated immune response. Antiviral Res., Suppl. 1: 267–271.

Berger, R., Florent, G. and Just, M. (1981) Decrease of the lymphoproliferative response to varicella-zoster virus antigen in the aged. Infect. Immun., 32: 24–27.

Berger, R., Luescher, D. and Just, M. (1984) Enhancement of varicella-zoster-specific immune responses in the elderly by boosting with varicella vaccine. J. Infect. Dis., 149: 647–648.

Berger, R., Luescher, D. and Just, M. (1985b) Restoration of varicella-zoster virus cell-mediated immune response after varicella booster vaccination. Postgrad. Med. J., 61: 143–145.

Bergen, R.E., Diaz, P.S. and Arvin, A.M. (1990) The immunogenicity of the Oka/Merck varicella vaccine in relation to infectious varicella-zoster virus and relative viral antigen content. J. Infect. Dis., 162: 1049–1054.

Bruusgaard, E. (1932) The mutual relation between zoster and varicella. Br. J. Dermatol., 44: 1.

Burke, B.L., Steele, R.W. and Beard, O.W. (1982) Immune responses to varicella-zoster in the aged. Arch. Intern. Med., 142: 291–293.

Clarke, P., Beer, T., Cohrs, R. and Gilden, D.H. (1995) Configuration of latent varicella-zoster virus DNA. J. Virol., 69: 8151–8154.

Cleeland, C.S. (1990) Assessment of pain in cancer: measurement issues. Adv. Pain Res. Ther., 16: 47–55.

Cohrs, R.J., Barbour, M.B. and Mahalingam, R. et al. (1995) Varicella-zoster virus (VZV) transcription during latency in human ganglia: prevalence of VZV gene 21 transcripts in latently infected human ganglia. J. Virol., 69: 2674–2678.

Cohrs, R.J., Barbour, M. and Gilden, D.H. (1996) Varicella-Zoster virus (VZV) transcription during latency in human ganglia: Detection of transcripts mapping to genes 21, 29, 62, and 63 in a cDNA library enriched for VZV RNA. J. Virol., 70: 2789–2796.

Colebunders, R., Mann, J.M. and Francis, H. et al. (1988) Herpes zoster in Africans: a clinical predictor of human immunodeficiency virus infection. J. Infect. Dis., 157: 314–318.

Croen, K.D., Ostrove, J.M., Dragovic, L.J. and Straus, S.E. (1988) Patterns of gene expression and sites of latency in human nerve ganglia are different for varicella-zoster and herpes simplex viruses. Proc. Natl. Acad. Sci. USA, 85: 9773–9777.

Debrus, S., Sadzot-Delvaux, C. and Nikkels, A.F. et al. (1995) Varicella-zoster virus gene 63 encodes an immediate-early protein that is abundantly expressed during latency. J. Virol., 69: 3240–3245.

Derryck, A., LaRussa, P. and Steinberg, S. et al. (1998) Varicella and zoster in children with human immunodeficiency virus infection. Pediatr. Infect. Dis. J., 17: 931–933.

Dolin, R., Reichman, R.C., Mazur, M.H. and Whitely, R.J. (1978) Herpes zoster-varicella infections in immunosuppressed patients. Ann. Intern. Med., 89: 375–388.

Feldman, S., Hughes, W.T. and Kim, H.Y. (1973) Herpes zoster in children with cancer. Am. J. Dis. Child., 126: 178–184.

Furuta, Y., Takasu, T. and Fukuda, S. et al. (1992) Detection of varicella-zoster virus DNA in human geniculate ganglia by polymerase chain reaction. J. Infect. Dis., 166: 1157–1159.

Furuta, Y., Takasu, T. and Suzuki, S. et al. (1997) Detection of latent varicella-zoster virus infection in human vestibular and spiral ganglia. J. Med. Virol., 51: 214–216.

Garnett, G.P. and Grenfell, B.T. (1992) The epidemiology of varicella-zoster virus infections: the influence of varicella on the prevalence of herpes zoster. Epidemiol. Infect., 108: 513–528.

Gelb, L.D., Dohner, D.E. and Gershon, A.A. et al. (1987) Molecular epidemiology of live, attenuated varicella virus vaccine in children with leukemia and in normal adults. J. Infect. Dis., 155: 633–640.

Gershon, A.A. and Steinberg, S.P. (1981) Antibody responses to varicella-zoster virus and the role of antibody in host defense. Am. J. Med. Sci., 282: 12–17.

Gershon, A.A., Steinberg, S.S. and Borkowsky, W. et al. (1982) IgM to varicella-zoster virus: demonstration in patients with and without clinical zoster. Pediatr. Infect. Dis. J., 1: 164–167.

Gershon, A.A., Steinberg, NIAID Varicella Vaccine Collaborative Study Group (1990) Live attenuated varicella vaccine: protection in healthy adults compared with leukemic children. J. Infect. Dis., 161: 661–666.

Gershon, A.A., LaRussa, P. and Steinberg, S. et al. (1996) The protective effect of immunologic boosting against zoster: An analysis in leukemic children who were vaccinated against chickenpox. J. Infect. Dis., 173: 450–453.

Gilden, D.H., Wright, R.R. and Schneck, S.A. et al. (1994) Zoster sine herpete, a clinical variant. Ann. Neurol., 35: 530–533.

Gilden, D.H., Kleinschmidt-DeMasters, B.K. and LaGuardia, J.J. et al. (2000) Neurologic complications of the reactivation of varicella-zoster virus. New Engl. J. Med., 342: 635–645.

Hardy, L., Gershon, A.A., Steinberg, S.P. and LaRussa, P. (1991) The incidence of zoster after immunization with live attenuated varicella vaccine. New Engl. J. Med., 325: 1545–1550.

Hata, S. (1980) Skin test with varicella-zoster virus antigen on herpes zoster patients. Arch. Dermatol. Res., 268: 65–70.

Hayakawa, Y., Torigoe, S. and Shiraki, K. et al. (1984) Biologic and biophysical markers of a live varicella vaccine strain (Oka): identification of clinical isolates from vaccine recipients. J. Infect. Dis., 149: 956–963.

Hayward, A., Levin, M.J. and Wolf, W. et al. (1991) Varicella-zoster virus-specific immunity after herpes zoster. J. Infect. Dis., 163: 873–875.

Hayward, A.R., Buda, K. and Levin, M.J. (1994a) Immune response to secondary immunization with live or inactivated VZV vaccine in elderly adults. Viral Immunol., 7: 31–36.

Hayward, A.R., Zerbe, G.O. and Levin, M.J. (1994b) Clinical application of responder cell frequency estimates with four years of follow up. J. Immunol. Methods, 170: 27–36.

Hayward, A.R., Buda, K. and Jones, M. et al. (1996) VZV specific cytotoxicity following secondary immunization with live or killed vaccine. Clin. Immunol., 9: 241–245.

Hayward, A.R., Cosyns, M. and Jones, M. et al. (1998) Cytokine production in varicella-zoster virus-stimulated cultures of human blood lymphocytes. J. Infect. Dis., 178 (Suppl. 1): S95–S98.

Hope-Simpson, R.E. (1965) The nature of herpes zoster: a long-term study and a new hypothesis. Proc. R. Soc. Med., 58: 9–20.

Hyman, R.W., Ecker, J.R. and Tenser, R.B. (1983) Varicella-zoster RNA in human trigeminal ganglia. Lancet, 2: 814–816.

Kawasaki, H., Takayama, J. and Ohira, M. (1996) Herpes zoster infection after bone marrow transplantation in children. J. Pediatr., 128: 353–356.

Kennedy, P.G.E., Grinfeld, E. and Gow, J.W. (1998) Latent varicella-zoster virus is located predominantly in neurons in human trigeminal ganglia. Proc. Natl. Acad. Sci. USA, 95: 4658–4662.

Kennedy, P.G.E., Grinfeld, E. and Gow, J.W. (1999) Latent varicella zoster virus in human dorsal root ganglia. Virology, 258: 451–454.

Krause, P.R. and Klinman, D.M. (1995) Efficacy, immunogenicity, safety, and use of live attenuated chickenpox vaccine. J. Pediatr., 127: 518–525.

LaGuardia, J.J., Cohrs, R.J. and Gilden, D.H. (1999) Prevalence of varicella-zoster DNA in dissociated human trigeminal ganglion neurons and nonneuronal cells. J. Virol., 73: 8571–8577.

Levin, M.J. and Hayward, A.R. (1996) Prevention of herpes zoster. Infect. Dis. Clin. North Am., 10: 657–675.

Levin, M.J., Murray, M. and Zerbe, G.O. et al. (1994) Immune responses of elderly persons 4 years after receiving a live attenuated varicella vaccine. J. Infect. Dis., 170: 522–526.

Levin, M.J., Barber, D. and Goldblatt, E. et al. (1998) Use of live attenuated varicella vaccine to boost varicella-specific immune responses in seropositive people 55 years of age and older: duration of booster effect. J. Infect. Dis., 178 (Suppl. 1): S109–S112.

Levin, M.J., Ellison, M.C. and Zerbe, G.O. et al. (2000) Comparison of a live attenuated and an inactivated varicella vaccine to boost the varicella-specific immune response in seropositive people 55 years of age and older. Vaccine, 18: 2915–2920.

Liedtke, W., Opalka, B., Zimmermann, C.W. and Lignitz, E. (1993) Age distribution of latent herpes simplex virus 1 and varicella-zoster virus genome in human nervous tissue. J. Neurol. Sci., 116: 6–11.

Lieu, T.A., Black, S.B. and Rieser, N. et al. (1994) The cost of childhood chickenpox: parents' perspective. Pediatr. Infect. Dis. J., 13: 173–177.

Ljungman, R., Lonnqvist, B. and Gahrton, G. et al. (1986) Clinical and subclinical reactivations of varicella-zoster virus in immunocompromised patients. J. Infect. Dis., 153: 840–847.

Lungu, O., Annunziato, P.W. and Gershon, A. et al. (1995) Reactivated and latent varicella-zoster virus in human dorsal root ganglia. Proc. Natl. Acad. Sci. USA, 92: 10980–10984.

Mahalingam, R., Wellish, M. and Wolf, W. et al. (1990) Latent varicella-zoster viral DNA in human trigeminal and thoracic ganglia. New Engl. J. Med., 323: 627–631.

Mahalingam, R., Wellish, M.C. and Dueland, A.N. et al. (1992) Localization of herpes simplex and varicella zoster virus DNA in human ganglia. Ann. Neurol., 31: 441–448.

Mahalingam, R., Wellish, M. and Cohrs, R. et al. (1996) Expression of protein encoded by varicella-zoster virus open reading frame 63 in latently infected human ganglionic neurons. Proc. Natl. Acad. Sci. USA, 93: 2122–2124.

Meier, J.F., Holman, R.P. and Croen, K.D. et al. (1993) Varicella-Zoster transcription in human trigeminal ganglia. Virology, 193: 193–200.

Miller, A.E. (1980) Selective decline in cellular immune response to varicella-zoster in the elderly. Neurology, 30: 582–587.

Redman, R.L., Nader, S. and Zerboni, L. et al. (1997) Early reconstitution of immunity and decreased severity of herpes zoster in bone marrow transplant recipients immunized with inactivated varicella vaccine. J. Infect. Dis., 176: 578–585.

Rotbart, H.A., Levin, M.J. and Hayward, A.R. (1993) Immune responses to varicella zoster virus infections in healthy children. J. Infect. Dis., 167: 195–199.

Somekh, E. and Levin, M.J. (1993) Identification of human dorsal root neurons with wild type varicella virus and the Oka strain varicella vaccine. J. Med. Virol., 40: 241–243.

Sperber, S.J., Smith, B.V. and Hayden, F.G. (1992) Serologic response and reactogenicity to booster immunization of healthy seropositive adults with live or inactivated varicella vaccine. Antiviral Res., 17: 214–222.

Starr, S.E., Tinklepaugh, C., Bocks, E. et al. (1987) Immunization of healthy seropositive middle aged and elderly adults with varicella-zoster virus (VZV) vaccine. In: Programs and Abstracts of the Twenty-Seventh Interscience Conference on Antimicrobial Agents and Chemotherapy, New York, p. 313, abstract 1237.

Straus, S.E., Reinhold, W. and Smith, H.A. et al. (1984) Endonuclease analysis of viral DNA from varicella and subsequent zoster infections in the same patient. New Engl. J. Med., 311: 1362–1364.

Trannoy, E., Berger, R. and Hollander, G. et al. (2000) Vaccination of immunocompetent elderly subjects with a live attenuated Oka strain of varicella zoster virus: a randomized, controlled, dose–response trial. Vaccine, 18: 1700–1706.

Weller, T.H. and Witton, H.M. (1958) The etiologic agents of varicella and herpes zoster: serologic studies with the viruses as propagated in vitro. J. Exp. Med., 108: 869–890.

Wilson, A., Sharp, M. and Koropchak, C.M. et al. (1992) Subclinical varicella-zoster virus viremia, herpes zoster, and T lymphocyte immunity to varicella-zoster antigens after bone marrow transplantation. J. Infect. Dis., 165: 119–126.

Yawn, B.P., Yawn, R.A. and Lydick, E. (1997) Community impact of childhood varicella infections. J. Pediatr., 130: 759–765.

Zhang, Y., Cosyns, M., Levin, M.J. and Hayward, A.R. (1994) Cytokine production in varicella zoster virus stimulated limiting dilution lymphocyte cultures. Clin. Exp. Immunol., 98: 128–133.

Herpes Zoster and Postherpetic Neuralgia, 2nd Revised and Enlarged Edition
Pain Research and Clinical Management, Vol. 11
Edited by C.P.N. Watson and A.A. Gershon
© 2001 Elsevier Science B.V. All rights reserved

CHAPTER 13

Pain, sensory change, and allodynia in postherpetic neuralgia

David Bowsher[*]

Pain Research Institute, Clinical Sciences Building, University Hospital Aintree, Liverpool L9 7AL, UK

1. Introduction

Postherpetic neuralgia (PHN) is the commonest form of neuropathic pain (Bowsher, 1988, 1991a,b; Bowsher and Miles, 1991). It may be defined as pain persisting or recurring at the site of acute herpes zoster (HZ) three or more months after the onset of acute HZ (Dworkin and Portenoy, 1996); however, some authors prefer to use a 6-month interval. The important point is that any pain of less than 3 months duration after the onset of HZ should not be regarded as PHN. PHN may be regarded as a somewhat different entity from HZ, not a continuation of it (Bowsher, 1992); indeed it may be considered to be a disease *caused* as a result of having had HZ (Bowsher, 1995).

By the age of 80, 25% of the UK population will have had HZ, equally distributed between the sexes; 15% of them (two thirds women) will have developed PHN (Bowsher, 1999). Hope-Simpson (1975) found that 14% of HZ sufferers developed PHN. The condition is of course particularly common in people who contract HZ in old age (De Moragas and Kierland, 1957). There is evidence that just over half of PHN patients recover within 12 months, due to spontaneous remission or treatment (Bowsher, 1999). But at any one time, it has been estimated that some 200,000 UK citizens out of a total population of 58 million are suffering from PHN (Bowsher, 1999).

Common features of PHN include the following.
(1) Pain, frequently of a burning character, especially in younger patients; episodes of spontaneous stabbing pain may also occur.
(2) A partial sensory deficit, with thresholds raised particularly to sharpness, warmth, and cold.
(3) Allodynia, exhibited by more than 90% of our patients.
(4) Autonomic instability, exacerbation of pain by physical or mental stress, and alleviation by relaxation. The latter means that patients with even the most severe pain are able to *fall* asleep, even though they may wake in/be woken by pain. Objective autonomic instability is seen as changes in skin blood flow and sweating.

2. The nature of pain in HZ and PHN

The McGill Pain Questionnaire (Melzack, 1975) has been used to investigate the quality of pain in HZ and in PHN. Pain was found to be of a different nature in PHN than in acute HZ, and the quality of the

[*] Correspondence to: Dr. D. Bowsher, Pain Research Institute, Clinical Sciences Building, University Hospital Aintree, Liverpool L9 7AL, UK. Phone: + 44 (151) 529-5820; Fax: +44 (151) 529-5821; E-mail: pri@liv.ac.uk or bowsher@liv.ac.uk

TABLE I

Sensory words (groups 1–9) most frequently chosen from McGill Questionnaire by patients with acute HZ (from Bhala et al., 1988), and PHN in patients treated and not treated with acyclovir (ACV) for acute HZ [1]

Acute HZ (N = 64)	Non-ACV-treated PHN (N = 80)	ACV-treated PHN (N = 25)
Sharp 42 (66)	Burning 39 (49)	Throbbing 8 (32)
Stabbing 35 (55)	Throbbing 32 (40)	Stabbing 8 (32)
Shooting 30 (47)	Stabbing 32 (40)	Sharp 7 (28)
Throbbing 30 (47)	Shooting 30 (37.5)	Shooting 6 (24)
Itching 23 (36)	Sharp 29 (36)	Aching 6 (24)
Hot 22 (34)	Aching 15 (19)	Burning 5 (20)
	Whole of group 7 (hot, burning, scalding, searing): 62 (77.5%)	Whole of group 7 (hot, burning, scalding, searing): 7 (28%)

[1] The words chosen are given in absolute and (percentage) numbers. Patients could choose up to nine words out of a possible 38 words.

pain in PHN was changed by the treatment (or not) of acute HZ with an antiviral (acyclovir) (Bowsher, 1992). These differences are tabulated in Table I, which also shows that in PHN there are, in addition to allodynia (see below), two types of spontaneous pain: (a) a more or less constant background pain, most frequently described as burning or throbbing; and (b) paroxysms of stabbing or shooting pain. The stabbing or shooting episodes do not occur in every case.

3. Sensory change in acute herpes zoster

Nurmikko et al. (1990) examined somatosensory perception thresholds in 31 patients with acute herpes zoster. They found that, although there was a significant elevation of vibration threshold ($P < 0.0002$) in comparison with the unaffected mirror-image area on the opposite side, the warm–cold limen was the most significantly changed parameter ($P < 0.00005$). The patients were followed up at 3, 6, and 12 months, at which time 7, 3, and 2 patients, respectively, still had pain (PHN). The authors reported that thermal threshold abnormalities in acute HZ were significantly associated with persistence of pain beyond 3 months.

In a later publication (Haanpää et al., 2000), reduction of sharpness sensitivity in acute zoster was also found to be predictive of later PHN.

Nurmikko and Bowsher (1990) had earlier found that in established PHN, thresholds for thermal as well as mechanical modalities were greatly raised.

4. Allodynia in PHN

Allodynia (pain produced by a non-noxious stimulus), or extreme tenderness, was found in 55% of acute zoster patients by Haanpää et al. (2000). The majority of patients exhibiting no allodynia in acute zoster did not go on to develop PHN.

The vast majority (~90%) of PHN patients have allodynia (see Table II), which is indeed usually their most prominent complaint. In almost all cases, dynamic mechanical allodynia (sensitivity to a low-

TABLE II

Types of allodynia in PHN: 223 patients (151 female [1]) of whom 198 (89%) had allodynia

Allodynia type	All (%)
No allodynia	25 (11)
Dynamic mechanical	194 (87)
Cold only	2 (0.9)
Dynamic mechanical + cold	2 (0.9)
All allodynia	198 (89)

[1] The 2 : 1 female : male ratio for the prevalence of PHN in these hospital patients was also found in a population survey of 1071 elderly subjects (Bowsher, 1999).

intensity moving tactile stimulus) is by far the commonest form, causing patients to be agonised by the slightest movement of their clothes or bedclothes over the affected region, or of a breeze on exposed areas. Skin-stretch and static mechanical allodynia is also (but less frequently) encountered, and cold allodynia occurs in some patients. The frequency of allodynia in our patients is shown in Table II.

Tactile allodynia in PHN patients fades almost instantly following stimulation, and occurs following each stimulus on repetitive stimulation at rates of 6 Hz. This is a distinct difference from allodynia (triggering) in trigeminal neuralgia, in which each stimulus is followed by an appreciable refractory period, during which allodynia cannot be elicited (Kugelberg and Lindblom, 1959).

The classification of Fields et al. (1998) recognises a category without allodynia, seen in 11% of our patients.

Nurmikko et al. (1991) injected local anaesthetic into the supraorbital nerve of 10 subjects with (allodynic) ophthalmic PHN and paravertebrally in two subjects with cervical PHN accompanied by dynamic mechanical allodynia. In 8 of the 12, allodynia was abolished by the block, but returned as the effect on Aβ fibres wore off and before small-fibre modalities (temperature and sharpness) recovered. Sympathetic blockade had no effect. This is a powerful argument for at least three-quarters of cases of allodynia being subserved by large (Aβ) fibres.

Fields et al. (1998) argue that some cases of allodynia are subserved by C fibres, which they call 'irritable nociceptors'. Patients with this type of allodynia have minimal sensory deficit, and their pain is relieved by local anaesthetic infiltration of the skin, while subjects with marked sensory loss are not relieved by intradermal infiltration of local anaesthetic. In this respect, it is interesting that coagulation of the dorsal root entry zone in 10 PHN patients failed to relieve pain in eight of them; but in two, it did so (Rath et al., 1997). Did these patients have 'irritable nociceptors' transmitting pain through unmyelinated primary afferents? Rowbotham et al. (1996) looked at skin biopsies from non-scarred areas in 18 cases of PHN and found that the reduction in free nerve

endings in the skin correlated with thermal sensory loss, but was inversely correlated with allodynia, suggesting "that surviving cutaneous primary afferent nociceptors that are spontaneously active and/or sensitized contribute to PHN pain and allodynia". However, Rowbotham et al. (1998) describe a PHN patient who, over 10 years, changed from sensory loss with no allodynia to sensory loss with severe allodynia. But Fields et al. (1998) state that more than one of the three pathophysiological mechanisms which they describe can co-exist within the same patient. While it is true that a patient will be aware as to whether allodynia exists *anywhere* within the affected region, the presence, absence, or intensity of the sensory deficit will depend upon the particular area of affected body surface the investigator happens to examine.

The desire to explain PHN and other neuropathic pains as being conducted encephalopetally by classical 'pain pathways' is a curious atavism. In the half-century between about 1920 and 1970, before the differences between nociceptive and neuropathic pain were recognised, anterolateral cordotomy (section of the crossed fibres ascending to the reticular formation and thalamus) was carried out on many thousands of patients. This procedure very effectively (if adequately performed) raised pain thresholds above perception level in most cases of nociceptively painful malignant disease. However, as a survey of the literature shows, in the large number of operations carried out on subjects with PHN and similar conditions, allodynia was unaltered. The fact that a very similar allodynia occurs in many cases of central post-stroke pain where of course there is no peripheral nerve damage or ongoing excitation, also casts doubt on such a proposition.

When PHN is treated with tricyclics, many clinicians are of the opinion that the drug has a greater effect on ongoing pain (including spontaneous stabbing episodes) than on allodynia which is often the last thing to disappear in most successfully treated cases. Sometimes the allodynia persists even after ongoing pain has been abolished. It will be interesting to see whether gabapentin or *N*-methyl D-aspartate (NMDA) antagonists will be shown to have a greater effect on allodynia. To date, ongoing pain and allodynia have not been separately examined in published accounts of the effects of treatment of PHN. Interestingly, treatment of acute zoster with acyclovir, while reducing the incidence of sensory deficit in PHN (see above), has little effect on the proportion of patients exhibiting allodynia in this author's experience.

5. Autonomic instability

In addition to the subjective factors listed in the introduction (exacerbation and alleviation of pain by stress and relaxation), there are also objective signs of autonomic change (Rowbotham and Fields, 1989). Changes in sweating are sometimes reported by the patient, of which, in our own experience, hyperhidrosis in the affected dermatome(s) is the commonest. Sometimes when hyperhidrosis occurs concomitantly with exacerbations of pain, the affected area may become red and even present an evanescent rash. Our observations on skin temperature with liquid crystal thermography, like those of Rowbotham and Fields (1989) and Baron and Saguer (1993) with telethermography, have given inconclusive results. This is in contrast to the situation in trigeminal neuralgia (Hardy and Bowsher, 1989) and central post-stroke pain (Bowsher, 1996), in which cutaneous vasoconstriction invariably occurs.

There has been an unfortunate tendency to refer to the autonomic instability found in PHN as 'sympathetic-dependent pain'. This is a tautologous expression which means that if a pain is relieved by sympathectomy, it must have been sympathetic-dependent. While autonomic instability is undoubtedly present in PHN, there is no evidence that the pain or allodynia are in any way sympathetic-dependent. Confirming the finding of Nurmikko et al. (1991) that stellate ganglion block does not affect pain or allodynia in trigeminal or upper cervical cases, a survey of more than 50 case-sheets from our clinic of patients with ophthalmic or upper cervical PHN in whom stellate ganglion blockade had been performed for therapeutic purposes revealed only

one patient in whom the procedure could conceivably have been beneficial for more than a few hours.

More scientific is the evidence obtained by Nurmikko and Hietaharju (1992). They studied the effect of prolonged sauna heat on (among others) 61 patients with peripheral neuropathy, of whom 9 had PHN. The heat, near hot pain threshold, can be presumed to have activated both afferent (nociceptive) and efferent (sympathetic) C fibres; it produced both perspiration and vasodilation in the patients, and in young healthy volunteers a tripling of plasma noradrenaline levels (Kukkonen-Harjula et al., 1989). Pain or allodynia were increased in 9 of the patients; clinical and instrumental examination suggested that only 3 of them demonstrated signs of sympathetic instability, and only one subsequently benefitted from repeated sympathetic blockade. Pain or allodynia decreased in nearly 30% of these patients on exposure to sauna heat.

6. Conclusion

PHN, which can be said to be present three or more months after the onset of acute zoster, is characterised by ongoing (background) pain, sensory deficit, and allodynia; the two latter are to some extent independently variable. There is a suggestion that a minority of cases exhibit a type of allodynia subserved by peripheral C fibres ('irritable nociceptors', Fields et al., 1998), although in most cases large Aβ fibres are responsible for the allodynia. The pathophysiology of PHN is a dynamic process which changes with time (it becomes less responsive to tricyclics as a function of duration (Bhala et al., 1988), and the type of sensory deficit may alter). Allodynia is the bugbear of PHN, and may persist after background pain has disappeared, resisting most current therapeutic efforts to a far greater extent than other features of the disease.

References

Baron, R. and Saguer, M. (1993) Postherpetic neuralgia. Are C-nociceptors involved in signalling and maintenance of tactile allodynia? Brain, 116: 1477–1496.

Bhala, B.B., Ramamoorthy, C., Bowsher, D. and Yelnoorker, K.N. (1988) Shingles and postherpetic neuralgia. Clin. J. Pain, 4: 169–174.

Bowsher, D. (1988) Pain as a neurological emergency. In: D. Bowsher (Ed.), Neurological Emergencies in Medical Practice. Croom Helm, Beckenham, pp. 218–236.

Bowsher, D. (1991a) Clinical anatomy and physiology of pain. In: M. Swash and J.M. Oxbury (Eds.), Clinical Neurology, Vol. 1. Churchill Livingstone, Edinburgh, pp. 627–627.

Bowsher, D. (1991b) Neurogenic pain syndromes and their management. Br. Med. Bull., 47: 644–666.

Bowsher, D. (1992) Acute shingles and postherpetic neuralgia: Effects of acyclovir and outcome of treatment. Br. J. Gen. Pract., 42: 244–246.

Bowsher, D. (1995) Pathophysiology of postherpetic neuralgia: towards a rational treatment. Neurology, 45(Suppl. 8): 56–57.

Bowsher, D. (1996) Central pain: clinical and physiological characteristics. J. Neurol. Neurosurg. Psychiatry, 61: 62–69.

Bowsher, D. (1999) The lifetime occurrence of Herpes Zoster and prevalence of post-herpetic neuralgia: a retrospective survey in an elderly population. Eur. J. Pain, 3: 335–342.

Bowsher, D. and Miles, J.B. (1991) Chronic pain syndromes. In: M. Swash and J.M. Oxbury (Eds.), Clinical Neurology, Vol. 1. Churchill Livingstone, Edinburgh, pp. 649–657.

De Moragas, J.M. and Kierland, R.R. (1957) The outcome of patients with herpes zoster. Arch. Dermatol., 75: 193–196.

Dworkin, R.H. and Portenoy, R.K. (1996) Pain and its persistence in herpes zoster. Pain, 67: 241–252.

Fields, H.L., Rowbotham, M. and Baron, R. (1998) Postherpetic neuralgia: Irritable nociceptors and deafferentation. Neurobiol. Dis., 5: 209–227.

Haanpää, M., Laippala, P. and Nurmikko, T. (2000) Allodynia and pinprick hypesthesia in acute herpes zoster, and the development of postherpetic neuralgia. J. Pain Symptom Manage., 20: 50–58.

Hardy, P.A.J. and Bowsher, D. (1989) Contact thermography in idiopathic trigeminal neuralgia and other facial pains. Br. J. Neurosurg., 3: 399–402.

Hope-Simpson, R.E. (1975) The nature of herpes zoster: a long-term study and a new hypothesis. Proc. R. Soc. Med., 58: 9–20.

Kugelberg, E. and Lindblom, U. (1959) The mechanisms of pain in trigeminal neuralgia. J. Neurol. Neurosurg. Psychiatry, 22: 36–43.

Kukkonen-Harjula, K., Oja, P., Laustiola, K., Vuori, I., Jolkkonen, J., Siitonen, S. and Vapaatalo, H. (1989) Haemodynamic and hormonal responses to heat exposure in a Finnish sauna bath. J. Appl. Physiol., 58: 543–550.

Melzack, R. (1975) The McGill Pain Questionnaire: major properties and scoring methods. Pain, 1: 277–299.

Nurmikko, T. and Bowsher, D. (1990) Somatosensory findings in postherpetic neuralgia. J. Neurol. Neurosurg. Psychiatry, 49: 135–141.

Nurmikko, T. and Hietaharju, A. (1992) Effect of exposure to sauna heat on neuropathic and rheumatoid pain. Pain, 49: 43–51.

Nurmikko, T.J., Räsänen, A. and Häkkinen, V. (1990) Clinical and neurophysiological observations on acute herpes zoster. Clin. J. Pain, 6: 284–290.

Nurmikko, T., Wells, C. and Bowsher, D. (1991) Pain and allodynia in postherpetic neuralgia: role of somatic and sympathetic systems. Acta Neurol. Scand., 84: 146–152.

Rath, S.A., Seitz, K., Soliman, N., Kahamba, J.F., Antoniadis, G. and Richter, H.F. (1997) DREZ coagulations for deafferentation pain related to spinal and peripheral nerve lesions; indication and results of 79 consecutive procedures. Stereotact. Funct. Neurosurg., 68: 161–167.

Rowbotham, M.C. and Fields, H.L. (1989) Post-herpetic neuralgia: the relation of pain complaint, sensory disturbance, and skin temperature. Pain, 39: 129–144.

Rowbotham, M.C., Yosipovitch, G., Kari Connolly, M., Finlay, D., Forde, G. and Fields, H.L. (1996) Cutaneous innervation density in the allodynic form of postherpetic neuralgia. Neurobiol. Dis., 3: 205–214.

Rowbotham, M.C., Petersen, K.L. and Fields, H.L. (1998) Is postherpetic neuralgia more than one disorder? Pain Forum, 7: 231–237.

Herpes Zoster and Postherpetic Neuralgia, 2nd Revised and Enlarged Edition
Pain Research and Clinical Management, Vol. 11
Edited by C.P.N. Watson and A.A. Gershon
© *2001 Elsevier Science B.V. All rights reserved*

Editorial comment on Chapter 14

Dr. Gerhard Fromm has died since the first edition of this book in 1993. His work remains thoughtful and helpful. His original chapter is reproduced in this volume as a tribute to him because it continues to be very relevant. It is followed by a commentary by Dr. Barry Sessle who was co-editor with him of a classic text on trigeminal neuralgia (Fromm and Sessle, 1991).

C. Peter N. Watson
Toronto, Ontario

Reference

Fromm G.H. and Sessle, B.J. (Eds.) (1991) Trigeminal Neuralgia. Butterworth-Heinemann, Stoneham.

Herpes Zoster and Postherpetic Neuralgia, 2nd Revised and Enlarged Edition
Pain Research and Clinical Management, Vol. 11
Edited by C.P.N. Watson and A.A. Gershon

Facial pain with herpes zoster and postherpetic neuralgia and a comparison with trigeminal neuralgia [1]

Gerhard H. Fromm [2]

Department of Neurology, University of Pittsburgh, School of Medicine, Pittsburgh, PA 15261, USA

1. Epidemiology, incidence and natural history

The herpes zoster virus has a particular predilection for the first (ophthalmic) division of the trigeminal nerve and the mid-thoracic dermatomes. In several reported series, ophthalmic herpes zoster accounted for 16.3–29.0% of all cases of herpes zoster (Burgoon et al., 1957; De Moragas and Kierland, 1957; Hope-Simpson, 1975; Harding et al., 1987; Watson et al., 1988b; Nurmikko et al., 1990), and the ophthalmic division is involved four times as often as either the second or third division of the trigeminal nerve (Selby, 1984). Not only is the first division of the trigeminal nerve a favorite site for the herpes zoster virus, but the incidence of postherpetic neuralgia is higher in these patients than in those with herpes zoster elsewhere, occurring in 20–50% of cases (Cobo et al., 1986, 1987; Harding et al., 1987; Nigam et al., 1991). It is most likely to occur in patients over 80 years of age and in those who have a lot of pain during the acute phase, and the rash tends to be more severe and to last longer in the patients who go on to develop postherpetic neuralgia (Harding et al., 1987). Thermal threshold abnormalities at 3 months also appear to be a predictor for the development of postherpetic neuralgia (Nurmikko et al., 1990). Some reports have suggested that postherpetic neuralgia affecting the trigeminal region lasts longer than postherpetic neuralgia affecting other dermatomes (De Moragas and Kierland, 1957; Hope-Simpson, 1975), but others have found that the prognosis is the same regardless of the affected area (Watson et al., 1991b).

2. Clinical features

Postherpetic neuralgia is associated with three different types of pain: (1) a constant deep aching or burning pain; (2) an intermittent, transient pain with a sharp, jabbing or electric shock-like quality; and (3) a sharp, radiating dysesthesia triggered by light tactile stimulation of specific trigger areas (allodynia). In some patients with ophthalmic postherpetic neuralgia, the allodynia occurs over the maxillary region and can be so prominent as to resemble the trigger zones in trigeminal neuralgia (Nurmikko and Bowsher, 1990). Perception of warm, cold, hot pain, touch, pinprick, two-point discrimination and vibration is diminished in the affected areas, indicating a

---

[1] Previously published in C.P.N. Watson (Ed.), Herpes Zoster and Postherpetic Neuralgia. Pain Research and Clinical Management, Vol. 8. Elsevier, Amsterdam, pp. 109–122.

[2] Deceased.

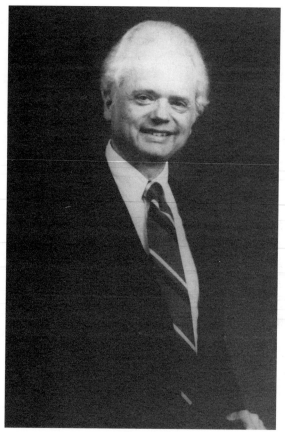

Dr. Gerhard Fromm

and ophthalmic herpes zoster (Reske-Nielsen et al., 1986). Patients with thoracic postherpetic neuralgia have also been found to have dorsal horn atrophy while patients without persistent pain do not (Watson et al., 1988a, 1991a), but there is so far no similar data for ophthalmic postherpetic neuralgia.

4. Neuropharmacological observations

Several double-blind controlled studies have documented that amitriptyline and desipramine provide good to excellent pain relief in 47–67% of patients suffering from postherpetic neuralgia (Watson et al., 1982; Watson and Evans, 1985; Max et al., 1988; Kishore-Kumar et al., 1990). The i.v. administration of 1.0–4.0 mg/kg amitriptyline to cats anesthetized with α-chloralose significantly enhances the segmental inhibition of wide dynamic range neurons in the spinal trigeminal nucleus caudalis (Fig. 1), but has little or no effect on low-threshold mechanoceptive neurons (Fig. 2) (Fromm et al., 1991). Amitriptyline also facilitated the segmental inhibition of some nociceptive specific neurons (Fig. 2), but this effect was not statistically significant. These doses of amitriptyline had little effect on excitatory transmission in the trigeminal nucleus as evidenced by the fact that there was only a small change in the neuron response to the unconditioned stimulus (Fig. 1). It would appear from these findings that amitriptyline exerts its antineuralgic action by enhancing the ability of segmental inhibition to prevent the excessive firing of wide dynamic range neurons which may be responsible for neuropathic pain.

It has been proposed that neuropathic pain is caused by an alteration in the functioning of wide dynamic range neurons resulting from deafferentation or chronic irritation (Roberts, 1986; Dubner et al., 1987; Sessle, 1987). This hypothesis proposes that peripheral nerve injury leads to an impairment of segmental or afferent inhibition resulting in an overreaction of wide dynamic range neurons which mimics the activity normally produced by noxious stimuli. This notion would be supported by the fact that peripheral nerve injuries producing

deficit of sensory functions mediated by both large and small diameter primary afferent fibers (Nurmikko and Bowsher, 1990). It has also been reported that areas of dense sensory loss with predominantly continuous pain and without allodynia are usually cooler than the rest of the skin, and that allodynia is localized in areas with relatively preserved sensation which are often warmer than the rest of the skin on infrared thermography (Rowbotham and Fields, 1989).

3. Pathology

Post-mortem studies have demonstrated marked loss of myelin and axons in the nerve and/or root following both spinal (Watson et al., 1988a, 1991a)

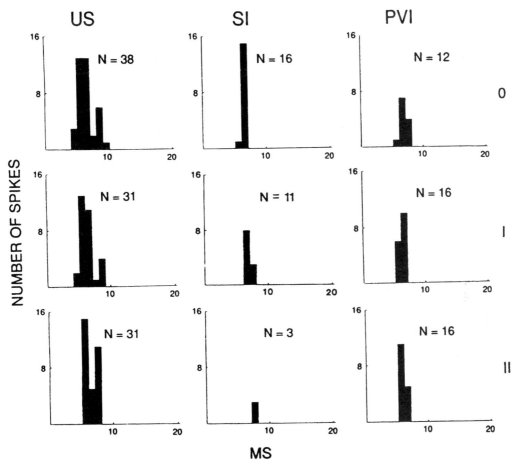

Fig. 1. Poststimulus histograms (16 stimuli at 0.5 Hz, 1 ms bin width) of the response of a wide dynamic range neuron in the trigeminal nucleus caudalis: US, an unconditioned stimulus to the infraorbital nerve; SI, stimulation of the infraorbital nerve 100 ms after a conditioning stimulus to this nerve; and PVI, stimulation of the infraorbital nerve 100 ms after a conditioning stimulus to the periventricular gray matter. Recordings obtained just prior to the injection of amitriptyline (top row, 0), 10 min after the injection of 2 mg/kg amitriptyline (middle row, I), and 10 min after a second injection of 2 mg/kg amitriptyline (bottom row, II). N is the total number of spikes. (From Fromm et al. (1991), with permission.)

neuropathic-like pain in experimental animals cause the degeneration of presumed inhibitory interneurons (Sugimoto et al., 1989, 1990). Clinical studies in postherpetic neuralgia (Nurmikko and Bowsher, 1990) and in other neuropathic pains (Lindblom and Verillo, 1979; Noordenbos and Wall, 1981) also suggest that neuropathic pain is due to dysfunction in the central nervous system. The observation that there is dorsal horn atrophy in patients suffering from postherpetic neuralgia, but not in patients without persistent pain (Watson et al., 1988a, 1991a), provides further evidence in favor of an involvement of neu-

rons in the central nervous system in the pathogenesis of postherpetic neuralgia. Amitriptyline's lack of effect on low-threshold mechanoceptive neurons contrasts with the observations that baclofen and carbamazepine markedly facilitate the segmental inhibition of low-threshold mechanoceptive neurons (Fromm et al., 1980, 1981, 1982). Similarly, the clinical experience has been that amitriptyline can alleviate the pain of postherpetic neuralgia, but not of trigeminal neuralgia. Baclofen and carbamazepine, on the other hand, are effective against the paroxysmal attacks of trigeminal neuralgia, but not against

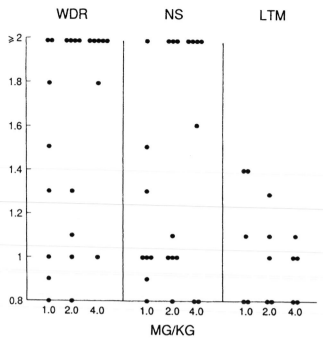

Fig. 2. Changes in the magnitude of the segmental inhibition observed in wide dynamic range (WDR), nociceptive specific (NS) and low-threshold mechanoceptive (LTM) neurons in the trigeminal nucleus caudalis 10 min after administration of total doses of 1.0, 2.0 and 4.0 mg/kg amitriptyline. (From Fromm et al. (1991), with permission.)

the chronic burning pain of postherpetic neuralgia or other neuropathic pain.

Allodynia appears to occur in areas of relatively preserved sensation (Rowbotham and Fields, 1989), and can be so prominent as to resemble the trigger zones in trigeminal neuralgia (Nurmikko and Bowsher, 1990). Like the attacks of trigeminal neuralgia, the allodynia in postherpetic neuralgia can be alleviated by lidocaine (Rowbotham and Fields, 1989). Moreover, baclofen may also relieve the allodynia and the sharp, jabbing pains of ophthalmic postherpetic neuralgia in some patients (Terrence et al., 1985).

5. Pathophysiology of postherpetic neuralgia: comparison with trigeminal neuralgia

Viewed collectively, these clinical and experimental observations suggest that the paroxysmal pains of trigeminal neuralgia may be due to impairment of segmental inhibition and hyperactivity of low-threshold mechanoceptive neurons which intermittently cause paroxysmal discharges of wide dynamic range neurons that are perceived as the excruciating attacks of pain (Fromm, 1991). The chronic pain of postherpetic neuralgia, on the other hand, may be due to impaired segmental inhibition of the wide dynamic range neurons themselves, causing them to continually overreact and mimic the activity normally elicited only by noxious stimuli (Fromm et al., 1991).

The type of trigeminal dysfunction would thus depend on the degree of damage to the afferent fibers. The compression of the trigeminal roots by a blood vessel or small tumor that appears to cause trigeminal neuralgia (Fromm, 1991) leads to only minimal sensory impairment (Altenmüller et al., 1990; Cruccu et al., 1990; Ackermann-Körner and Draeger, 1991; Nurmikko, 1991) and pathological changes (Beaver et al., 1965; Kerr and Miller, 1966) associated with dysfunction of segmental inhibition of low-threshold mechanoceptive neurons and ectopic neural pacemakers (Devor, 1991). Tactile stimulation of the face can then result in hyperactivity of

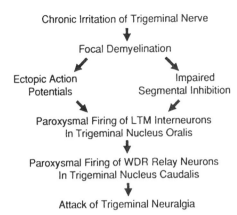

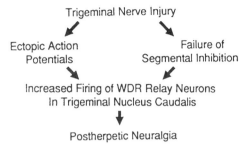

Fig. 4. The chronic burning pain of postherpetic neuralgia is caused by a combination of increased afferent activity and more extensive failure of segmental inhibition. This occurs when injury to the trigeminal nerve causes more extensive transsynaptic neuronal degeneration with loss of LTM neurons and a failure of segmental inhibition of WDR neurons. The combination of increased input from ectopic neural pacemakers with impaired segmental inhibition of WDR neurons leads these neurons to continually fire at frequencies normally associated with noxious stimuli and results in the perception of a chronic aching or burning sensation. (From Fromm (1993), with permission.)

Fig. 3. The painful paroxysms of trigeminal neuralgia are caused by a combination of increased afferent activity and decreased segmental inhibition of low-threshold mechanoceptive neurons. This occurs when chronic compression of the trigeminal nerve leads to degeneration of some inhibitory interneurons as well as the development of ectopic neural pacemakers. The combination of increased afferent activity with impaired segmental inhibition results in an excessive paroxysmal response of LTM neurons to tactile stimulation. The attacks of trigeminal neuralgia ensue when this paroxysmal discharge spreads to WDR neurons and causes them to fire at frequencies otherwise associated with intensely noxious stimuli. (From Fromm (1991), with permission.)

low-threshold mechanoceptive neurons due to this combination of increased afferent input and impaired segmental inhibition (Fig. 3). An attack of trigeminal neuralgia ensues when this paroxysmal activity spreads to wide dynamic range neurons in nucleus caudalis and causes them to fire at frequencies normally associated with intensely noxious stimulation.

In postherpetic neuralgia, the more extensive pathological changes caused by the herpes zoster virus (Watson et al., 1988a, 1991a) lead to more extensive sensory loss (Watson et al., 1988b; Nurmikko and Bowsher, 1990; Nurmikko et al., 1990) associated with destruction of low-threshold mechanoceptive neurons and a failure of segmental inhibition of wide dynamic range neurons. In this situation, the combination of increased afferent input from ectopic neural pacemakers and impaired segmental inhibition of wide dynamic range neurons causes these neurons to continually overreact (Fig. 4). This increased activity mimics the response normally elicited by noxious stimuli and results in the per-

ception of the chronic burning pain of postherpetic neuralgia.

In this scheme, postherpetic neuralgia with allodynia and jabbing, electric shock-like pain occupies an intermediate position. Allodynia mainly occurs in areas of relatively preserved sensation (Rowbotham and Fields, 1989). These episodic pains could thus be due to impaired segmental inhibition of relatively preserved low-threshold mechanoceptive neurons, resulting in their firing paroxysmally in response to tactile stimulation akin to the pathogenesis of the attacks of trigeminal neuralgia (Fig. 3).

The increased incidence of postherpetic neuralgia in elderly patients is probably related to the fact that aging is associated with a significant reduction in the axo-axonic synaptic complexes (Johnson et al., 1991) which mediate segmental inhibition. The similarity of these changes to those elicited by partial denervation suggests that the aging process would provide a favorable substrate for the pathogenesis of postherpetic neuralgia. On the other hand, the temporary nature of some denervation-induced changes (Sessle, 1991) indicates a considerable capacity for recovery in the trigeminal nuclei and could explain why postherpetic neuralgia ameliorates with time in many patients.

Prolonged topical application of capsaicin desensitizes C nociceptors (Westerman et al., 1988; Bjerring et al., 1990; LeVasseur et al., 1990; Peikert et al., 1991; Simone and Ochoa, 1991), decreasing their input to CNS neurons. This decrease in afferent activity would lessen the likelihood that the firing rate of wide dynamic range neurons would reach the level associated with the perception of pain even though segmental inhibition is impaired. The temporary improvement observed after the intravenous administration of lidocaine (Rowbotham et al., 1991) appears to be similarly due to a decrease in nociceptive input to wide dynamic range neurons (Sotgiu et al., 1991). The tricyclic antidepressants, on the other hand, keep the firing rate of wide dynamic range neurons rate below the level at which pain is perceived by enhancing the segmental inhibition.

6. Treatment of herpes zoster ophthalmicus and prevention of postherpetic neuralgia

The fact that postherpetic neuralgia is a common complication of herpes zoster ophthalmicus (De Moragas and Kierland, 1957; Cobo et al., 1986, 1987; Harding et al., 1987; Nigam et al., 1991) and continues to be a difficult therapeutic problem (Liesegang, 1991a,b) places a premium on the prevention of this complication if at all possible. It was initially reported that oral acyclovir reduces the zoster-related pain during the acute phase of herpes zoster ophthalmicus, but has no effect on the incidence, severity, or duration of postherpetic neuralgia (Cobo et al., 1986). However, a recent placebo-controlled study found that higher doses of oral acyclovir (800 mg instead of 600 mg five times a day) did reduce the severity and incidence of postherpetic pain, as well as protecting against long-term ocular complications (Harding and Porter, 1991). Stellate ganglion blocks too have been shown to relieve the acute pain in herpes zoster ophthalmicus in a randomized prospective controlled trial (Harding et al., 1986). However, it appears that sympathetic blocks do not affect the development of postherpetic neuralgia even with very early intervention (Yanagida et

al., 1987; Nurmikko et al., 1990), despite anecdotal reports regarding its ability to prevent postherpetic neuralgia (Currey and Dalsania, 1991).

7. Treatment of ophthalmic postherpetic neuralgia

The tricyclic antidepressants and the topical application of capsaicin constitute the mainstay of treatment once ophthalmic postherpetic neuralgia develops. The effectiveness of amitriptyline, desipramine and maprotiline has been documented in several double-blind, randomized studies (Watson et al., 1982, 1982; Max et al., 1988; Kishore-Kumar et al., 1990). However, only about one-half to two-thirds of the patients benefit from these medications. Of note, the serotonergic agents buspirone, m-chlorophenylpiperazine and zimelidine do not relieve the pain of postherpetic neuralgia (Watson and Evans, 1985; Kishore-Kumar et al., 1989), and the noradrenergic antidepressant maprotiline is less effective than amitriptyline (Watson et al., 1992, p. 241). Therapy should therefore start with amitriptyline at 10–25 mg at bedtime and increasing by 10–25 mg at weekly intervals until pain relief is achieved or side effects occur. If amitriptyline fails, desipramine or maprotiline should be tried next.

The topical application of capsaicin has been reported to relieve the pain of ophthalmic, as well as spinal, postherpetic neuralgia in half to three-quarters of the patients in several open studies (Bernstein et al., 1987; Bucci et al., 1988; Watson et al., 1988) and one double-blind study (Bernstein et al., 1989). The use of this medication requires careful supervision and patient education (Watson et al., 1988). Capsaicin has to be applied 4–5 times per day for as long as 4 weeks as the onset and best response may be delayed until that time. Accidental contact of capsaicin with the eye needs to be meticulously avoided. Post-capsaicin burning can be decreased by applying 5% xylocaine ointment prior to the capsaicin application. The application of a suspension of aspirin in chloroform or diethyl ether has also been reported to relieve postherpetic neuralgia (King, 1988; De

Benedittis et al., 1992). Care must be exercised to avoid the chloroform evaporating near the eye lest the cornea be damaged.

8. Conclusions

Ophthalmic postherpetic neuralgia thus continues to be a difficult therapeutic problem for which there is no generally effective treatment at this time. In view of its relatively frequent occurrence, especially in elderly patients, and its debilitating character, it appears that the best approach is to try to prevent its development by the early administration of high-dose oral acyclovir (Harding and Porter, 1991; Liesegang, 1991a,b). The tricyclic antidepressants amitriptyline, desipramine and maprotiline or the careful application of capsaicin are the most effective therapeutic modalities currently available for the treatment of ophthalmic postherpetic neuralgia, but they are by no means always effective.

9. Summary

Herpes zoster ophthalmicus is a common manifestation of herpes zoster, accounting for about one-fifth of all cases. Moreover, postherpetic neuralgia is a frequent complication in these patients, especially in the elderly. Three different types of pain are associated with postherpetic neuralgia: a chronic burning pain, an intermittent lancinating or electric shock-like pain, and a sharp dysesthesia evoked by light touch (allodynia). The clinical and experimental data currently available suggest that the chronic burning pain of postherpetic neuralgia occurs when the attack of herpes zoster causes the loss of inhibitory neurons in the trigeminal nucleus or dorsal horn and the development of ectopic neural pacemaker sites, leading to a more or less continual overactivity of wide dynamic range neurons mimicking the activity normally elicited by noxious stimuli. The pathophysiology of the intermittent lancinating pain and allodynia is probably akin to that of trigeminal neuralgia, involving intermittent paroxysmal discharges of low-threshold mechanoceptive neurons as an intermediate step. Oral acyclovir (800 mg five times a day) has been reported to reduce the incidence and severity of postherpetic neuralgia, as well as alleviating many of the acute symptoms of herpes zoster ophthalmicus. The tricyclic antidepressants and the topical administration of capsaicin are the main therapeutic modalities once postherpetic neuralgia has developed, but these are only effective in about one-half to two-thirds of the cases.

Reference

Ackermann-Körner, M. and Draeger, J. (1991) Quantitative Messungen der Hornhautsensibilität bei idiopathischer Trigeminusneuralgie und nach neurochirurgischen Eingriffen am N. trigeminus. Klin. Mbl. Augenheilk., 199: 84–90.

Altenmüller, E., Cornelius, C.P. and Buettner, U.W. (1990) Somatosensory evoked potentials following tongue stimulation in normal subjects and patients with lesions of the afferent trigeminal system. Electroencephalogr. Clin. Neurophysiol., 77: 403–415.

Beaver, D.L., Moses, H.L. and Ganote, C.E. (1965) Electron microscopy of the trigeminal ganglion. III. Trigeminal neuralgia. Arch. Pathol., 79: 571–582.

Bernstein, J.E., Bickers, D.R., Dahl, M.V. and Roshal, J.Y. (1987) Treatment of chronic postherpetic neuralgia with topical capsaicin. J. Am. Acad. Dermatol., 17: 93–96.

Bernstein, J.E., Korman, N.J., Bickers, D.R., Dahl, M.V. and Millikan, L.E. (1989) Topical capsaicin in chronic postherpetic neuralgia. J. Am. Acad. Dermatol., 21: 265–270.

Bjerring, P., Arendt-Nielsen, L. and Sderberg, U. (1990) Argon laser induced cutaneous sensory and pain thresholds in post-herpetic neuralgia. Quantitative modulation by topical capsaicin. Acta. Dermatol. Venereol. (Stockholm), 70: 121–125.

Bucci, F.A. Jr., Gabriels, C.F. and Krohel, G.B. (1988) Successful treatment of postherpetic neuralgia with capsaicin. Am. J. Ophthalmol., 106: 758–759.

Burgoon, C.F. Jr., Burgoon, J.S. and Baldridge, G.D. (1957) The natural history of herpes zoster. J. Am. Med. Assoc., 164: 265–269.

Cobo, L.M., Foulks, G.N., Liesegang, T., Lass, J., Sutphin, J.E., Wilhelmus, K., Jones, D.B., Chapman, S., Segreti, A.C. and King, D.H. (1986) Oral acyclovir in the treatment of acute herpes zoster ophthalmicus. Ophthalmology, 93: 763–770.

Cobo, L.M., Foulks, G.N., Liesegang, T., Lass, J., Sutphin, T., Wilhelmus, K. and Jones, D.B. (1987) Observations on the natural history of herpes zoster ophthalmicus. Curr. Eye Res., 6: 195–199.

Cruccu, G., Leandri, M., Feliciani, M. and Manfredi, M. (1990) Idiopathic and symptomatic trigeminal pain. J. Neurol. Neurosurg. Psychiatr., 53: 1034–1042.

Currey, T.A. and Dalsania, J. (1991) Treatment of herpes zoster ophthalmicus: Stellate ganglion block as a treatment for acute pain and prevention of postherpetic neuralgia. Ann. Ophthalmol., 23: 188–189.

De Benedittis, G., Besana, F. and Lorenzetti, A. (1992) A new topical treatment for acute herpetic neuralgia and post-herpetic neuralgia: The aspirin/diethyl ether mixture. An open-label study plus a double-blind controlled trial. Pain, 48: 383–390.

De Moragas, J.M. and Kierland, R.R. (1957) The outcome of patients with herpes zoster. Arch. Dermatol., 75: 193–196.

Devor, M. (1991) Neuropathic pain and injured nerve: peripheral mechanisms. Br. Med. Bull., 47: 619–630.

Dubner, R., Sharav, Y., Gracely, R.H. and Price, D.D. (1987) Idiopathic trigeminal neuralgia: sensory features and pain mechanisms. Pain, 31: 23–33.

Fromm, G.H. (1991) Pathophysiology of trigeminal neuralgia. In: G.H. Fromm and B.J. Sessle (Eds.), Trigeminal Neuralgia: Current Concepts Regarding Pathogenesis and Treatment. Butterworth-Heinemann, Boston, pp. 105–130.

Fromm, G.H. (1993) Physiological rationale for the treatment of neuropathic pain. APS J., 2: 1–7.

Fromm, G.H., Terrence, C.F., Chattha, A.S. and Glass, J.D. (1980) Baclofen in trigeminal neuralgia: its effect on the spinal trigeminal nucleus: a pilot study. Arch. Neurol., 37: 768–771.

Fromm, G.H., Chattha, A.S., Terrence, C.F. and Glass, J.D. (1981) Role of inhibitory mechanisms in trigeminal neuralgia. Neurology, 31: 683–687.

Fromm, G.H., Chattha, A.S., Terrence, C.F. and Glass, J.D. (1982) Do phenytoin and carbarnazepine depress excitation and/or facilitate inhibition? Eur. J. Pharmacol., 78: 403–409.

Fromm, G.H., Nakata, M. and Kondo, T. (1991) Differential action of amitriptyline on neurons in the trigeminal nucleus. Neurology, 41: 1932–1936.

Fromm, G.H., Aumentado, D. and Terrence, C.F. (1993) A clinical and experimental investigation of the effects of tizanidine in trigeminal neuralgia. Pain, in press.

Harding, S.P. and Porter, S.M. (1991) Oral acyclovir in herpes zoster ophthalmicus. Curr. Eye Res. 10 (Suppl): pp. 177–182.

Harding, S.P., Lipton, J.R., Wells, J.C.D. and Campbell, J.A. (1986) Relief of acute pain in herpes zoster ophthalmicus by stellate ganglion block. Br. Med. J., 292: 1428.

Harding, S.P., Lipton, J.R. and Wells, J.C.D. (1987) Natural history of herpes zoster ophthalmicus: predictors of postherpetic neuralgia and ocular involvement. Br. J. Ophthalmol., 71: 353–358.

Hope-Simpson, R.E. (1975) Postherpetic neuralgia. J. R. Coll. Gen. Pract., 25: 571–575.

Johnson, L.R., Westrum, L.E. and Henry, M.A. (1991) Anatomic organization of the trigeminal system and the effects of deafferentation. In: G.H. Fromm and B.J. Sessle (Eds.), Trigemi-

nal Neuralgia: Current Concepts Regarding Pathogenesis and Treatment. Butterworth-Heinemann, Boston, pp. 27–69.

Kerr, F.W.L. and Miller, R.H. (1966) The pathology of trigeminal neuralgia. Electron microscopic studies. Arch. Neurol., 15: 308–319.

King, R.B. (1988) Concerning the management of pain associated with herpes zoster and of postherpetic neuralgia. Pain, 33: 73–78.

Kishore-Kumar, R., Schafer, S.C., Lawlor, B.A., Murphy, D.L. and Max, M.B. (1989) Single doses of the serotonin agonists busiprone and m-chlorophenylpyperazine do not relieve neuropathic pain. Pain, 37: 223–227.

Kishore-Kumar, R., Max, M.B., Schafer, S.C., Gaughan, A.M., Smoller, B., Gracely, R.H. and Dubner, R. (1990) Desipramine relieves postherpetic neuralgia. Clin. Pharmacol. Ther., 47: 305–312.

LeVasseur, S.A., Gibson, S.J. and Helme, R.D. (1990) The measurement of capsaicin-sensitive sensory nerve fiber function in elderly patients with pain. Pain, 41: 19–25.

Liesegang, T.J. (1991a) Diagnosis and therapy of herpes zoster ophthalmicus. Ophthalmology, 98: 1216–1229.

Liesegang, T.J. (1991b) Ophthalmic herpes zoster: diagnosis and antiviral therapy. Geriatrics, 46: 64–71.

Lindblom, U. and Verillo, R.T. (1979) Sensory functions in chronic neuralgia. J. Neurol. Neurosurg. Psychiatry, 42: 422–435.

Max, M.B., Schafer, S.C., Culnane, M., Smoller, B., Dubner, R. and Gracely, R.H. (1988) Amitriptyline, but not lorazepam, relieves postherpetic neuralgia. Neurology, 38: 1427–1432.

Nigam, P., Kumar, A., Kapoor, K.K., Sarkari, N.B., Gupta, A.K., Lal, B.B. and Mukhija, R.D. (1991) Clinical profile of herpes zoster ophthalmicus. J. Indian Med. Assoc., 89: 117–119.

Noordenbos, W. and Wall, P.D. (1981) Implications of the failure of nerve resection and graft to cure chronic pain produced by nerve lesions. J. Neurol. Neurosurg. Psychiatry, 44: 1068–1073.

Nurmikko, T. and Bowsher, D. (1990) Somatosensory findings in postherpetic neuralgia. J. Neurol. Neurosurg. Psychiatry, 53: 135–141.

Nurmikko, T.J. (1991) Altered cutaneous sensation in trigeminal neuralgia. Arch. Neurol., 48: 523–527.

Nurmikko, T.J., Räsänen, A. and Häkkinen, V. (1990) Clinical and neurophysiological observations on acute herpes zoster. Clin. J. Pain, 6: 284–290.

Peikert, A., Hentrich, M. and Ochs, G. (1991) Topical 0.025% capsaicin in chronic post-herpetic neuralgia: efficacy, predictors of response and long-term course. J. Neurol., 238: 452–456.

Reske-Nielsen, E., Oster, S. and Pedersen, B. (1986) Herpes zoster ophthalmicus and the mesencephalic nucleus. Acta Pathol. Microbiol. Immunol. Scand. Sect. A, 94: 263–269.

Roberts, W.J. (1986) A hypothesis on the physiological basis for causalgia and related pains. Pain, 24: 297–311.

Rowbotham, M.C. and Fields, H.L. (1989) Post-herpetic neuralgia: The relation of pain complaint, sensory disturbance, and skin temperature. Pain, 39: 129–144.

Rowbotham, M.C., Reisner-Keller, L.A. and Fields, H.L. (1991) Both intravenous lidocaine and morphine reduce the pain of postherpetic neuralgia. Neurology, 41: 1024–1028.

Selby, G. (1984) Diseases of the fifth cranial nerve. In: P.J. Dyck, P.K. Thomas, E.H. Lambert and R. Bunge (Eds.), Peripheral Neuropathy. WB Saunders, Philadelphia, PA, pp. 1224–1265.

Sessle, B.J. (1987) The neurobiology of facial and dental pain: Present knowledge, future directions. J. Dent. Res., 66: 962–981.

Sessle, B.J. (1991) Physiology of the trigeminal system. In: G.H. Fromm and B.J. Sessle (Eds), Trigeminal Neuralgia: Current Concepts Regarding Pathogenesis and Treatment. Butterworth-Heinemann, Boston, pp. 71–104.

Simone, D.A. and Ochoa, J. (1991) Early and late effects of prolonged topical capsaicin on cutaneous sensibility and neurogenic vasodilatation in humans. Pain, 47: 285–294.

Sotgiu, M.L., Lacerenza, M. and Marchettini, P. (1991) Selective inhibition by systemic lidocaine of noxious evoked activity in rat dorsal horn neurons. NeuroReport, 2: 425–428.

Sugimoto, T., Bennett, G.J. and Kajander, K.C. (1989) Strychnine-enhanced transsynaptic degeneration of dorsal horn neurons in rats with an experimental painful peripheral neuropathy. Neurosci. Lett., 98: 139–143.

Sugimoto, T., Bennett, G.J. and Kajander, K.C. (1990) Transsynaptic degeneration in the superficial dorsal horn after sciatic nerve injury: Effects of a chronic constriction injury, transection, and strychnine. Pain, 42: 205–213.

Terrence, C.F., Fromm, G.H. and Tenicela, R. (1985) Baclofen as an analgesic in chronic peripheral nerve disease. Eur. Neurol., 24: 380–385.

Watson, C.P., Evans, R.J., Reed, K., Merskey, H., Goldsmith, L. and Warsh, J. (1982) Amitriptyline versus placebo in postherpetic neuralgia. Neurology, 32: 671–673.

Watson, C.P.N., Evans, R.J. and Watt, V.R. (1988) Post-herpetic neuralgia and topical capsaicin. Pain, 33: 333–340.

Watson, C.P.N. and Evans, R.J. (1985) A comparative trial of amitriptyline and zimelidine in post-herpetic neuralgia. Pain, 23: 387–394.

Watson, C.P.N., Morshead, C., Van der Kooy, D., Deck, J. and Evans, R.J. (1988a) Post-herpetic neuralgia: Post-mortem analysis of a case. Pain, 34: 129–138.

Watson, C.P.N., Evans, R.J., Watt, V.R. and Birkett, N. (1988b) Post-herpetic neuralgia: 208 cases. Pain, 35: 289–297.

Watson, C.P.N., Deck, J.H., Morshead, C., Van der Kooy, D., Evans, R.J. (1991a) Post-herpetic neuralgia: further post-mortem studies of cases with and without pain. Pain, 44: 105–117.

Watson, C.P.N., Watt, V.R., Chipman, M., Birkett, N. and Evans, R.J. (1991b) The prognosis with postherpetic neuralgia. Pain, 46: 195–199.

Watson, C.P.N., Chipman, M., Reed, K., Evans, R.J. and Birkett, N. (1992) Amitriptyline versus maprotiline in postherpetic neuralgia: a randomized, double-blind, crossover trial. Pain, 48: 29–36.

Westerman, R.A., Roberts, R.G., Kotzmann, R.R., Westerman, D.A., Delaney, C., Widdop, R.E. and Carter, B.E. (1988) Effects of topical capsaicin on normal skin and affected dermatomes in herpes zoster. Clin. Exp. Neurol., 25: 71–84.

Yanagida, H., Suwa, K. and Corssen, G. (1987) No prophylactic effect of early sympathetic blockade on postherpetic neuralgia. Anesthesiology, 66: 73–76.

Herpes Zoster and Postherpetic Neuralgia, 2nd Revised and Enlarged Edition
Pain Research and Clinical Management, Vol. 11
Edited by C.P.N. Watson and A.A. Gershon
© 2001 Elsevier Science B.V. All rights reserved

Commentary on Gerhard Fromm's 1993 chapter

Barry J. Sessle [*]

Faculty of Dentistry, University of Toronto, 124 Edward Street, Toronto, ON M5G 1G6, Canada

1. Introduction

My comments on Gerhard Fromm's chapter (which was also published about 10 years ago in the previous edition of this book) will focus on his proposals to account for the pathogenesis of trigeminal neuralgia (VN) and postherpetic neuralgia (PHN) in the orofacial region, and particularly their status in light of subsequent research. His chapter emphasized the integral involvement of both peripheral and central neural factors. Dr. Fromm proposed that these neuropathic pain conditions occur when chronic irritation or damage of afferent fibers produces increased afferent activity that leads to the degeneration of presumed inhibitory interneurons, with the consequent failure of the presynaptic and postsynaptic inhibitory mechanisms that normally serve to control the level of activity of wide dynamic range (WDR) neurons in the spinal dorsal horn and trigeminal brainstem sensory nuclear complex. He indicated that the degree of damage to afferent fibers is the significant factor in determining whether PHN or VN develops.

2. Pathophysiological mechanisms

2.1. Current concepts

Dr. Fromm's concept of the eventual involvement of WDR neurons in the pathogenesis of these two conditions is indeed consistent with earlier proposals (Dubner et al., 1987; Sessle, 1987; Dubner, 1991; Woolf, 1991) suggesting that the basis for the development of several pain conditions is injury-induced interference with central inhibitory mechanisms that normally modulate nociceptive neurons. The involvement of altered inhibitory mechanisms in VN is also suggested by the clinical features of this condition, e.g. the pain of VN that is usually evoked by a tactile stimulus can show summation and a variable refractory period, persist beyond the stimulation period, and be radiated or referred to more distant sites. More recently, espoused concepts related to PHN (Bennett, 1994; Rowbotham et al., 1999) also continue to emphasize the loss of central inhibitory mechanisms in some forms of PHN, and usually link this loss of inhibition to the development of a central neuroplasticity, with ensuing 'hyperexcitability' or 'sensitization' in the central nociceptive pathways. Emphasis is also being placed in some types of PHN on the presence of peripheral nociceptor sensitization or 'irritation' or on central reorganization due to central sprouting of undamaged afferents. The afferent nerve fiber, or the dorsal root or trigeminal ganglion, is also a site of particular emphasis in some concepts of both PHN and VN, where peripheral nerve damage or direct interference with ganglion cell functions is considered to lead to physiological and chemical changes in the injured axons or ganglion cells that is reflected in ectopic firing and

[*] Correspondence to: Dr. B.J. Sessle, Faculty of Dentistry, University of Toronto, 124 Edward Street, Toronto, ON M5G 1G6, Canada. Phone: +1 (416) 979-4910; Fax: +1 (416) 979-4936; E-mail: barry.sessle@utoronto.ca

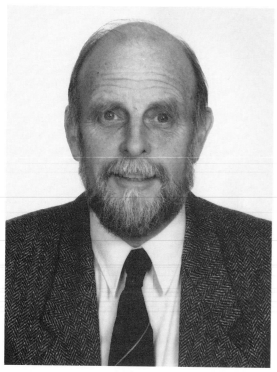

Dr. Barry J. Sessle

abnormal sensory inputs into the central nervous system that can induce alterations in central nociceptive pathways (see Bennett, 1994; Rappaport and Devor, 1994; Devor and Seltzer, 1999). The chapters in this book by Dr. Wall (Chapter 17) and by Dr. Rowbotham et al. (Chapter 16) provide detailed outlines of these various concepts.

2.2. The role of WDR, NS and LTM neurons

In his proposals for VN and for PHN involving the craniofacial region, Dr. Fromm outlined an integral role for brainstem WDR neurons, and specifically those in trigeminal subnucleus caudalis. The evidence for the involvement of caudalis WDR neurons in trigeminal pain mechanisms is substantial and includes anatomical, clinical, physiological and neurochemical data (for review, see Sessle, 1999, 2000). Let me first consider the features of WDR neurons in general, and then consider in the next section the role of subnucleus caudalis per se. The WDR

neurons have been known for many years to be involved in the discrimination and encoding of noxious stimuli, to receive both large-fiber (e.g. tactile) and small-fiber (e.g. nociceptive) afferent inputs, and to have a complex mechanoreceptive field, with zones having gradients of sensitivity to these inputs (for review, see Dubner and Bennett, 1983; Sessle, 2000). One especially noteworthy feature of these neurons is their remarkable neuroplasticity and capability of manifesting central sensitization in certain circumstances, in keeping with some of the current concepts of PHN and VN noted above. Peripheral deafferentation, injury, or inflammation can lead to changes in central inhibitory mechanisms that appear to result in an unmasking of relatively ineffective convergent afferent inputs and that are reflected in an increase in the numbers of neurons responding as WDR neurons as well as an increase in their mechanoreceptive field size and an increase in their excitability to peripheral afferent inputs (Dubner, 1991; Woolf, 1991; Doubell et al., 1999; Ren and Dubner, 1999; Sessle, 2000). In the case of trigeminal WDR neurons, such changes include an increased excitability to orofacial stimuli and expansion of the tactile component of the receptive field of trigeminal WDR neurons into regions of the face and mouth that previously were sensitive only to noxious stimuli (Hu et al., 1992; Chiang et al., 1998). These changes would mean that a tactile stimulus of the type that triggers, for example, a paroxysm of neuralgic pain will activate more WDR neurons than normal and produce a level of activity that mimics a level of central excitability normally only achieved by noxious stimuli, and as a consequence pain is experienced (e.g. see Dubner et al., 1987).

However, these neuroplastic changes are not limited to WDR neurons: some peripheral injuries or inflammation can lead to excitability changes not only in WDR neurons, but also in low-threshold mechanoreceptive (LTM) neurons and especially in nociceptive-specific (NS) neurons in subnucleus caudalis and oralis (Hu et al., 1986, 1990, 1992; Chiang et al., 1998). For example, following the application of inflammatory agents to craniofacial tissues, NS neurons as well as WDR neurons develop an expanded mechanoreceptive field and an increased responsiveness to peripheral noxious stimuli. Furthermore, neurons that previously could only be excited by noxious stimuli (i.e. NS neurons) may become responsive also to tactile stimulation and thereby take on the features of WDR neurons. Thus, it is possible that peripheral damage or inflammation may lead to impairment of central inhibitory mechanisms that lead not only to increased excitability of NS as well as WDR neurons to nociceptive afferent inputs but also to unmasking of normally inhibited tactile inputs that become effective in exciting NS neurons (or become more effective in the case of WDR neurons). Thus, I do not believe NS neurons can be discounted in the pathogenesis of PHN and VN.

Dr. Fromm also invoked LTM neurons in the pathogenesis of both PHN and VN. While LTM neurons can be activated by tactile stimuli of the type than may evoke pain in PHN and VN and do show a propensity for neuroplastic changes following some forms of peripheral insult, I see a more crucial role for the WDR neurons and NS neurons in the early stages of PHN or VN, for several reasons. As noted earlier, the functional properties and potential for neuroplasticity of WDR neurons in normal and injured states are consistent with the clinical features and likely pathogenic mechanisms underlying PHN and VN. In addition, NS neurons also have properties consistent with a generally accepted role for them in nociceptive processing and in localization and discrimination of noxious stimuli. Furthermore, as noted above, NS neurons also can undergo neuroplastic changes, including the manifestation of a tactile receptive field, after peripheral tissue damage or inflammation. Many NS neurons as well as WDR neurons in the trigeminal brainstem complex have a mechanoreceptive field localized to intraoral and perioral regions where the trigger sites occur and the pain is experienced in VN. It is also clear from Dr. Fromm's own investigations that the features in LTM neurons of segmental inhibition and sensitivity of this inhibition to neuralgic-relieving drugs are also characteristic of nociceptive neurons.

2.3. The role of trigeminal subnucleus oralis and subnucleus caudalis

Dr. Fromm appears to have suggested that neuronal changes within trigeminal subnucleus caudalis lies at the heart of the development of PHN, whereas an integral component of his hypothesis of the pathogenesis of VN is that the trigeminal neuronal changes start in subnucleus oralis, and not in subnucleus caudalis. On one hand, this latter concept is not in itself unreasonable. While subnucleus caudalis has traditionally been viewed as the essential brainstem nociceptive relay in the trigeminal system, it is now clear that nociceptive processing involving WDR and NS neurons also occurs in the more rostral components of the trigeminal brainstem complex, such as subnucleus oralis (e.g. Dallel et al., 1990; Hu et al., 1992; for review, see Sessle, 1987, 2000). These nociceptive oralis neurons, as well LTM neurons in subnucleus oralis, have mechanoreceptive fields localized to orofacial regions (intraoral and perioral) that encompass the usual sites for the tactile trigger points of VN and those parts of the maxillary and mandibular divisions where the excruciating pain is usually experienced. Furthermore, tooth pulp deafferentation can produce increased excitability of LTM neurons within subnucleus oralis with little evidence of such changes occurring in caudalis neurons (Sessle, 1991) (although it might be argued that the pulp deafferentation-induced changes in oralis are too mild to 'spill over' into caudalis). Dr. Fromm, moreover, reported that drugs effective against VN enhance segmental inhibitory mechanisms modulating the properties of LTM neurons in subnucleus oralis. In addition, the efficacy of trigeminal tractotomy in relieving VN is not incompatible with a primary role of subnucleus oralis in the pathogenesis of this disorder, since this procedure would reduce the predominantly ascending facilitatory effect that subnucleus caudalis normally exerts on the relay of tactile inputs to neurons in subnucleus oralis (for review, see Dubner et al., 1978; Sessle, 1987, 2000).

On the other hand, there is increasing evidence that peripherally induced excitability changes in nociceptive neurons in subnucleus oralis are dependent on changes first occurring within subnucleus caudalis (for review, see Dallel et al., 1998; Sessle, 2000). Thus, it is very possible that the initial injury-induced changes in VN as well as in PN occur first in subnucleus caudalis, and then by way of its ascending modulatory influences on more rostral neurons (see above), other components of the trigeminal brainstem complex would become involved. Further investigation of these caudal–rostral interactions should help clarify the relative importance of the different elements of the trigeminal brainstem complex in the pathogenesis of both PHN and VN.

3. Future research directions

In view of Dr. Fromm's proposals and the recent data outlined above of the neuronal properties of the rostral and caudal components of the trigeminal brainstem complex, several research directions are suggested. More study is needed of peripheral mechanisms that may be associated with PHN and VN, given the proposed involvement of ectopic peripheral pacemakers and recent evidence bearing on a number of peripherally acting chemicals, such as the excitatory amino acids, opioids, cytokines and GABA (see Bennett, 1994; Rappaport and Devor, 1994; Devor and Seltzer, 1999; Rowbotham et al., 1999; Sessle, 2000). These include further study of the properties of trigeminal ganglion cells to determine whether changes specifically in these cells may contribute to the development and pathogenesis of VN and PHN in the orofacial region. Future studies of central mechanisms should, as noted above, investigate in more detail the interactions between subnuclei oralis and caudalis, and also consider the possibility that neurons in parts of the central nervous system other than subnuclei oralis and caudalis are implicated in PHN and VN. A limitation with Dr. Fromm's own studies is they were carried out in 'normal' animals, and a major drawback in testing many aspects of such proposals in the past has been the paucity of appropriate models for these conditions expressing pain in the orofacial region in particular. However, recent advances in the develop-

ment of animal models of acute and chronic pain hold promise of the acquisition of models that mimic the features of some types of PHN and VN and that provide for exploration of peripheral and central changes in the trigeminal system. Future studies also need to take account of clinical data revealing that not all patients with peripheral nerve damage develop these conditions, and the recent emphasis on the role of gender, genetic and environmental factors in the development of chronic pain conditions points to another area warranting investigation in PHN and VN.

Another important area of current research is the neurochemical mechanisms in the spinal cord and trigeminal brainstem complex that contribute to acute and chronic pain conditions. The application of this knowledge to the VN and PHN fields is important not only for the clarification of the pathogenesis of these two conditions, but also for the development of improved pharmacological approaches to these conditions. Further studies of the specificity and differential effects of drugs effective in relieving neuropathic pain states on LTM, WDR and NS neurons in oralis as well as in caudalis in normal animals and in experimental models of peripheral and central injury also represent crucial steps for future research in this area. In addition, the longer term effects of these drugs on these neurons warrant investigation, in view of the long-term clinical usage and efficacy of several of the drugs used to manage PHN and VN.

Reference

Bennett, G.J. (1994) Hypotheses on the pathogenesis of Herpes Zoster-associated pain. Ann. Neurol. 35: S38–S41.

Chiang, C.Y., Park, S.J., Kwan, C.L., Hu, J.W. and Sessle, B.J. (1998) NMDA receptor mechanisms contribute to neuroplasticity induced in caudalis nociceptive neurons by tooth pulp stimulation. J. Neurophysiol., 80: 2621–2631.

Dallel, R., Raboisson, P., Woda, A. and Sessle, B.J. (1990) Properties of nociceptive and nonnociceptive brainstem neurons in trigeminal subnucleus oralis of the rat. Brain Res., 521: 95–106.

Dallel, R., Duale, C. and Molat, J.-L. (1998) Morphine administered in the substantia gelatinosa of the spinal trigeminal nucleus caudalis inhibits nociceptive activities in the spinal trigeminal nucleus oralis. J. Neurosci., 18: 3529–3536.

Devor, M. and Seltzer, Z. (1999) Pathophysiology of damaged nerves in relation to chronic pain. In: P.D. Wall and R. Melzack (Eds.), Textbook of Pain, 4th edn. Churchill Livingstone, Edinburgh, pp. 129–164.

Doubell, T.P., Mannion, R.J. and Woolf, C.J. (1999) The dorsal horn: state-dependent sensory processing, plasticity and the generation of pain. In: P.D. Wall and R. Melzack (Eds.), Textbook of Pain, 4th edn., Churchill Livingstone, Edinburgh, pp. 165–181.

Dubner, R. (1991) Neuronal plasticity and pain following peripheral tissue inflammation or nerve injury. In: M.R. Bond, J.E. Charlton and C.J. Woolf (Eds.), Proceedings of the VIth World Congress on Pain. Pain Research and Clinical Management, Vol. 4. Elsevier, Amsterdam, pp. 263–276.

Dubner, R. and Bennett, G.J. (1983) Spinal and trigeminal mechanisms of nociception. Annu. Rev. Neurosci., 6: 381–418.

Dubner, R., Sessle, B.J. and Storey, A.T. (1978) The Neural Basis of Oral and Facial Function. Plenum, New York.

Dubner, R., Sharav, Y., Gracely, R.H. and Price, D.D. (1987) Idiopathic trigeminal neuralgia: sensory features and pain mechanisms. Pain, 31: 23–33.

Hu, J.W., Dostrovsky, J., Lenz, Y., Ball, G. and Sessle, B.J. (1986) Tooth pulp deafferentation is associated with functional alterations in the properties of neurons in the trigeminal spinal tract nucleus. J. Neurophysiol., 56: 1650–1668.

Hu, J.W., Sharav, Y. and Sessle, B.J. (1990) Effects of one or two-staged deafferentation of mandibular and maxillary tooth pulps on the functional properties of trigeminal brainstem neurones. Brain Res., 516: 271–279.

Hu, J.W., Sessle, B.J., Raboisson, P., Dallel, R. and Woda, A. (1992) Stimulation of craniofacial muscle afferents induces prolonged facilitatory effects in trigeminal nociceptive brainstem neurones. Pain, 48: 53–60.

Rappaport, Z.H. and Devor, M. (1994) Trigeminal neuralgia: the role of self-sustaining discharge in the trigeminal ganglion (TG). Pain, 56: 127–138.

Ren, K. and Dubner, R. (1999) Central nervous system plasticity and persistent pain. J. Orofacial Pain 13: 155–163.

Rowbotham, M.C., Petersen, K.L. and Fields, H.L. (1999) Is postherpetic neuralgia more than one disorder? IASP Newsletter, Fall, 3–7.

Sessle, B.J. (1987) The neurobiology of orofacial and dental pain. J. Dent. Res., 66: 962–981.

Sessle, B.J. (1991) Physiology of the trigeminal system. In: G.H. Fromm and B.J. Sessle (Eds.), Trigeminal Neuralgia: Current Concepts Regarding Pathogenesis and Treatment. Butterworths, Stoneham, pp. 71–104.

Sessle, B.J. (1999) The neural basis of temporomandibular joint and masticatory muscle pain. J. Orofacial Pain, 13: 238–245.

Sessle, B.J. (2000) Acute and chronic craniofacial pain: brainstem mechanisms of nociceptive transmission and neuroplasticity, and their clinical correlates. Crit. Rev. Oral Biol. Med., 11: 57–91.

Woolf, C.J. (1991) Central mechanisms of acute pain. In: M.R. Bond, J.E. Charlton and C.J. Woolf (Eds.), Proceedings of the VIth World Congress on Pain. Pain Research and Clinical Management, Vol. 4. Elsevier, Amsterdam, pp. 25–34.

Herpes Zoster and Postherpetic Neuralgia, 2nd Revised and Enlarged Edition
Pain Research and Clinical Management, Vol. 11
Edited by C.P.N. Watson and A.A. Gershon
© *2001 Elsevier Science B.V. All rights reserved*

CHAPTER 15

The neuropathology of herpes zoster with particular reference to postherpetic neuralgia and its pathogenesis

C. Peter N. Watson [1,*], Anne Louise Oaklander [2] and John H. Deck [3]

[1] *Department of Medicine, University of Toronto, Toronto, Ontario, Canada,* [2] *Departments of Anesthesiology, Neurology and Pathology, Massachusetts General Hospital, Harvard Medical School, Boston, MA, USA and* [3] *Department of Pathology, University of Toronto, Toronto, Ontario Canada*

1. Introduction

Since the first edition of this book much has been learned about the pathology of cutaneous nerve endings in postherpetic neuralgia (PHN). As well, a single case of ophthalmic PHN has been autopsied with new pathological findings. Evidence from both of these lines of work as well as previous data suggest that unilateral shingles has bilateral effects. The chief objective of this book and this chapter is to collect information about the acute and chronic pain resulting from herpes zoster (HZ). This chapter's focus remains on the pathological findings in the spinal cord, nerve root, ganglion, and peripheral nerves extending to their cutaneous termination. Cerebral involvement is mentioned briefly with references for the interested reader.

2. Encephalitis and delayed hemiplegia

Varicella-zoster (VZV) can cause encephalitis (Rose et al., 1964; McCormick et al., 1969; Horten et al., 1981; Jemsek et al., 1983), vasculitis (Linnemann and Alvira, 1980; Eidelberg et al., 1986) and granulomatous angiitis (Rosenblum and Hadfield, 1972). Information on the pathology of delayed hemiplegia following ophthalmic zoster is also available (Doyle et al., 1983). Encephalitis unassociated with skin lesions has been described with AIDS (Morgello et al., 1988) as well as progressive AIDS-related encephalitis (Gilden et al., 1988). These conditions will not be discussed in any detail here; however, clinical aspects of these disorders are discussed in earlier chapters. MRI studies have suggested that central nervous system (CNS) involvement occurs more frequently than previously appreciated (Chapter 8) and that PHN occurs much more frequently in shingles patients with MRI abnormalities involving the CNS (Haanpää et al., 1998).

3. Early pathological studies

Reports of the pathological features associated with HZ extend back to the nineteenth century. Although Bright (1831) suggested the association of HZ with the nervous system, Von Barensprung (1861, 1862)

---

* Correspondence to: C.P.N. Watson, Department of Medicine, University of Toronto, Toronto, Ontario, Canada.

first described the haemorrhagic involvement of a dorsal root ganglion (DRG). Subsequent cases in the latter part of the century consisted of two cases of trigeminal zoster with haemorrhage and inflammation in the gasserian ganglion (Wyss, 1871; Sattler, 1875) and four cases with haemorrhage, inflammation, and ganglion cell destruction in thoracic and cervical ganglia (Lesser, 1881, 1883; Dubler, 1884). Chandelux (1879) described one chronic case with ganglionic connective tissue and cell loss.

4. Head and Campbell (1900)

In 1900 Henry Head (Fig. 1) and A.W. Campbell added a further twenty-one cases in their landmark

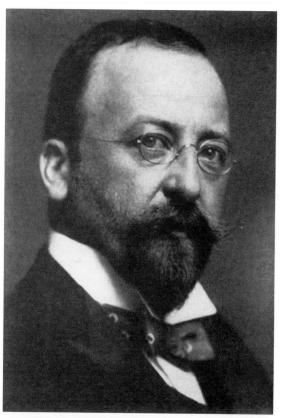

Fig. 1. Henry Head (1861–1940), neurologist, physiologist, poet and literary critic. He wrote exhaustive early works on the clinical and pathological features of herpes zoster.

study, *The pathology of herpes zoster and its bearing on sensory localization*, published in the journal *Brain* (Fig. 2; Head and Campbell, 1900; Oaklander, 1999). These were a mix of 8 acute cases (death occurring 4–30 days after the rash) of herpes zoster and 13 more chronic ones (death 57–790 days after onset). Only one of these chronic cases was clearly noted to have had pain at the time of death. Head and Campbell corroborated the ganglionic changes found earlier, that is, the acute infiltration of small round inflammatory cells, the extravasation of blood and the destruction of sensory neurons and axons, and satellite cells in acute cases (Fig. 3) with scarring in the affected portion of the ganglion and thickening of its sheath in the chronic ones (Fig. 4). The authors established that only one ganglion was affected and that these findings were usually located in the dorsal part of this structure (Figs. 3 and 4). They also pointed out that if the eruption had not been severe the ganglion could appear normal. Their detailed studies also showed no evidence for overt infection in ganglia contralateral to the shingles-affected ganglia. suggesting that later discoveries of bilateral damage after unilateral shingles do not merely reflect direct involvement of contralateral DRG by zoster. Head and Campbell added new information about the time, course and nature of degeneration and subsequent sclerosis with fibrous connective tissue in the sensory root and peripheral nerve. They considered these changes to be secondary to the ganglionic lesion in most cases although in two cases they found inflammation and haemorrhage in the peripheral nerve as well as the ganglion. They described in detail the location, onset, slower resolution and complete disappearance of secondary degenerative change in the ipsilateral posterior column of the spinal cord. Degenerating central axons appeared as early as the ninth day after onset of HZ and persisted as long as 5 and 9 months following the rash. By tracing degenerating tracts with Marchi stains, they helped establish the anatomy of somatosensory systems and mapping of the dermatomes.

Of particular note, in light of more recent autopsy findings on cases with PHN (Watson et al., 1991), is the lack of Head and Campbell's documentation of

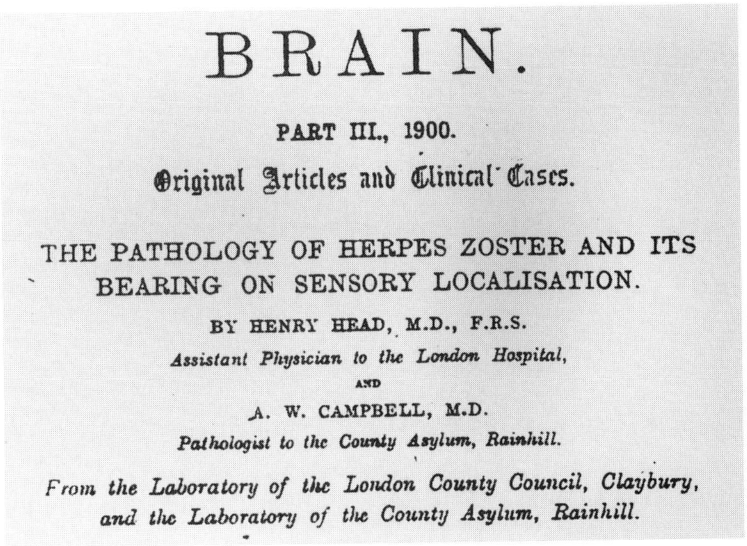

BRAIN.

PART III., 1900.

Original Articles and Clinical Cases.

THE PATHOLOGY OF HERPES ZOSTER AND ITS BEARING ON SENSORY LOCALISATION.

BY HENRY HEAD, M.D., F.R.S.

Assistant Physician to the London Hospital,

AND

A. W. CAMPBELL, M.D.

Pathologist to the County Asylum, Rainhill.

From the Laboratory of the London County Council, Claybury,
and the Laboratory of the County Asylum, Rainhill.

Fig. 2. The title page from Head and Campbell's very detailed study of the pathology of herpes zoster published in the journal *Brain* in 1900.

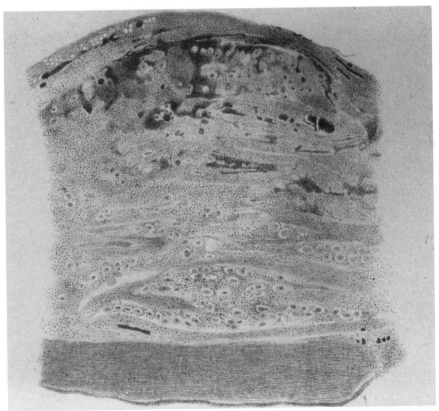

Fig. 3. From a coloured drawing of a longitudinal section of the 7th dorsal ganglion of the right side in a case that died eight days after the outburst of the eruption. This section is stained with haematoxylin and eosin. (From Head and Campbell, 1900.)

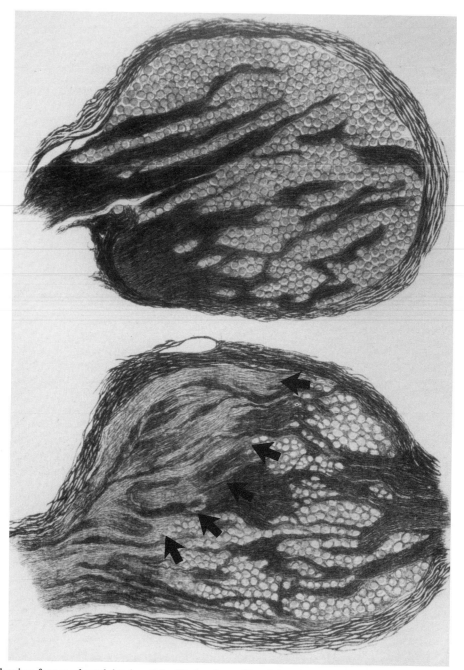

Fig. 4. Upper drawing: from a coloured drawing of the 7th dorsal ganglion of the normal (left) side. Death occurred 153 days after the outburst of the eruption. Stained by Marchi's method, and counterstained by van Gieson's picro-haematoxylin method. Lower drawing: the 7th dorsal ganglion of the abnormal (right) side in the same case, stained by the same methods. The scarred area is outlined with arrows. (From Head and Campbell, 1900.)

changes in the posterior horn of the spinal cord, since they studied this area carefully. Two of their cases were trigeminal, one in the mandibular division occurring 30 days prior to death, the other the more typical ophthalmic involvement 6 months before death. At autopsy the pathological changes in the gasserian ganglion were similar to those observed in spinal ganglia. Secondary central degenerative changes were present only in the mandibular case and were found in the root and spinal tract of the fifth nerve.

Although Head laboured in ignorance of the nature of the causative agent, we still cannot answer any more clearly his questions as to the reasons for the preference for sensory ganglia at certain levels (ophthalmic and thoracic), why only one ganglion is affected and why the dorsal aspect of the ganglion is favoured.

5. Denny-Brown et al. (1944): myelitis and the Ramsay–Hunt syndrome

Denny-Brown et al. (1944) reported the pathology of three cases: two with acute thoracic zoster (one with and one without pain) and one of the rare Ramsay–Hunt syndrome (facial nerve paralysis with cranial zoster). These authors corroborated the haemorrhagic thoracic ganglionic inflammation with one ganglion containing a curious cystic structure. They found in all three cases inflammatory central nervous system changes of zoster myelitis, findings previously reported but hitherto relatively inaccessible in the French (Lhermitte and Nicolas, 1924; Faure-Beaulieu and Lhermitte, 1929) and German literature (Wohlwill, 1924). They described 'poliomyelitis' (inflammation in the gray matter) of the anterior and posterior horns accompanied by a leptomeningitis producing pleocytosis in the spinal fluid. They also found a true peripheral mononeuritis in nerves distal to the ganglion and in the anterior root. They used this to explain the facial paralysis in their case of the Ramsay–Hunt syndrome since the geniculate ganglion was completely spared, with a ganglionitis in this case involving the second cervical ganglion. In that same year another case of direct cellular infiltration of the facial nerve during herpetic infection was described (Adams, 1944).

6. Noordenbos: 'Fast blocks slow' and gate control

Noordenbos (1959) (Fig. 5) examined four intercostal nerve biopsies from patients with PHN and found an increase in unmyelinated nerve fibres. He analysed the size distribution of myelinated axons and demonstrated a great reduction in numbers of large fibres and an increase in the smaller myelinated population. He postulated that zoster might preferentially damage the larger cells of the posterior root ganglion with consequent loss of thicker myelinated fibres and that "remaining sensibility was subserved by fibers of the slowest conduction rate." These find-

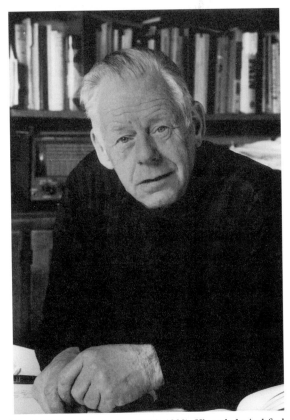

Fig. 5. William Noordenbos (1910–1990). His pathological findings in four nerve biopsies from patients with postherpetic neuralgia, showing a preponderance of small fibres and loss of larger myelinated fibres, led him to the concept that 'fast blocks slow'. The impact of this on Ronald Melzack and Patrick Wall helped them towards formulating the gate control theory of pain.

ings led Noordenbos towards the development of his idea that interactions between different types of fibres might influence pain, and the concept that 'fast blocks slow.' These observations helped to stimulate Ronald Melzack and Patrick Wall to propose the gate control theory of pain (Melzack and Wall, 1965).

Although Noordenbos interpreted his microscopic analyses as demonstrating relative preservation of small fibres over large, the pathology within previously shingles-affected DRG makes it clear that no one type of neuron is preferentially preserved within the focal area affected by shingles. It is more likely that the increase in small calibre axons documented by Noordenbos represents sprouts from damaged axons. All types of peripheral neurons emit small-diameter unmyelinated sprouts after axonal injury. These would not be distinguishable from preserved small-diameter axons using microscopy alone.

7. Fibrosis in peripheral cases

Zacks et al. (1964) studied four peripheral nerve biopsies from patients following HZ, two with and two without pain. They found evidence for wallerian degeneration, which they presumed was secondary to damage to neuronal perikarya, and also direct inflammatory changes within the nerve bundle. They found small fibres present in the early stage but eventually lost. Later collagen proliferation transformed the nerve into a nearly solid mass of fibrous tissue containing rare small myelinated fibres. They were not able to correlate the presence and severity of fibrosis with postherpetic neuralgia. Although they suggested that a central pain mechanism was involved because of the paucity of surviving fibres, it is obvious from the clinical features (the presence of allodynia, hyperesthaesia and dysesthaesia in most patients) that peripheral mechanisms are important as well.

8. Varicella-zoster virus in sensory ganglia

Esiri and Tomlinson (1972) demonstrated varicella-zoster virus within the trigeminal nerve and gan-

glion of a patient with ophthalmic zoster using immunofluorescence and electron microscopy. Ghatak and Zimmerman (1973) described the virus particles in affected spinal ganglia of a case of HZ associated with Hodgkin's disease, as well as intranuclear inclusions in ganglionic neurons as described earlier by Cheatham (1953) and McCormick et al. (1969). Ghatak and Zimmerman also found multinucleated giant cells and alterations suggestive of mitosis within neurons in the sensory ganglia, but speculated that these changes might reflect an altered expression of HZ superimposed on Hodgkin's disease.

9. Ophthalmic zoster (see also Chapter 11)

The gasserian ganglion has been infrequently examined in cases of HZ affecting the fifth nerve territory (Wyss, 1871; Sattler, 1875; Head and Campbell, 1900). These reports described the changes within the gasserian ganglion as being similar to spinal ganglionic findings. Reske-Nielsen et al. (1986) autopsied three cases of ophthalmic zoster with death 22–117 days after the eruption. The pain status of these patients was not mentioned. They found lesions in the ophthalmic part of the gasserian ganglion and were the first to describe involvement of the mesencephalic trigeminal nucleus which they considered to be a primary phenomenon, remarking on its structural resemblance to spinal and trigeminal sensory ganglia.

10. Attempts to describe the pathology of postherpetic neuralgia

Relatively few autopsied cases were documented as having significant pain close to the time of death (case 7 of Head and Campbell, case 2 of Denny-Brown, cases 2 and 3 of Zacks, the 4 biopsies of Noordenbos). Only Noordenbos (1959) and Zacks et al. (1964) focused on this issue and attempted to explain the pathogenesis of PHN. Watson et al. (1988a,b) described in detail the pathology in a case of severe thoracic PHN for 5 years. The most striking finding was the atrophy of the dorsal horn over

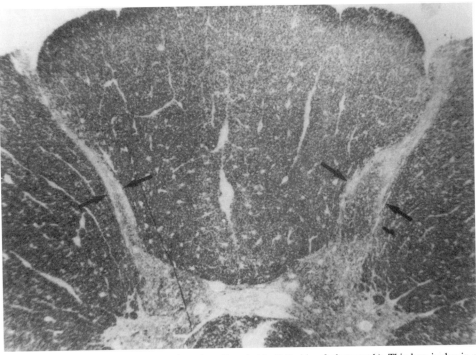

Fig. 6. Atrophy of the dorsal horn of the spinal cord on the affected side (left side of photograph). This loss is due in part to loss of myelin as evidenced by the reduced darker staining of the central area of the dorsal horn compared with the control (unaffected side) (MBP × 2.5).

five segments (Fig. 6) with only one ganglion affected by fibrosis and cellular loss (Fig. 7) and with only the roots at that level involved. The more extensive spinal pathology may help to explain clinical findings (Fig. 15) which are often more extensive than can be explained by the involvement of a single ganglion. The spinal atrophy extending over several segments is compatible with the known branching of primary afferents in Lissauer's tract. Neurotransmitter staining of the dorsal horn revealed no difference from the contralateral mirror site for substance P (Fig. 8). This was initially interpreted as confirming the integrity of small primary afferents; however, recovery of substance P after deafferentation has been described by Tessler et al. (1981). Staining for serotonin (Fig. 9) and dopamine-beta-hydroxylase (DBH) (Fig. 10) (a marker for noradrenaline) similarly showed no difference from the control side so these studies did not provide evidence for a deficiency of inhibitory neurotransmitters utilised by descending inhibitory pathways from the brainstem

to the dorsal horn. Opiate receptor binding studies revealed no difference between the affected side and the contralateral sides (Fig. 11) The persistence of opioid receptors is compatible with opioid responsivity seen in many PHN patients (Watson and Babul, 1998). A comparison of neurotransmitters and opioid receptors between the affected and contralateral dorsal horn may not reveal changes that are bilateral. The lack of posterior column degeneration was quite compatible with Henry Head's observation that this disappears by 9 months after acute zoster.

Further studies (Watson et al., 1991) of five cases corroborated the dorsal horn atrophy and ganglionic changes described above. Again, the lack of a reduction in dorsal horn staining for substance P and for CGRP was noted despite a complete loss of cell bodies and staining in the affected ganglia. A marked inflammatory reaction was seen in the dorsal horn in one acute case. Loss of axons and myelin in the sensory root and peripheral nerve was present in cases with and without persistent pain. A peripheral

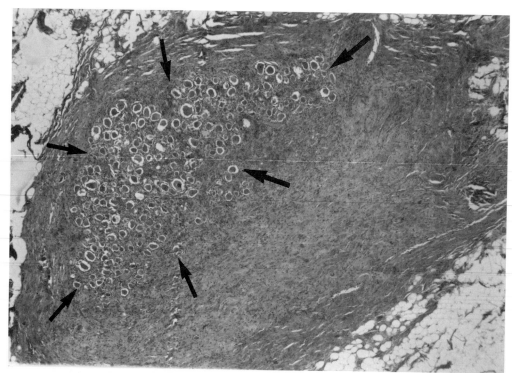

Fig. 7. Dorsal root ganglion at T8 on the right shows fibrosis occupying a significant portion of this structure. Residual normal appearing ganglion is outlined by arrows (Masson trichrome × 10).

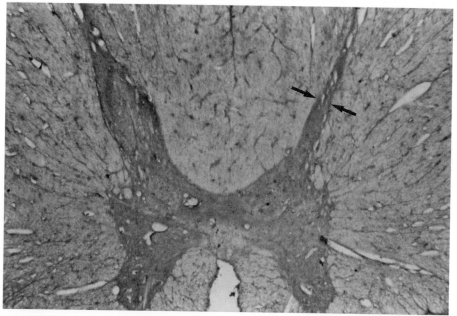

Fig. 8. Substance P. Coronal sections of formaldehyde fixed spinal cord at T7 levels were processed for substance P using immunocyto-chemistry. At T7 one can observe the shrinkage of the dorsal horn on the affected side (arrow); however, there is no obvious difference with respect to the density of substance P in the substantia gelatinosa when the two dorsal horns are compared.

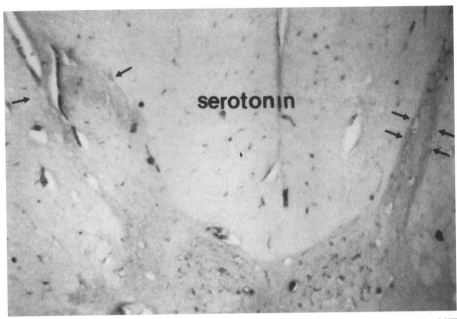

Fig. 9. Serotonin. Coronal sections at T8 were immunostained for serotonin (5-HT). There is no difference in 5-HT staining in the substantia gelatinosa regardless of the level and side of the spinal cord. One can observe shrinkage of the dorsal horn at T8 on the affected side (double arrows) on the right side of the illustration.

nerve histogram (Fig. 12) corroborated the findings of Noordenbos (1959) (Fig. 13) (increased small and reduced large myelinated fibres). The preponderance of unmyelinated and small myelinated fibres must be interpreted with caution. These could be regenerating motor or autonomic fibres and may not correlate with the pain of PHN. The presence of inflammatory changes at multiple levels bilaterally affecting roots, ganglia and nerves in a case of 2 years duration, raised the possibility of ongoing generalised inflammation as a pathogenetic mechanism in some cases. One case (case 4) of only 5 weeks duration had substantial collagen present suggesting a process of much longer duration which may have been clinically occult.

An autopsied case of ophthalmic PHN presented several features that were surprising in light of the literature on spinal PHN (Watson et al., 2000). First, despite documented shingles, residual V_1 facial scarring, and severe pain for more than 10 years, the central nervous system showed no significant morphological abnormalities. Second, severe pathological involvement of the ophthalmic and supra-

orbital nerves included fibrosis, demyelination, loss of myelinated fibres, and a shift in the fibre diameter spectrum toward small-diameter axons. This occurred without prominent pathology in the gasserian ganglion or the trigeminal root and raised the possibility of a dying-back type of pathology expressed mostly in the periphery. The lack of prominent findings in the ganglion, root, and central nervous system is strikingly different from cases of spinal PHN where most have cell loss in the DRG and atrophy of the dorsal horn of the spinal cord (Watson et al., 1988a,b, 1991).

The third outstanding finding in this case was the obvious pathological involvement of the contralateral ophthalmic and supra-orbital nerves, despite the lack of obvious clinical contralateral symptoms and signs. This finding supports other recently published information on bilateral involvement as noted in the introduction (Baron and Saguer, 1994; Oaklander et al., 1998). Previous spinal cases that we have autopsied also demonstrated that the myelinated fibre spectrum of the patient's contralateral ('non-affected') side differs from that of age-matched controls (cases 1

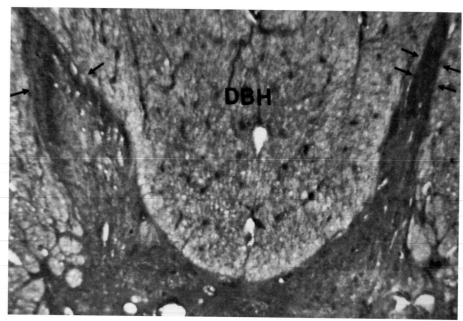

Fig. 10. DBH. T7 sections were stained for dopamine-B-hydroxylase (DBH), a marker for norepinephrine in the spinal cord. There is obvious shrinkage of the dorsal horn on the affected side at T7 (arrow); yet no obvious difference is apparent in the staining in the substantia gelatinosa when comparing the affected and unaffected dorsal horns in the same section.

and 2: Watson et al., 1991) and that an imbalance of myelinated fibres may favour fibres of small diameter. Furthermore, one of our previous cases (case 5: Watson et al., 1991) had contralateral inflammatory changes in nerves of the affected segment and also bilaterally in segments above and below. Ophthalmic division cases are of particular interest with regard to PHN because V_1 is purely sensory whereas the spinal nerves also have a motor component.

Although it is clearly inappropriate to draw firm conclusions from a single case that might not be representative of V_1 PHN in general, our observations raise the question of whether the pathology of some cases of trigeminal PHN is primarily peripheral. Pain mechanisms could include an imbalance of small-diameter versus large-diameter input as predicted by the gate control theory. Alternatively, pain may be due to ectopic firing of peripherally injured axons, in association with central sensitisation (Devor and Seltzer, 1999). Finally, pain could result from abnormal response properties of residual, uninjured fibres. There is also the possibility of biomechanical or electrophysiologic CNS abnormalities not visible by

light microscopy. Each of these mechanisms, which are not mutually exclusive, may have a threshold below which symptoms and signs do not manifest clinically. This situation would account for the observation of neural pathology on the right side in our patient despite the absence of obvious pain. It is not unlikely that sensory abnormalities would have been detected on the right side through detailed, quantitative sensory testing methods. Further studies of spinal and trigeminal cases will be required to fully describe the pathological features and differences between PHN and pain free cases.

11. Herpes zoster myelitis

In the 1920s, reports in the French and German literature documented HZ myelitis (Lhermitte and Nicolas, 1924; Wohlwill, 1924; Faure-Beaulieu and Lhermitte, 1929). Denny-Brown et al. (1944) added to this. More recently, Devinsky et al. (1991) reported the autopsy findings in nine patients with herpes zoster myelitis associated with immunosuppressive

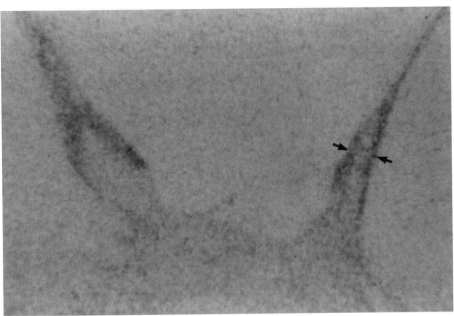

Fig. 11. Opiate receptors. Fresh frozen sections of spinal cord at T8 were processed for the autoradiographic demonstration of opiate receptor distribution ([³H]etorphine). The results indicate no variation in opiate receptor density between the two substantiae gelatinosae at T8 although the shrinkage of the dorsal horn at T8, the affected side, is obvious (arrows).

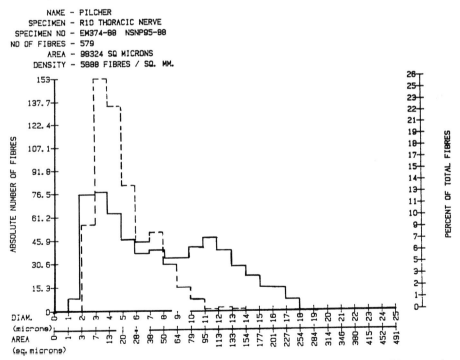

```
NAME - PILCHER
SPECIMEN - R10 THORACIC NERVE
SPECIMEN NO - EM374-88  NSNP95-88
NO OF FIBRES - 579
AREA - 98324 SQ MICRONS
DENSITY - 5888 FIBRES / SQ. MM.
```

Fig. 12. Superimposed myelinated fibre spectra of the abnormal 10th intercostal nerve (dashed line) with a normal age-matched 10th intercostal nerve (solid line). The numbers of fibres are expressed on the vertical axis as percentage of total fibres for the purpose of comparison.

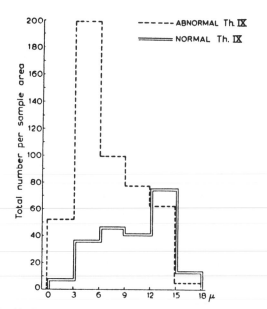

Fig. 13. Superimposed fibre spectra of an abnormal 9th inter-costal nerve (dashed line) from a case of postherpetic neuralgia and a normal 9th intercostal nerve (double solid line). (Reproduced from William Noordenbos' (1959) book *Pain*, with permission.)

illnesses. Involvement was most severe in the dorsal root entry zone and posterior horn of the spinal cord corresponding to the involved dermatome, with variable spread horizontally and vertically. They found evidence of viral invasion, particularly of demyelination. Four patients had evidence of vasculitis associated with leptomeningitis and haemorrhagic necrosis. Because of the presence of inclusion bodies in Schwann cells and fibroblasts in the posterior root, they suggested that central spread of the virus from dorsal root ganglion to the spinal cord caused the myelitis. Because there was a prolonged interval for central versus peripheral spread, despite the shorter distance, cell to cell contact was suggested as the mechanism for the myelitis versus axoplasmic transport for the skin lesions. They went on to say that immunosuppression may have facilitated this type of spread to cause cord involvement in these patients. Evidence of virus in the gracilis and cuneate nuclei of the brainstem suggested axoplasmic transport within the cord.

12. Cutaneous neuropathology

The ability to label punch skin biopsies with the pan-axonal marker antiPGP9.5 has created a window into the peripheral sensory nervous system. This immunohistochemical method labels neural processes coursing through non-neural tissue and makes them visible using light microscopy (Thompson et al., 1983; Karanth et al., 1991). The neural identity of PGP9.5-immunopositive cutaneous fibres has been confirmed by electron microscopy (Hilliges et al., 1995). Unlike most other neural markers, PGP9.5 appears to label all types of neurons. In the dermis, the densities of somatic and autonomic innervation can be assessed qualitatively, but the axons run in bundles, precluding quantitation. In contrast, virtually all epidermal neurites consist of individual free nociceptive C and A delta nerve endings (Simone et al., 1998). These can be visualised and quantitated using light microscopy (Kennedy et al., 1999). Since these epidermal nociceptors are the transducers for pain sensation, the ability to visualise them directly has contributed significantly to our understanding of the pathophysiology of PHN pain. Previous psychophysical studies of the function of these cutaneous nerve endings provided complex and sometimes contradictory results (Baron and Saguer, 1994; Rowbotham et al., 1996; Pappagallo et al., 2000).

Two laboratories have studied the density of PGP9.5 immunolabelled neurites in previously shingles-affected skin. Although there had been earlier reports of loss of cutaneous innervation after shingles, Ebert (1949) and Rowbotham et al. (1996) were the first to quantitate the density of dermal and epidermal innervation in allodynic PHN-affected skin. They found no correlation between density of remaining epidermal innervation and severity of PHN pain. Oaklander et al. (1998) compared neurite densities within PHN-affected skin to densities from previously shingles-affected skin without PHN, and included biopsies contralateral to the shingles, and from a site distant from the area of shingles involvement. The addition of these two control groups highlighted that PHN occurred only in patients with the fewest epidermal and dermal neurites remain-

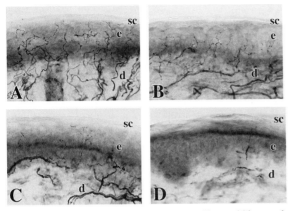

Fig. 14. PGP 9.5 immunolabeling of nerve fibers within punch skin biopsies. Representative labeled skin-biopsy-sections from subjects with and without PHN. In all panels, the stratum corneum (sc) is uppermost, followed by the epidermis (e), with the dermis (d) at the bottom. Individual neurites are visible in the epidermis, and neurite bundles are visible in the superficial dermis. The top panels show biopsies from the contralateral (A) and shingles-affected (B) sites on the back of a 75-year-old woman without PHN. She had 1952 epidermal neurites/mm^2 of skin surface area at the contralateral site, and 1672 epidermal neurites/mm^2 at the shingles site. The bottom panels show biopsies from the contralateral (C) and shingles-affected (D) sites on top of the shoulders of a 72-year-old woman with PHN who rated her pain level as 8 on a 0 to 10 scale. She had 812 epidermal neurites/mm^2 at the contralateral site, and 145 epidermal neurites/mm^2 at the shingles site. (Reprinted from Oaklander et al. (1998), with permission.)

ing after shingles. Subjects with PHN had a mean density of 339 ± 97 neurites/mm^2 of skin surface area in previously shingles-affected epidermis compared with a density of 1661 ± 262 neurites/mm^2 for subjects without PHN pain.

The inclusion of biopsies from a site on the upper back distant from the area involved by shingles also led to the discovery that there is bilateral damage to sensory neurons in patients with typical unilateral shingles on the torso (Fig. 14). Surprisingly, there was significant correlation between severity of PHN pain, and severity of loss of epidermal neurites at the mirror-image contralateral side. Contralateral damage occurred despite the lack of contralateral shingles eruptions or pain, and did not extend to the distant site. In light of these findings, other authors have appreciated that their data indicated bilateral effects of unilateral shingles as well (Watson et al.,

1991, 2000; Baron and Saguer, 1994). There are currently two hypotheses to explain the contralateral neural damage. One is that it may represent an indirect transcellular effect akin to those that often occur after unilateral injuries restricted to peripheral nerves (Koltzenburg et al., 1999). The other is that contralateral damage to primary afferents may be a marker for the presence of spinal cord injury after shingles. This appears to occur more often in shingles than previously realised, and may be a fundamental anatomical difference between patients with and without PHN after shingles (Watson et al., 1991; Haanpää et al., 1998). Alternatively, it is conceivable that the loss of contralateral cutaneous innervation contributes directly to the presence of PHN after shingles, perhaps by influencing descending modulation of the dorsal horn.

13. Conclusions

The pathological findings described above give clues about the pathogenesis and pathophysiology of the pain of HZ and PHN. When combined with clinical information, we can form a rough concept of what might be amiss, recognising that pain mechanisms may differ amongst patients, amongst sites of shingles, and that a patient may have more than one cause for discomfort. Most patients have allodynia, hyperesthaesia or hyperalgesia (Watson et al., 1988b) often over areas of skin much greater than the area involved with scarring or a single dermatome (Fig. 15). This indicates the importance of peripheral input. Woolf et al. (1992) have suggested that the anatomical basis of tactile allodynia is sprouting of A-beta fibres into nociceptive lamina of the superficial dorsal horn. The imbalance in fibre types seen in peripheral nerves, if relevant to pain, provides a basis for increased small fibre (excitatory) input and decreased large fibre (inhibiting) input to the dorsal horn; however, it may simply represent irrelevant sprouting. Loss of peripheral input and loss of inhibition, rather than increased input, may be the major peripheral pathology. We can postulate that ectopic generators or activity might exist at the site of regen-

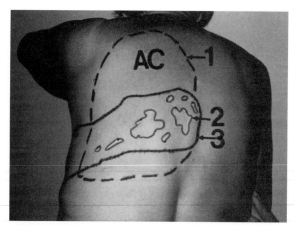

Fig. 15. Patient AC: (1) margin of area of allodynia to skin stroking; (2) postherpetic scarring; (3) margin of area of reduced sensation to pinprick, cold and touch.

erating axonal sprouts in the peripheral nerve or in the scarred dorsal root ganglion.

Conversely, there is also evidence of pain generators within the CNS. The atrophy of the dorsal horn of the spinal cord and the general failure of surgical peripheral deafferentation procedures to relieve PHN as well as the relief in some patients by DREZ (dorsal root entry zone) lesions provides evidence for a central pain mechanism. Hyperreactive nociceptive neurons in this area with expanded receptive fields responding to non-nociceptive input may account for the clinical features found on examination of the affected skin. Totally or partially deafferented wide-dynamic-range (WDR) neurons may become hyperexcitable as has been shown in animals and in humans after root avulsions. Ongoing occult inflammation in nerve, ganglia, root and cord could account for progressively resistant pain in some cases.

Sympathetic interruption has not proven a satisfactory treatment for most cases of PHN and has not been proven by controlled trial in the pain of HZ. Physical signs of sympathetic overactivity are usually not present in most patients in our experience.

14. Summary

With HZ, varicella-zoster virus erupts, favouring specific dorsal root ganglia, to cause a haemorrhagic inflammation which usually spreads distally into the nerve, skin and other tissues. Degeneration also extends centrally in the dorsal columns as the central axons of affected primary afferent neurons degenerate and may spread to other areas of the spinal cord, meninges and brain. After the acute disorder subsides, its footprint remains usually in one ganglion, the skin, the nerve, nerve roots and spinal cord. This injury may or may not lead to PHN. Both clinical and pathological information support the concept that both central and peripheral mechanisms can be important in the genesis of PHN. More is known about the neuropathology of PHN than any other neuropathic pain syndrome. Because PHN is caused by a single, well-defined disease entity and the neurological lesions can be precisely localised based on their cutaneous lesions, PHN is ideal for scientific study into pain mechanisms. Efforts to obtain autopsy material should be continued. It is likely that insights gained from PHN will be applicable to mechanisms of other neuropathic pain syndromes.

References

Adams, R.D. (1944) Herpes zoster: pathologic features. Bull. N. Engl. Med. Center, 6: 12.

Baron, R. and Saguer, M. (1994) Axon-reflex reactions in affected and homologous contralateral skin after unilateral peripheral injury of thoracic segmental nerves in humans. Neurosci. Lett., 165: 97–100.

Bright, R. (1831) Reports of medical cases. London, 2(Part 1): 383.

Chandelux (1879) Observation pour servir a l'histoire des lesions nerveuses dans le zona. Arch. Physiol., XI: 674.

Cheatham, W.J. (1953) The relation of heretofore unreported lesions to pathogenesis of herpes zoster. Am. J. Pathol., 29: 401–412.

Denny-Brown, D., Adams, R.D. and Fitzgerald, P.J. (1944) Pathologic features of herpes zoster: a note on 'geniculate herpes'. Arch. Neurol. Psychiatr. (Chicago), 57: 216.

Devinsky, O., Cho, E., Petite, C.K. and Price, R.W. (1991) Herpes zoster myelitis. Brain, 114: 1181–1196.

Devor, M. and Seltzer, Z. (1999) Pathophysiology of damaged nerves in relation to chronic pain. In: P.D. Wall and R. Melzack (Eds.), Textbook of Pain, 4th ed. Churchill Livingston, New York, pp. 129–164.

Doyle, P.W., Gibson, G. and Dobman, C.L. (1983) Herpes zoster ophthalmicus with contralateral hemiplegia: identification of cause. Ann. Neurol., 14: 84–95.

Dubler (1884) Ueber Neuritis bei Herpes Zoster. Virchows Arch., XCVI: 195.

Ebert, M.H. (1949) Histologic changes in sensory nerves of the skin in herpes zoster. Arch. Dermatol. Syphil., 60: 641–648.

Eidelberg, D., Sotrel, A., Horoupian, D.S., et al. (1986) Thrombotic cerebral vasculopathy associated with herpes zoster. Ann. Neurol., 19: 7–14.

Esiri, M.M. and Tomlinson, A.H. (1972) Herpes zoster: demonstration of virus in trigeminal nerve and ganglion by immunofluorescence and electron microscopy. J. Neurol. Sci., 14: 35–48.

Faure-Beaulieu, M. and Lhermitte, J. (1929) Les lesions medullaires du zona idiopathique: la myelite zosterienne. Rev. Neurol., 1: 1250–1258.

Ghatak, N.R. and Zimmerman, H.M. (1973) Spinal ganglion in herpes zoster: a light and electron microscopic study. Arch. Pathol., 95: 411–415.

Gilden, D.H., Murray, R.S., Wellish, M., Kleinschmidt-DeMasters, B.K. and Vafai, A. (1988) Chronic progressive varicella-zoster virus encephalitis in an AIDS patient. Neurology, 38: 1150.

Haanpää, M., Dastidar, P. and Weinberg, A. (1998) CSF and MRI findings in patients with acute herpes zoster. Neurology, 51: 1045–1411.

Head, H. and Campbell, A.W. (1900) The pathology of herpes zoster and its bearing on sensory localization. Brain, 23: 353–523.

Hilliges, M., Wang, L. and Johansson, O. (1995) Ultrastructural evidence for nerve fibers within all vital layers of the human epidermis. J. Invest. Dermatol., 104: 134–137.

Horten, B., Price, R.W. and Jimenez, D. (1981) Multifocal varicella-zoster virus leukoencephalitis temporally remote from herpes zoster. Ann. Neurol., 9: 251–266.

Jemsek, J., Greenberg, S.B., Taber, I. et al. (1983) Herpes zoster-associated encephalitis: clinicopathologic report of 12 cases and review of the literature. Medicine, 62: 81–97.

Karanth, S., Springall, D.R., Kuhn, D.M., Levene, M.M. and Black, J.M. (1991) An immunocytochemical study of cutaneous innervation and the distribution of neuropeptides and protein gene product 9.5 in man and animals. Am. J. Anat., 191: 368–383.

Kennedy, W.R., Wendelschafter-Crabb, G. and Lindall, A.W. (1999) Quantitative epidermal nerve analysis in skin blister and skin biopsies. Ann. Neurol., 46: 461–462.

Koltzenburg, M., Wall, P.D. and McMahon, S.B. (1999) Does the right side know what the left side is doing? TINS, 22: 122–127.

Lesser (1881) Beitrage zur Lehre vom Herpes Zoster. Virchows Arch., XXXVI: 391.

Lesser (1883) Weitere Beitrage zur Lehre vom Herpes Zoster. Virchows Arch., XCIII: 506.

Lhermitte, J. and Nicolas, P. (1924) Les lesions spinales du zona: la myelite zosterienne. Rev. Neurol., 1: 361–364.

Linnemann, C.C. and Alvira, M.M. (1980) Pathogenesis of varicella-zoster angiitis in the CNS. Arch. Neurol., 37: 239–240.

McCormick, W.F., Rodnitzky, R.L., Schochet, S.S. et al. (1969) Varicella-zoster encephalomyelitis: a morphologic and virologic study. Arch. Neurol., 21: 559–570.

Melzack, R. and Wall, P.W. (1965) Pain mechanisms: A new theory. Science, 150: 971–979.

Morgello, S., Block, G.A., Price, R.W. and Petito, C.K. (1988) Varicella-zoster virus leukoencephalitis and cerebral vasculopathy. Arch. Pathol. Lab. Med., 112: 173.

Noordenbos, W. (1959) Pain: problems pertaining to the transmission of nerve impulses which give rise to pain. Elsevier, Amsterdam, Ch. 1, pp. 4–10; Ch. 10, pp. 68–80.

Oaklander, A.L. (1999) The pathology of shingles; Head and Campbell's 1900 monograph. Arch. Neurol., 56(iv): 1292–1294.

Oaklander, A.L., Romans, K., Horasek, S., Stocks, A., Hauer, P. and Meyer, R.A. (1998) Unilateral postherpetic neuralgia is associated with bilateral sensory neuron damage. Ann. Neurol., 44: 789–795.

Pappagallo, M., Oaklander, A.L., Quatrano-Piacentini, A.L., Clark, M.R. and Raja, S.N. (2000) Heterogenous patterns of sensory dysfunction in postherpetic neuralgia suggest multiple pathophysiologic mechanisms. Anesthesiology, 92: 691–698.

Reske-Nielsen, E., Oster, S. and Pedersen, B. (1986) Herpes zoster ophthalmicus and the mesencephalic nucleus. Acta Pathol. Microbiol. Immunol. Scand., 94: 263–269.

Rose, F.C., Brett, E.M. and Burston, J. (1964) Zoster encephalomyelitis. Arch. Neurol., 11: 155–172.

Rosenblum, W.I. and Hadfield, M.G. (1972) Granulomatous angiitis of the nervous system in cases of herpes zoster and lymphosarcoma. Neurology, 22: 348–354.

Rowbotham, M.C., Yosipovitch, G., Connolly, M.K., Finlay, D., Forde, G. and Fields, H.L. (1996) Cutaneous innervation density in the allodynic form of postherpetic neuralgia. Neurobiol. Dis., 3: 205–214.

Sattler (1875) Ueber das Wesen des Herpes ophthalmicus. Anzeiger der K.K. Gesellschaft der Aertze in Wien. Protocoll der Sitzung (this will be found at the end of the Medizinische Jahrbuch von der K.K. Gesellschaft der Aertze).

Simone, D.A., Noland, M., Johnson, T., Wendelschafer-Crabb, G. and Kennedy, W.R. (1998) Intradermal injection of capsaicin in humans produces degeneration and subsequent reinnervation of epidermal nerve fibers. J. Neurosci., 18(21): 8947–8959.

Tessler, A., Himos, B.T., Hrtymyshyn, R., Murray, M. and Goldenberger, M.E. (1981) neurons mediate return of substance P following deafferentation of the cut spinal cord. Brain, 230: 263–281.

Thompson, R.J., Doran, J.F., Jackson, P., Dhillon, A.P. and Rode, J. (1983) PGP 9.5 — a new marker for vertebrate neurons and neuroendocrine cells. Brain Res., 278: 224–228.

Von Barensprung, F.G.F. (1861) Die Gurtelkrankheit. Ann. Char-Krankenh. Berlin, 9: 40–238.

Von Barensprung, F.G.F. (1862) Beitraege zur Kenntnis des Zoster. Ann. Char-Krankenh. Berlin, 10: 96–104.

Watson, C.P.N. and Babul, N. (1998) Oxycodone relieves neuropathic pain: A randomized trial in postherpetic neuralgia. Neurology, 50: 1837–1841.

Watson, C.P.N., Morshead, C., Van der Kooy, D., Deck, J.H. and Evans, R.J. (1988a) Postherpetic neuralgia: post-mortem analysis of a case. Pain, 34: 129–138.

Watson, C.P.N., Evans, R.J., Watt, V.R. and Birkett, N. (1988b) Postherpetic neuralgia: 208 cases. Pain, 35: 289–297.

Watson, C.P.N., Deck, J.H., Morshead, C., Van der Kooy, D. and Evans, R.J. (1991) Postherpetic neuralgia: further post-mortem studies of cases with and without pain. Pain, 44: 105–117.

Watson, C.P.N., Midha, R., Devor, M., Nag, S., Munro, C. and Dostrovsky, J.O. (2000) Trigeminal postherpetic neuralgia postmortem: Clinically unilateral, pathologically bilateral. In: M. Devor, M.C. Rowbotham and Z. Wiesenfeld-Hallin (Eds.), Proceedings of the 9th World Congress on Pain. Progress in Pain Research and Management, IASP Press, Seattle, WA.

Wohlwill, F. (1924) Zur pathologischen Anatomie des Nervensystems vom Herpes Zoster. Z. Ges. Neurol. Psychiatr., 89: 170–212.

Woolf, C.J., Shortland, P. and Coggeshall, R.E. (1992) Peripheral nerve injury triggers central sprouting of myelinated afferents. Nature, 355(6355): 75–78.

Wyss, O. (1871) Beitrag zur Kentniss des Herpes Zoster. Arch. Heilkd., XVI: 261.

Zacks, S.L., Langfitt, T.W. and Elliott, F.A. (1964) Herpetic neuritis: a light and electron microscopic study. Neurology, 14: 744–750.

Herpes Zoster and Postherpetic Neuralgia, 2nd Revised and Enlarged Edition
Pain Research and Clinical Management, Vol. 11
Edited by C.P.N. Watson and A.A. Gershon

CHAPTER 16

Spectrum of pain mechanisms contributing to PHN

Michael C. Rowbotham [1,2,*], Ralf Baron [4], Karin Lottrup Petersen [1] and Howard L. Fields [1,3]

UCSF Pain Clinical Research Center, Departments of [1] Neurology, [2] Anesthesia, and [3] Physiology,
University of California, San Francisco, CA 94115, USA and [4] Klinik für Neurophysiologie,
Christian-Albrechts-Universität Kiel, Kiel, Germany

1. Introduction

Nearly all patients with post-herpetic neuralgia (PHN) report continuous superficial and/or deep pain and many also report spontaneous lancinating pains (Noordenbos, 1959; Watson et al., 1988; Rowbotham and Fields, 1989a,b). Furthermore, the majority of patients with PHN experience dynamic mechanical allodynia, an unpleasant sensation produced by normally innocuous moving light mechanical stimulation of the skin (Nurmikko and Bowsher, 1990). For some patients allodynia is the most disabling symptom of PHN. The area of allodynia can be very large, affecting more than 1200 cm^2 of skin (Choi and Rowbotham, 1997).

Long considered a somewhat obscure and intractable pain problem limited to the elderly, interest in PHN has grown steadily within the pain community. PHN is particularly suitable for research; like animal models, PHN is a well defined nerve injury that occurs in a well defined population. PHN is common, strikes otherwise healthy individuals within a relatively restricted age range, is easy to diagnose, has a known etiology, and is rarely complicated by litigation and disability issues. The date

of onset is known with precision, typically only a single dorsal root ganglion is affected, and the unaffected contralateral side can serve as a control during sensory testing and other manipulations. Over the past decade there has been an explosion in our understanding of neuropathic pain. Much of this progress is due to the development of animal models of painful peripheral nerve injury, but the study of patients with post-herpetic neuralgia has also contributed to our understanding by providing an opportunity to exploit the knowledge gained from studies of animal models of neuropathic pain. One approach to designing and testing new therapeutic options for PHN is to identify each pain generating mechanism and then devise rational interventions to mitigate that mechanism.

2. Mechanisms of pain in acute herpes zoster and PHN

In the previous edition of this book, Wall posed a number of questions about the mechanisms of acute herpes zoster (AHZ) and PHN to clinicians and basic scientists to further our understanding of

* Correspondence to: M.C. Rowbotham, UCSF Pain Clinical Research Center, 1701 Divisadero Street, Suite 480, San Francisco, CA 94115, USA. Phone: +1 (415) 885-7899; Fax: +1 (415) 885-7855; E-mail: mcrwind@itsa.ucsf.edu

these conditions. Four possible pain mechanisms were proposed that were not mutually exclusive. First, totally deafferented central cells, that have lost their peripheral input become more excitable and increase their spontaneous firing, as is known from experimental peripheral nerve section. Second, it is known that in response to partial deafferentation, the cell's receptive field increases and the cell responds to input from nearby intact nerves. This occurs because of either increased excitability or reduced pre- and post-synaptic inhibition. Third, Wall suggested that PHN pain could be due to prolonged central effects of afferent impulses. The intense initial barrage during the initial AHZ outbreak likely induces prolonged increased central excitability. Wall asked if these changes can become permanent from the acute barrage or "if a central excited state can be sustained by a trickle of arriving impulses from the periphery". Finally, the central effects of changed peripheral tissue was discussed. Wall suggested that in the course of the AHZ, the environment around peripheral nociceptors may change (scarring, dying back, changes in supportive cells) and if not restored could maintain the peripheral nerves and their central targets in an excited state. Wall finally suggested that we target the underlying mechanisms in future treatment strategies by preventing destruction of DRG-cells, taking advantage of the inhibitory systems, blocking the increased central excitability, and by reducing scar formation.

In the following sections, we first review the current understanding of the function of the uninjured nociceptive system to elucidate the mechanisms of neuropathic pain. Second, the pathophysiology of PHN and the hypotheses for the underlying pain mechanisms are reviewed. These hypotheses are natural developments from our 1989 studies and the questions posed by Wall in 1993. Finally, we review the evidence for (1) the 'irritable nociceptor' hypothesis and (2) deafferentation and reorganization as a pain generating mechanism in PHN. For details on pathology of AHZ and PHN, we refer to other chapters in this book.

3. Normal physiology of primary afferent nociceptors and their central targets

The nociceptive transmission system is defined by its responses to stimuli that are noxious (i.e. produce pain in human subjects) and potentially injurious. In the absence of nerve damage, responses to noxious stimuli are reversible. In contrast, the development of *neuropathic pain* requires persistent injury or abnormal function of the peripheral or central nervous system. It is important to point out, however, that neuropathic pain can share some basic mechanisms with pain that is generated by a normally functioning pain transmission system in response to tissue injury. Because of these shared mechanisms, studies using physiological stimulation of intact nociceptors have contributed almost as much as those of experimental nerve injury to our understanding of neuropathic pain.

3.1. Normal physiology of primary afferent nociceptors

Pain sensations are normally elicited by activity in unmyelinated (C-) and thinly myelinated (Aδ-) primary afferent neurons. Our current knowledge about the contribution of nociceptive Aδ-fibers to neuropathic pain is limited. The following sections, therefore, concentrate on C-fibers. Normally, C-nociceptors are silent in the absence of stimulation and respond best to stimuli that are potentially noxious. Following *acute tissue injury or in the presence of an ongoing inflammatory state* nociceptors become *physiologically* sensitized. Characteristic features of sensitized nociceptors are: ongoing discharge, a lowered activation threshold for thermal and mechanical stimuli, and an enhanced discharge to suprathreshold stimulation (hyperalgesia). Cutaneous application of algesic chemicals (e.g. capsaicin or mustard oil) produces a transient burning pain and thermal and mechanical hyperalgesia. Capsaicin is of particular interest because it selectively activates nociceptive primary afferents (Lynn, 1990; Holzer, 1991). The pain and thermal hyperalgesia that occur within the area of capsaicin application (termed the primary zone, Lewis, 1942) are due to active and sensitized CMH-units (CMH = C-mechano heat) (LaMotte et al., 1991, 1992). Pain in this region can be elicited by steadily applying gentle, normally innocuous pressure with a blunt probe (static mechanical hyperalgesia). Static mechanical hyperalgesia is mediated by sensitized CMH-nociceptors (Koltzenburg et al., 1992; Kilo et al., 1994). Since the thermal and static mechanical hyperalgesia are present exclusively in the primary zone where the C-nociceptors are directly activated by the algesic substance, this phenomenon is also called primary hyperalgesia. A different form of hyperalgesia develops in the surrounding skin where the C-nociceptors have not been activated. This form of hyperalgesia (secondary hyperalgesia) depends on mechanisms within the central nervous system (see below).

3.2. Responses of the central nervous system to massive or prolonged C-nociceptor activity

Massive or prolonged C-nociceptor input produces dramatic, long-term changes in the response of the central nervous system to somatosensory inputs. When identical noxious stimuli are repeatedly applied to the skin at a certain rate, there is a progressive build-up in the response of spinal cord dorsal horn neurons, a phenomenon called *wind-up* (Mendell and Wall, 1965; Price et al., 1978). In fact, any prolonged or massive input from C-nociceptors enhances the response of dorsal horn neurons to all subsequent afferent inputs (Woolf and Wall, 1986; Woolf and Thompson, 1991; Dickenson, 1994, 1995). In addition, the size of the dorsal horn neuron's receptive field grows (McMahon and Wall, 1984; Cervero et al., 1992). This process, called *central sensitization*, occurs with any tissue damage. As with sensitization of primary afferent nociceptors this sensitization of central pain transmission is a *normal physiological response of the undamaged nervous system*.

In normal human subjects, slowly repeated noxious stimuli are associated with a progressive increase in intensity of perceived pain, provided that the stimuli are presented no more than three seconds apart (Price et al., 1977).

3.3. Central sensitization and dynamic allodynia

Large diameter low threshold mechanoreceptive primary afferents (Aβ-fibers) are normally sensitive to innocuous tactile stimuli and do not increase their discharge frequency with more intense stimuli. Furthermore, in humans they produce innocuous tactile sensations when activated by electrical stimulation (Torebjörk et al., 1987). However, when central sensitization is produced by C-fiber activity these large diameter fibers (Aβ-mechanoreceptors) become capable of activating central nervous system pain signalling neurons (Simone et al., 1991a).

Central sensitization can be produced in normal human subjects using selective C-fiber activation by capsaicin. As a consequence of ongoing discharge in C-nociceptors at the site of capsaicin application (primary zone), an area of enhanced cutaneous sensitivity develops and spreads beyond the boundaries of the region directly activated by capsaicin. In this outer (secondary) zone, normally innocuous tactile stimuli, e.g. gently brushing the skin, become capable of producing pain. This type of mechanical hyperalgesia expands well into the surrounding unaffected skin (secondary zone) and is therefore called secondary mechanical hyperalgesia. Since secondary hyperalgesia is easily elicited by *moving* mechanical stimuli it is also termed dynamic mechanical hyperalgesia to distinguish it from static mechanical hyperalgesia which is due to activating sensitized CMH-nociceptors. Selective blockade and stimulation studies have revealed that dynamic mechanical hyperalgesia is mediated by Aβ-low threshold mechanoreceptive afferents (Koltzenburg et al., 1992; LaMotte et al., 1992; Torebjörk et al., 1992). Although the mechanism underlying secondary hyperalgesia in humans is unknown, following capsaicin activation of C-fibers in primates, Aβ stimulation becomes capable of powerfully driving nociceptive dorsal horn neurons (Simone et al., 1991a). Both neural peptides such as substance P (Levine et al., 1993; Dougherty et al., 1994, 1995) and excitatory amino acids acting at the NMDA receptor (Davies and Lodge, 1987; Dougherty et al., 1992, 1993; Dickenson, 1994, 1995; Dickenson et al., 1997) contribute to this central sensitization.

Clearly, activation of C-fibers produces a change in the central nervous system. In addition to enhanced responses to nociceptors, gentle moving tactile stimuli which activate Aβ-fibers become capable of evoking pain (dynamic allodynia). Under physiological conditions this change is reversible.

4. Pathophysiology of PHN

Noordenbos (1959) was the first to combine sensory and pathological examinations in proposing a comprehensive theory of PHN pain. He demonstrated deficits in the perception of single light touches, pinprick, heat, and cold that were greatest in the center of the area reported as painful and faded toward the boundary with normal skin. In these patients, intercostal nerve biopsies showed a reduction in the number of large-diameter myelinated fibers. Noordenbos proposed that the predominant loss of large myelinated afferents lead to a loss of their central inhibitory effects on pain produced by small-diameter nociceptive afferents. Noordenbos' hypothesis that the unrestrained effects of C-fiber input into spinal cord is responsible for chronic pain was highly influential in the development of Melzack and Wall's gate-control hypothesis (Melzack and Wall, 1965). Critical to the Noordenbos concept is that nociceptor input is essential for the pain of PHN.

Using simple bedside tests, Watson et al. (1988) reported sensory loss in nearly all of the 208 patients in his series. Nurmikko and Bowsher (1990) used quantitative methods to compare sensation in the affected area with a contralateral control site in 42 PHN patients and 20 post-zoster patients without pain. Using abnormally elevated thresholds in at least two of six modalities (tactile, pinprick, vibration, warmth, cold and heat pain) as a criterion, 93% of the PHN group and 10% of the non-PHN group had sensory loss. In a second study, Nurmikko and colleagues examined 31 patients during acute zoster (Nurmikko et al., 1990). When re-examined 3 months later, only 7 still had pain. A stepwise

logistic regression analysis incorporating a variety of variables showed that only thermal sensory loss during zoster was significantly associated with PHN development. Baron and Saguer used the histamine flare method to assess the relationship of C-fiber loss to pain in 10 patients with PHN and allodynia (Baron and Saguer, 1993). Iontophoresed histamine activates a subset of unmyelinated primary afferents. The loss of the flare reaction was positively correlated with the severity of ongoing pain, leading them to conclude that cutaneous nociceptors were not involved in the signaling and maintenance of allodynia. The conclusion from the above studies was that because PHN is associated with sensory loss, deafferentation is the cause of the pain.

In an earlier study, we categorized patients with PHN into two distinct clinical presentations based on pain complaint and sensory examination (Rowbotham and Fields, 1989b). Patients with marked sensory loss and minimal or no allodynia were usually unresponsive to local anesthetic skin infiltration. Patients with moderate to severe allodynia but little or no sensory loss typically experienced dramatic relief with local anesthetic skin infiltration. Using thermal sensory testing and skin biopsies to quantify cutaneous nerve damage, we have shown that in PHN patients with allodynia, those with relatively preserved sensory function and cutaneous innervation had the most severe pain and allodynia (Rowbotham and Fields, 1996; Rowbotham et al., 1996b). Both the severity of the thermal sensory deficit and the *loss* of epidermal nerve fibers were *inversely* correlated with the severity of pain and allodynia. These findings led to the hypothesis that preserved primary afferent nociceptors can contribute significantly to PHN pain and allodynia (Fields et al., 1998; Rowbotham et al., 1998). According to this hypothesis ongoing or recurrent input from these abnormal primary afferent nociceptors produces pain and maintains sensitization of central pain transmitting neurons in a way analogous to experimental secondary hyperalgesia. In a recent study we tested this hypothesis by selectively activating primary afferent nociceptors using topical application of capsaicin (Petersen et al., 2000). Eleven 'capsaicin responders' were characterized by higher average daily pain, higher allodynia ratings, and relatively preserved sensory function at baseline compared to seven non-responders. In three of the 'capsaicin responders' the area of allodynia expanded into previously non-allodynic and non-painful skin that had normal sensory function and cutaneous innervation. These observations support the hypothesis that allodynia in some PHN patients is a form of chronic secondary hyperalgesia maintained by input from intact and possibly 'irritable' primary afferent nociceptors to a sensitized CNS.

5. Evidence for the irritable nociceptor as a pain generating mechanism

5.1. Pathological sensitization and ectopic impulse generation after nerve damage

Abnormal nociceptor sensitization, i.e. sensitization in the absence of acute tissue injury or inflammation, and abnormal spontaneous afferent activity have been demonstrated in a variety of rodent peripheral nerve injury models. When the sciatic nerve is transected and allowed to regenerate and form a neuroma, the regenerating tips ('sprouts') of damaged axons acquire abnormal properties. They develop spontaneous activity (ectopic discharge) and increased sensitivity to chemical, thermal and mechanical stimuli (Wall and Gutnick, 1974; Scadding, 1981; Michaelis et al., 1995, 1997). A clear example of this is that within hours of being damaged the small-diameter nociceptive axons innervating the cornea become spontaneously active (Tanelian and MacIver, 1991). Furthermore, rats with experimental diabetic neuropathy become hyperalgesic and their C-nociceptors become sensitized to mechanical stimuli (Ahlgren and Levine, 1993). When a peripheral nerve is damaged, in addition to the sensitized peripheral terminals, a region near the dorsal root ganglion (which is distant from the site of injury) begins to generate 'spontaneous' impulses (Burchiel, 1984; Devor and Rappaport, 1990; Rappaport and Devor, 1990).

Ectopic impulse generation following experimental nerve injury is associated with enhanced expression of messenger RNA for certain voltage gated sodium channels in primary afferent neurons (Cummins and Waxman, 1997; Okuse et al., 1997; Novakovic et al., 1998). The accumulation of sodium channels at sites of ectopic impulse generation would lower the action potential threshold and has been postulated to be the underlying cause of spontaneous activity in damaged primary afferents (Devor et al., 1993; Matzner and Devor, 1994; Omana-Zapata et al., 1997).

An important advance in the field of experimental neuropathic pain is the development of *partial* nerve injury models (Bennett and Xie, 1988; Seltzer et al., 1990; Kim and Chung, 1992; Bennett, 1994a; Kim et al., 1997). These partial nerve damage models more closely resemble human painful nerve injuries than do the complete transection models. Importantly, spontaneous (ectopic) activity in small diameter primary afferents is a common feature (Tanelian and MacIver, 1991; Kajander and Bennett, 1992; Kajander et al., 1992; Koltzenburg et al., 1994).

In accordance with these animal data, microelectrode recordings from transected nerves in human amputees with phantom limb pain revealed spontaneous afferent activity (Nystrom and Hagbarth, 1981). Moreover, tapping the neuroma augmented the pain and induced afferent discharge in small and large afferent fibers. Interestingly, blocking the neuroma with lidocaine completely abolished the tap-induced nerve activity and the associated evoked pain but did not change spontaneous pain or neural activity. Therefore, the source of the latter is located more proximal, e.g. spontaneous impulses arising in or near dorsal root ganglion cells. Injection of a potassium channel blocker, which exacerbates a sprout's ongoing discharge, is intensely painful in patients with stump neuromas (Chabal et al., 1989). Interestingly, this phenomenon was found in several cases that were of more that 20 years' duration, which indicates that abnormal primary afferent hyperactivity in humans can be persistent.

The concept that abnormally activated C-fibers contribute to neuropathic pain in human subjects is also supported by clinical reports of patients with spontaneous pain and thermal and static mechanical hyperalgesia. The thermal and static mechanical hyperalgesia are similar to what is observed in the primary zone after capsaicin application. Ochoa and colleagues (Ochoa, 1986; Cline et al., 1989) have reported patients with a chronic peripheral neuropathy and mechanical hyperalgesia. Direct microneurographic recordings in these patients demonstrated sensitized C-nociceptors innervating the painful region. As will be discussed below, we feel that ectopic impulse generation in intact but abnormally functioning primary afferent nociceptors is a major contributing factor to pain in many patients with PHN.

5.2. Central nervous system consequences of hyperactive primary afferents: central sensitization

Centrally propagated activity of nociceptors produces a prolonged and significant enhancement of responses to both noxious and innocuous somatic stimuli, i.e. central sensitization. Animal studies indicate that this type of central mechanism plays a significant role in neuropathic pain. Partial peripheral nerve injury leads to an increase in the general excitability of spinal cord neurons similar to that observed after prolonged C-nociceptor stimulation (Kim and Chung, 1992; Palecek et al., 1992; Laird and Bennett, 1993; Tal and Bennett, 1994). This neuropathic central sensitization is probably due to activity in pathologically sensitized C-fibers, which sensitize spinal cord dorsal horn neurons by releasing glutamate and the neuropeptide substance P (Qian et al., 1996). Also comparable to the physiological condition, after partial nerve lesion, normally innocuous tactile stimuli become capable of activating spinal cord pain signalling neurons via Aβ-low threshold mechanoreceptors (Tal and Bennett, 1994). Similar abnormal sensitization also develops in thalamic and cortical neurons after partial nerve lesions (Guilbaud et al., 1990, 1992).

Human studies support the idea that Aβ activity can contribute to neuropathic pain. First, reaction time measurements have shown that dynamic hyperalgesia (allodynia) is signalled by afferents with conduction velocities appropriate for large myelinated axons (Lindblom and Verrillo, 1979; Campbell et al., 1988). Second, transcutaneous stimulation of nerves innervating the hyperalgesic skin can evoke pain at stimulus intensities which produce only tactile sensations in normally innervated skin (Price et al., 1989). Third, differential nerve blocks reveal that dynamic hyperalgesia is abolished concurrently with loss of innocuous tactile sensation at a time when Aδ- and C-fiber mediated modalities (pain and temperature) are unaffected (Ochoa and Yarnitsky, 1993; Koltzenburg et al., 1994).

Once central sensitization is established, activity in C-nociceptors can maintain the central processes that cause allodynia. In chronic neuropathic pain patients selective block of Aβ-fibers eliminates allodynia (Gracely et al., 1992; Koltzenburg et al., 1994) (see above), but ongoing burning pain persists indicating that it is mediated by C-nociceptors. Conversely, stepwise heating of the skin (which selectively activates C-fibers) produces a graded increase of both ongoing pain and allodynia intensity. These data indicate that C-nociceptor input from the periphery can dynamically maintain central sensitization which results in Aβ-mediated dynamic allodynia. Further evidence that central sensitization is present in PHN is the evidence that the NMDA antagonist ketamine has been shown to both relieve the pain and to reduce summation in patients with PHN (Eide et al., 1994).

6. Deafferentation and reorganization as a pain generating mechanism

Damage to primary afferents in peripheral nerves can result in deafferentation, sprouting of the central processes of surviving afferent axons and the development of aberrant connections in the spinal cord. Under these circumstances, surviving dorsal root axons can make functional contact with spinal cord neurons that have been deprived of their normal input (Devor and Wall, 1981; LaMotte et al., 1989). The type of anatomical reorganization that might enhance pain or produce allodynia has recently been described in a rodent neuropathic model. Neurons in lamina II (substantia gelatinosa) of the spinal cord dorsal horn normally receive direct input from small-diameter (Aδ-, C-) fibers and respond best to noxious stimulation (Ralston and Ralston, 1979; Wall et al., 1979; Sugiura et al., 1986; Hylden et al., 1986). Peripheral nerve damage results in a substantial degeneration of C-fiber primary afferent terminals in lamina II (Jänig and McLachlan, 1984; Lisney, 1989). As a consequence of this loss of synaptic contacts normally made by C-fiber afferents onto pain signalling neurons in lamina II (Castro-Lopes et al., 1990), the central terminals of Aβ-mechanoreceptive afferents which normally terminate in deeper laminae (III and IV) grow into lamina II and directly contact the deafferented cells (Woolf et al., 1992; Shortland and Woolf, 1993). This sprouting of Aβ-terminals depends critically on the extent of C-fiber degeneration. Thus, application of the neurotrophin NGF, which prevents C-fibers from degenerating, prevents central Aβ-fiber sprouting (Bennett et al., 1996). After such reorganization, large diameter primary afferents including those which respond best to innocuous moving stimuli (Aβ) provide a major direct input to spinal neurons that normally have direct input exclusively from unmyelinated primary afferents. In fact, recording from dorsal horn neurons in rats with partial peripheral nerve injuries reveals a marked increase in responses to light tactile stimulation (Laird and Bennett, 1993). Such changes might be the neural correlate of the dynamic mechanical allodynia observed in some PHN patients who have loss of C-fiber function (see below). It could also explain allodynia in areas of skin without heat hyperalgesia.

7. Dynamic mechanical allodynia: irritable nociceptor or deafferentation?

We propose that there are at least two distinct mechanisms for dynamic mechanical (Aβ) allodynia in PHN patients: central sensitization and/or sprouting of the spinal terminals of Aβ primary afferents to innervate dorsal horn neurons following loss of their normal C-nociceptor input. These two forms of PHN are distinguishable on clinical examination. In those patients with the irritable nociceptor form of PHN, prolonged nociceptor input would lead to central sensitization of dorsal horn neurons and consequent secondary hyperalgesia or dynamic mechanical allodynia spreading outward from the zone of maximal pain. Further C-fiber activation in these patients (for example by heating or acute application of capsaicin) would be expected to worsen their pain and increase their allodynia. Cooling or locally anesthetizing the area of maximal pain, by reducing C-fiber input, would reduce pain and both the area and intensity of allodynia. In contrast, in those patients with anatomical reorganization of the dorsal horn secondary to C-fiber deafferentation, there is reduced C-fiber function in the area of maximal pain. In these deafferentation patients, neither heating and capsaicin nor local anesthetic application to the area of maximal pain would affect ongoing pain and/or allodynia in the immediately adjacent skin.

8. Pain and allodynia in hypoalgesic skin: alternative mechanisms

Although aberrant connections within the spinal cord seems a likely contributor to PHN, alternative explanations for pain and allodynia in the setting of impaired cutaneous C-fiber function must be considered.

(1) The origin of ongoing C-nociceptor activity might be tiny sub- or intracutaneous microneuromas. It is possible that small fascicles of regenerating axons do not grow through herpetic scars (Bennett, 1994b). In this case the peripheral terminals remain deep to the surface resulting in elevated sensory thresholds. This argument is supported by the clinical observation that areas of Aβ-allodynia often surround zones of scar tissue.

(2) The nociceptive C-fibers may degenerate exclusively in the peripheral branch leaving the dorsal root ganglion soma and the central axon branch intact. The cell bodies of these injured neurons could then generate ectopic impulse activity that would

maintain the pathologic central sensitization in the presence of analgesic skin (Devor et al., 1992).

(3) In theory, since most tests have only studied the function of *cutaneous* C-fibers, ongoing activity might originate in nociceptors of deep somatic tissues (e.g. muscle, ligaments, etc.; Wall and Woolf, 1984).

In all of these possible mechanisms, allodynia would be the result of activity in primary afferent nociceptors and thus should respond to NMDA antagonists, systemic local anesthetics or appropriate nerve root blockade.

9. Deafferentation: hyperactivity of central pain transmission neurons

In some patients with PHN, there is virtually complete cutaneous deafferentation of the painful area with no significant allodynia. Assuming that the dorsal root ganglion cells and the central connections of all afferents are lost in such patients, their pain must be the result of intrinsic CNS changes. In animal studies, following complete primary afferent loss of a spinal segment, many dorsal horn cells begin to fire spontaneously at high frequencies (Lombard and Larabi, 1983). Similar hyperactivity in dorsal horn neurons has been reported following partial nerve injury resulting in significant loss of function of unmyelinated primary afferents (Laird and Bennett, 1993). There is some evidence that a similar process may underlie the pain that follows extensive denervating injuries in human. For example, pain is a characteristic sequela of the deafferentation produced by brachial plexus avulsion (Wynn-Parry, 1980, 1984). Recordings of spinal neuron activity in a pain patient whose dorsal roots were injured by trauma to the cauda equina revealed high-frequency regular and paroxysmal bursting discharges (Loeser et al., 1967). That patient complained of spontaneous burning pain in a region rendered anesthetic by the lesion (anesthesia dolorosa). There is anecdotal evidence that pain after brachial plexus avulsion responds to a surgical DREZ (dorsal root entry zone) lesion which destroys nociceptive dorsal horn neu-

rons (Nashold and Ostdahl, 1979). This procedure has also been reported to be effective for patients with PHN (Friedman and Nashold, 1984); however, it is unclear what sensory abnormalities were present in the patients who responded. This procedure is currently rarely used except in cases of brachial plexus avulsions.

10. Differential loss of Aβ-afferents: disinhibition

Large-diameter primary afferents (Aβ-fibers) respond to light mechanical stimuli. In normal subjects, in the absence of central sensitization, Aβ-activity produces only innocuous tactile sensations (Torebjörk et al., 1987). Activity in Aβ-fibers excites interneurons that inhibit the second-order pain-transmission cell. Accordingly, when myelinated primary afferents are selectively blocked (e.g., by ischemic compression of a peripheral nerve), light mechanical or thermal stimuli in the innervation territory of the partially blocked nerve produce a sensation that has a poorly localized, tingly and/or burning dysesthetic quality (Landau and Bishop, 1953). Furthermore, skin stimuli which normally produce only mild pain produce exaggerated burning pain. These observations indicate that input from myelinated fibers has a significant inhibitory effect on central pain transmission cells. In fact, selective stimulation of large myelinated primary afferents in peripheral nerve (or their central processes in the dorsal columns) inhibits dorsal horn cells that are excited by noxious stimuli (Hillman and Wall, 1969). Noordenbos (1959) was the first to propose that the pain of PHN was due to predominant large-fiber loss combined with activity in surviving primary afferent nociceptors. Shortly thereafter, Melzack and Wall (1965) in their gate control hypothesis proposed that selective damage to pain-inhibiting large-diameter myelinated sensory axons was a general mechanism in neuropathic pain. Whether there is in fact a predominant loss of large-diameter myelinated primary afferents in PHN awaits pathological confirmation. However, the recent observation that a preexisting large-fiber polyneuropathy is a risk factor for developing chronic post-herpetic pain suggests that predominant large-fiber primary afferent loss could be a contributing factor in PHN (Baron et al., 1997).

11. Disinhibition: loss of inhibitory interneurons

Loss of large-fiber evoked inhibition could also be brought about if the central inhibitory interneurons were impaired. Many of the neurons in the spinal cord dorsal horn contain inhibitory neurotransmitters such as GABA and enkephalin (Hunt et al., 1981). In animal studies, peripheral damage of primary afferents leads to transsynaptic signs of degeneration of deafferented spinal neurons in dorsal horn lamina I–III (Sugimoto et al., 1990). Cells showing these changes have been named 'dark neurons'. It has been proposed that dark neurons appear secondary to the high incidence of ectopic discharge in injured primary afferent neurons indicating a excitotoxic effect mediated by NMDA-receptors (Sugimoto et al., 1990; Kajander and Bennett, 1992). If some dark neurons were inhibitory interneurons one would expect disinhibition of dorsal horn neurons (Wall and Devor, 1981; Woolf and Wall, 1982; Laird and Bennett, 1992).

If this loss of inhibitory interneurons occurs in herpes zoster it could lead to enhanced responsiveness to peripheral stimulation and an increase in spontaneous activity of central nervous system pain transmission neurons. In fact, significant shrinkage of the dorsal horn has been shown in PHN patients (Watson et al., 1991). However, it is unclear what types of neurons, if any, are lost.

12. Conclusion

We propose that there are at least two distinct mechanisms for dynamic mechanical (Aβ) allodynia in PHN patients: central sensitization and sprouting of the spinal terminals of Aβ primary afferents to innervate dorsal horn neurons following loss of their normal C-nociceptor input. Furthermore, upregulation of excitatory adrenergic receptors on primary affer-

ents after axonal damage and inflammation along its axon can produce a hyperexcitable state in a primary afferent (Choi and Rowbotham, 1997). The latter mechanisms have not been reviewed here.

The possibility of multiple mechanisms in the same patient may well explain why response to any single intervention (especially a selective one) is so often partial and opens the possibility that therapy can be targeted to underlying mechanisms in individual patients (Bennett, 1994b). There is evidence in favor of using pharmacologic probes such as i.v. lidocaine infusion to select patients for longer-term therapy with analogous sodium channel blocking drugs (Galer et al., 1996). The same is believed true for opioids, though controlled data are lacking. Treatment of PHN should address the dominant presumed underlying pathophysiological mechanism in each patient. In the clinic, simple tests of capsaicin and lidocaine response could help determine underlying mechanisms. To the extent that pain is due to input from preserved and possibly 'irritable' primary afferent nociceptors and central sensitization, patients would experience increased pain and allodynia to a single application of topical capsaicin cream and relief with application of local anesthetic in the most painful skin. In these patients, treatment should be aimed at reducing abnormal peripheral input and suppressing central sensitization. To the extent that deafferentation and central reorganization is the dominant mechanism, patients would experience no persistent change in pain or allodynia with either of the treatments. Treatment of these patients is less clear because the pharmacology of the deafferentation-altered CNS has not been specifically studied. The hypothesis of a spectrum of pain mechanisms underlying PHN has not been tested in clinical trials yet. The data to date suggest that the mechanisms are likely not mutually exclusive and may coexist in many patients.

Acknowledgements

Supported by Grants NS21445, NS39521, and NS02164 from the National Institute of Neurological

Disorders and Stroke. Dr. Petersen is supported by a fellowship from the Varicella Zoster Virus Research Foundation.

References

Ahlgren, S.C. and Levine, J.D. (1993) Mechanical hyperalgesia in streptozotocin-diabetic rats is not sympathetically maintained. Brain Res., 616: 171–175.

Baron, R., Haendler, G. and Schulte, H. (1997) Afferent large fiber polyneuropathy predicts the development of postherpetic neuralgia. Pain, 73: 231–238.

Baron, R. and Saguer, M. (1993) Postherpetic neuralgia: are C-nociceptors involved in signalling and maintenance of tactile allodynia? Brain, 116: 1477–1496.

Bennett, G.J. (1994a) Animal models of neuropathic pain. In: G.F. Gebhart, D.L. Hammond and T.S. Jensen (Eds.), Proceedings of the 7th World Congress on Pain. Progress in Pain Research and Management, Vol. 2, IASP Press, Seattle, WA, pp. 495–510.

Bennett, G.J. (1994b) Hypotheses on the pathogenesis of herpes zoster-associated pain. Ann. Neurol., 35: S38–41.

Bennett, G.J. and Xie, Y.K. (1988) A peripheral mononeuropathy in rat that produces disorders of pain sensation like those seen in man [see comments]. Pain, 33: 87–107.

Bennett, D.L., French, J., Priestley, J.V. and McMahon, S.B. (1996) NGF but not NT-3 or BDNF prevents the A fiber sprouting into lamina II of the spinal cord that occurs following axotomy. Mol. Cell Neurosci., 8: 211–220.

Burchiel, K.J. (1984) Effects of electrical and mechanical stimulation on two foci of spontaneous activity which develop in primary afferent neurons after peripheral axotomy. Pain, 18: 249–265.

Campbell, J.N., Raja, S.N., Meyer, R.A. and Mackinnon, S.E. (1988) Myelinated afferents signal the hyperalgesia associated with nerve injury. Pain, 32: 89–94.

Castro-Lopes, J.M., Coimbra, A., Grant, G. and Arvidsson, J. (1990) Ultrastructural changes of the central scalloped (C1) primary afferent endings of synaptic glomeruli in the substantia gelatinosa Rolandi of the rat after peripheral neurotomy. J. Neurocytol., 19: 329–337.

Cervero, F., Laird, J.M. and Pozo, M.A. (1992) Selective changes of receptive field properties of spinal nociceptive neurones induced by noxious visceral stimulation in the cat. Pain, 51: 335–342.

Chabal, C., Jacobson, L., Russell, L.C. and Burchiel, K.J. (1989) Pain responses to perineuromal injection of normal saline, gallamine, and lidocaine in humans. Pain, 36: 321–325.

Choi, B. and Rowbotham, M.C. (1997) Effect of adrenergic receptor activation on post-herpetic neuralgia pain and sensory disturbances. Pain, 69: 55–63.

Cline, M.A., Ochoa, J. and Torebjork, H.E. (1989) Chronic hyperalgesia and skin warming caused by sensitized C nociceptors. Brain, 112: 621–647.

Cummins, T.R. and Waxman, S.G. (1997) Downregulation of tetrodotoxin-resistant sodium currents and upregulation of a rapidly repriming tetrodotoxin-sensitive sodium current in small spinal sensory neurons after nerve injury. J. Neurosci., 17: 3503–3514.

Davies, S.N. and Lodge, D. (1987) Evidence for involvement of N-methylaspartate receptors in 'wind-up' of class 2 neurones in the dorsal horn of the rat. Brain Res., 424: 402–406.

Devor, M. and Rappaport, Z.H. (1990) Pain and pathophysiology of damaged nerves. In: H.L. Fields (Ed.), Pain Syndromes in Neurology, Butterworth, London, pp. 47–84.

Devor, M. and Wall, P.D. (1981) Plasticity in the spinal cord sensory map following peripheral nerve injury in rats. J. Neurosci., 1: 679–684.

Devor, M., Wall, P.D. and Catalan, N. (1992) Systemic lidocaine silences ectopic neuroma and DRG discharge without blocking nerve conduction. Pain, 48: 261–268.

Devor, M., Govrin-Lippmann, R. and Angelides, K. (1993) Na$^+$ channel immunolocalization in peripheral mammalian axons and changes following nerve injury and neuroma formation. J. Neurosci., 13: 1976–1992.

Dickenson, A.H. (1994) NMDA receptor antagonists as analgesics. In: H.L. Fields and J.C. Liebeskind (Eds.), Progress in Pain Management and Research, IASP Press, Seattle, pp. 173–187.

Dickenson, A.H. (1995) Central acute pain mechanisms. Ann. Med., 27: 223–227.

Dickenson, A.H., Chapman, V. and Green, G.M. (1997) The pharmacology of excitatory and inhibitory amino acid-mediated events in the transmission and modulation of pain in the spinal cord. Gen. Pharmacol., 28: 633–638.

Dougherty, P.M., Palecek, J., Paleckova, V., Sorkin, L.S. and Willis, W.D. (1992) The role of NMDA and non-NMDA excitatory amino acid receptors in the excitation of primate spinothalamic tract neurons by mechanical, chemical, thermal, and electrical stimuli. J. Neurosci., 12: 3025–3041.

Dougherty, P.M., Palecek, J., Zorn, S. and Willis, W.D. (1993) Combined application of excitatory amino acids and substance P produces long-lasting changes in responses of primate spinothalamic tract neurons. Brain Res. Brain Res. Rev., 18: 227–246.

Dougherty, P.M., Palecek, J., Paleckova, V. and Willis, W.D. (1994) Neurokinin 1 and 2 antagonists attenuate the responses and NK1 antagonists prevent the sensitization of primate spinothalamic tract neurons after intradermal capsaicin. J. Neurophysiol., 72: 1464–1475.

Dougherty, P.M., Palecek, J., Paleckova, V. and Willis, W.D. (1995) Infusion of substance P or neurokinin A by microdialysis alters responses of primate spinothalamic tract neurons to cutaneous stimuli and to iontophoretically released excitatory amino acids. Pain, 61: 411–425.

Eide, P.K., Jorum, E., Stubhaug, A., Bremnes, J. and

Breivik, H. (1994) Relief of post-herpetic neuralgia with the N-methyl-D-aspartic acid receptor antagonist ketamine: a double-blind, cross-over comparison with morphine and placebo. Pain, 58: 347–354.

Fields, H.L., Rowbotham, M.C. and Baron, R (1998) Postherpetic neuralgia: irritable nociceptors and deafferentation. Neurobiol. Disease, 5: 209–227.

Friedman, A.H. and Nashold Jr., B.S. (1984) Dorsal root entry zone lesions for the treatment of postherpetic neuralgia. Neurosurgery, 15: 969–970.

Galer, B.S., Harle, J. and Rowbotham, M.C. (1996) Response to intravenous lidocaine infusion predicts subsequent response to oral mexiletine: a prospective study. J. Pain Symptom Manage., 12: 161–167.

Gracely, R.H., Lynch, S.A. and Bennett, G.J. (1992) Painful neuropathy: altered central processing maintained dynamically by peripheral input. Pain, 51: 175–194.

Guilbaud, G., Benoist, J.M., Jazat, F. and Gautron, M. (1990) Neuronal responsiveness in the ventrobasal thalamic complex of rats with an experimental peripheral mononeuropathy. J. Neurophysiol., 64: 1537–1554.

Guilbaud, G., Benoist, J.M., Levante, A., Gautron, M. and Willer, J.C. (1992) Primary somatosensory cortex in rats with pain-related behaviours due to a peripheral mononeuropathy after moderate ligation of one sciatic nerve: neuronal responsivity to somatic stimulation. Exp. Brain Res., 92: 227–245.

Hillman, P. and Wall, P.D. (1969) Inhibitory and excitatory factors influencing the receptive fields of lamina 5 spinal cord cells. Exp. Brain Res., 9: 284–306.

Holzer, P. (1991) Capsaicin: cellular targets, mechanisms of action, and selectivity for thin sensory neurons. Pharmacol. Rev., 43: 143–201.

Hunt, S.P., Kelly, J.S., Emson, P.C., Kimmel, J.R., Miller, R.J. and Wu, J.Y. (1981) An immunohistochemical study of neuronal populations containing neuropeptides or gamma-aminobutyrate within the superficial layers of the rat dorsal horn. Neurosci., 6: 1883–1898.

Hylden, J.L., Hayashi, H., Dubner, R. and Bennett, G.J. (1986) Physiology and morphology of the lamina 1 spinomesencephalic projection. J. Comp. Neurol., 247: 505–515.

Jänig, W. and McLachlan, E. (1984) On the fate of sympathetic and sensory neurons projecting into a neuroma of the superficial peroneal nerve in the cat. J. Comp. Neurol. 225: 302–311.

Kajander, K.C. and Bennett, G.J. (1992) Onset of a painful peripheral neuropathy in rat: a partial and differential deafferentation and spontaneous discharge in A beta and A delta primary afferent neurons. J. Neurophysiol., 68: 734–744.

Kajander, K.C., Wakisaka, S. and Bennett, G.J. (1992) Spontaneous discharge originates in the dorsal root ganglion at the onset of a painful peripheral neuropathy in the rat. Neurosci. Lett., 138: 225–228.

Kilo, S., Schmelz, M., Koltzenburg, M. and Handwerker, H.O. (1994) Different patterns of hyperalgesia induced by experimental inflammation in human skin. Brain, 117: 385–396.

Kim, S.H. and Chung, J.M. (1992) An experimental model for peripheral neuropathy produced by segmental spinal nerve ligation in the rat. Pain, 50: 355–363.

Kim, K.J., Yoon, Y.W. and Chung, J.M. (1997) Comparison of three rodent neuropathic pain models. Exp. Brain Res., 113: 200–206.

Koltzenburg, M., Lundberg, L.E.R. and Torebjörk, H.E. (1992) Dynamic and static components of mechanical hyperalgesia in human hairy skin. Pain, 51: 207–219.

Koltzenburg, M., Kees, S., Budweiser, S., Ochs, G. and Toyka, K.V. (1994) The properties of nociceptive primary afferents change in a painful chronic constriction neuropathy. In: G.F. Gebhart, D.L. Hammond and T.S. Jensen (Eds.), Proceedings of the 7th World Congress on Pain. IASP Press, Seattle, pp. 134–141.

Laird, J.M. and Bennett, G.J. (1992) Dorsal root potentials and afferent input to the spinal cord in rats with an experimental peripheral neuropathy. Brain Res., 584: 181–190.

Laird, J.M. and Bennett, G.J. (1993) An electrophysiological study of dorsal horn neurons in the spinal cord of rats with an experimental peripheral neuropathy. J. Neurophysiol., 69: 2072–2085.

LaMotte, C.C., Kapadia, S.E. and Kocol, C.M. (1989) Deafferentation-induced expansion of saphenous terminal field labelling in the adult rat dorsal horn following pronase injection of the sciatic nerve. J. Comp. Neurol., 288: 311–325.

LaMotte, R.H., Shain, C.N., Simone, D.A. and Tsai, E.F. (1991) Neurogenic hyperalgesia: psychophysical studies of underlying mechanisms. J. Neurophysiol., 66: 190–211.

LaMotte, R.H., Lundberg, L.E.R. and Torebjörk, H.E. (1992) Pain, hyperalgesia and activity in nociceptive C units in humans after intradermal injection of capsaicin. J. Physiol., 448: 749–764.

Landau, W. and Bishop, G.G. (1953) Pain from dermal, periostal and fascial endings and from inflammation. Arch. Neurol. Psychiatry, 69: 490–504.

Levine, J.D., Fields, H.L. and Basbaum, A.I. (1993) Peptides and the primary afferent nociceptor. J. Neurosci., 13: 2273–2286.

Lewis, T. (1942) Pain. Macmillan, New York.

Lindblom, U. and Verrillo, R.T. (1979) Sensory functions in chronic neuralgia. J. Neurol. Neurosurg. Psychiatry, 42: 422–435.

Lisney, S.J. (1989) Regeneration of unmyelinated axons after injury of mammalian peripheral nerve. Q. J. Exp. Physiol., 74: 757–784.

Loeser, J.D., Ward, A.A. and White, L.E. (1967) Chronic deafferentation of human spinal cord neurons. J. Neurosurg., 29: 48–50.

Lombard, M.C. and Larabi, Y. (1983) Electrophysiological study of cervical dorsal horn cells in partially deafferented rats. In: J.J. Bonica, (Ed.), Advances in Pain Research and Therapy, Raven Press, New York, pp. 147–154.

Lynn, B. (1990) Capsaicin: actions on nociceptive C-fibres and therapeutic potential. Pain, 41: 61–69.

Matzner, O. and Devor, M. (1994) Hyperexcitability at sites of nerve injury depends on voltage-sensitive Na$^+$ channels. J. Neurophysiol., 72: 349–359.

McMahon, S.B. and Wall, P.D. (1984) Receptive fields of rat lamina 1 projection cells move to incorporate a nearby region of injury. Pain, 19: 235–247.

Melzack, R. and Wall, P.D. (1965) Pain mechanisms: a new theory. Science, 150: 971–978.

Mendell, L.M. and Wall, P.D. (1965) Responses of single dorsal cord cells to peripheral cutaneous unmyelinated fibers. Nature, 206: 97–99.

Michaelis, M., Blenk, K.H., Jänig, W. and Vogel, C. (1995) Development of spontaneous activity and mechanosensitivity in axotomized afferent nerve fibers during the first hours after nerve transection in rats. J. Neurophysiol., 74: 1020–1027.

Michaelis, M., Vogel, C., Blenk, K.H. and Jänig, W. (1997) Algesics excite axotomised afferent nerve fibres within the first hours following nerve transection in rats. Pain, 72: 347–354.

Nashold Jr., B.S. and Ostdahl, R.H. (1979) Dorsal root entry zone lesions for pain relief. J. Neurosurg., 51: 59–69.

Noordenbos, W. (1959) Pain. Elsevier, Amsterdam, pp. 68–80.

Novakovic, S.D., Tzoumaka, E., McGivern, J.G., Haraguchi, M., Sangameswaran, L., Gogas, K.R., Eglen, R.M. and Hunter, J.C. (1998) Distribution of the tetrodotoxin-resistant sodium channel PN3 in rat sensory neurons in normal and neuropathic conditions. J. Neurosci., 18: 2174–2187.

Nurmikko, T.J. and Bowsher, D. (1990) Somatosensory findings in postherpetic neuralgia. J. Neurol. Neurosurg. Psychiatry, 53: 135–141.

Nurmikko, T.J., Räsänen, A. and Häkkinen, V. (1990) Clinical and neurological observations on acute herpes zoster. Clin. J. Pain, 6: 284–290.

Nystrom, B. and Hagbarth, K.E. (1981) Microelectrode recordings from transected nerves in amputees with phantom limb pain. Neurosci. Lett., 27: 211–216.

Ochoa, J. (1986) The newly recognized painful ABC syndrome: thermographic aspects. Thermology, 2: 65–107.

Ochoa, J.L. and Yarnitsky, D. (1993) Mechanical hyperalgesias in neuropathic pain patients: dynamic and static subtypes. Ann. Neurol., 33: 465–472.

Okuse, K., Chaplan, S.R., McMahon, S.B., Luo, Z.D., Calcutt, N.A., Scott, B.P., Akopian, A.N. and Wood, J.N. (1997) Regulation of expression of the sensory neuron-specific sodium channel SNS in inflammatory and neuropathic pain. Mol. Cell Neurosci., 10: 196–207.

Omana-Zapata, I., Khabbaz, M.A., Hunter, J.C., Clarke, D.E. and Bley, K.R. (1997) Tetrodotoxin inhibits neuropathic ectopic activity in neuromas, dorsal root ganglia and dorsal horn neurons. Pain, 72: 41–49.

Palecek, J., Dougherty, P.M., Kim, S.H., Paleckova, V., Lekan, H., Chung, J.M., Carlton, S.M. and Willis, W.D. (1992) Re-

sponses of spinothalamic tract neurons to mechanical and thermal stimuli in an experimental model of peripheral neuropathy in primates. J. Neurophysiol., 68: 1951–1966.

Petersen, K.L., Fields, H.L., Brennum, J., Sandroni, P. and Rowbotham, M.C. (2000) Capsaicin activation of 'irritable' nociceptors in post-herpetic neuralgia. Pain, 88: 125–133.

Price, D.D., Bennett, G.J. and Rafii, A. (1989) Psychophysical observations on patients with neuropathic pain relieved by a sympathetic block. Pain, 36: 273–288.

Price, D.D., Hayes, R.L., Ruda, M. and Dubner, R. (1978) Spatial and temporal transformations of input to spinothalamic tract neurons and their relation to somatic sensations. J. Neurophysiol., 41: 933–947.

Price, D.D., Hu, J.W., Dubner, R. and Gracely, R.H. (1977) Peripheral suppression of first pain and central summation of second pain evoked by noxious heat pulses. Pain, 3: 57–68.

Qian, Y., Chao, D.S., Santillano, D.R., Cornwell, T.L., Nairn, A.C., Greengard, P., Lincoln, T.M. and Bredt, D.S. (1996) cGmp-dependent protein kinase in dorsal root ganglion: relationship with nitric oxide synthase and nociceptive neurons. J. Neurosci., 16: 3130–3138.

Ralston, H.J. and Ralston, D.D. (1979) Identification of dorsal root synaptic terminals on monkey ventral horn cells by electron microscopic autoradiography. J. Neurocytol., 8: 151–166.

Rappaport, Z.H. and Devor, M. (1990) Experimental pathophysiological correlates of clinical symptomatology in peripheral neuropathic pain syndromes. Stereotact. Funct. Neurosurg., 54: 90–95.

Rowbotham, M.C. and Fields, H.L. (1989) Post-herpetic neuralgia: the relationship of pain complaint, sensory disturbance, and skin temperature. Pain, 39: 129–144.

Rowbotham, M.C. and Fields, H.L. (1989) Topical lidocaine reduces pain in post-herpetic neuralgia. Pain, 38: 297–301.

Rowbotham, M.C. and Fields, H.L. (1996) The relationship of pain, allodynia and thermal sensation in post-herpetic neuralgia. Brain, 119: 437–354.

Rowbotham, M.C., Davies, P.S., Verkempinck, C. and Galer, B.S. (1996a) Lidocaine patch: double- blind controlled study of a new treatment method for post-herpetic neuralgia. Pain, 65: 39–44.

Rowbotham, M.C., Harden, N., Stacey, B., Bernstein, P. and Magnus-Miller. L. (1998) Gabapentin for the treatment of postherpetic neuralgia. JAMA, 280: 1837–1842.

Rowbotham, M.C., Yosipovitch, G., Connolly, M.K., Finlay, D., Forde, G. and Fields, H.L. (1996b) Cutaneous innervation density in the allodynic form of postherpetic neuralgia. Neurobiol. Dis., 3: 205–214.

Scadding, J.W. (1981) Development of ongoing activity, mechanosensitivity, and adrenaline sensitivity in severed peripheral nerve axons. Exp. Neurol., 73(2): 345–364.

Seltzer, Z., Dubner, R. and Shir, Y. (1990) A novel behavioral model of neuropathic pain disorders produced in rats by partial sciatic nerve injury. Pain, 43: 205–218.

Shortland, P. and Woolf, C.J. (1993) Chronic peripheral nerve section results in a rearrangement of the central axonal arborizations of axotomized A beta primary afferent neurons in the rat spinal cord. J. Comp. Neurol., 330: 65–82.

Simone, D.A., Sorkin, L.S., Oh, U., Chung, J.M., Owens, C., LaMotte, R.H. and Willis, W.D. (1991a) Neurogenic hyperalgesia: central neural correlates in responses of spinothalamic tract neurons. J. Neurophysiol., 66: 228–246.

Sugimoto, T., Bennett, G.J. and Kajander, K.C. (1990) Transsynaptic degeneration in the superficial dorsal horn after sciatic nerve injury: effects of a chronic constriction injury, transection, and strychnine. Pain, 42: 205–213.

Sugiura, Y., Lee, C.L. and Perl, E.R. (1986) Central projections of identified, unmyelinated (C) afferent fibers innervating mammalian skin. Science, 234: 358–361.

Tal, M. and Bennett, G.J. (1994) Extra-territorial pain in rats with a peripheral mononeuropathy: mechano-hyperalgesia and mechano-allodynia in the territory of an uninjured nerve. Pain, 57: 375–382.

Tanelian, D.L. and MacIver, M.B. (1991) Analgesic concentrations of lidocaine suppress tonic A-delta and C fiber discharges produced by acute injury. Anesthesiol., 74: 934–936.

Torebjörk, H.E., Lundberg, L.E.R. and LaMotte, R.H. (1992) Central changes in processing of mechanoreceptive input in capsaicin-induced secondary hyperalgesia in humans. J. Physiol., 448: 765–780.

Torebjörk, H.E., Vallbo, A.B. and Ochoa, J.L. (1987) Intraneural microstimulation in man. Its relation to specificity of tactile sensations. Brain, 110: 1509–1529.

Wall, P.D. and Devor, M. (1981) The effect of peripheral nerve injury on dorsal root potentials and on transmission of afferent signals into the spinal cord. Brain Res., 209: 95–111.

Wall, P.D. and Gutnick, M. (1974) Ongoing activity in peripheral nerves: the physiology and pharmacology of impulses originating from a neuroma. Exp. Neurol., 43(3): 580–593.

Wall, P.D. and Woolf, C.J. (1984) Muscle but not cutaneous C-afferent input produces prolonged increases in the excitability of the flexion reflex in the rat. J. Physiol. (London), 356: 443–458.

Wall, P.D., Merrill, E.G. and Yaksh, T.L. (1979) Responses of single units in laminae 2 and 3 of cat spinal cord. Brain Res., 160: 245–260.

Watson, C.P.N., Evans, R.J., Watt, V.R. and Birkett, N. (1988) Postherpetic neuralgia: 208 cases. Pain, 35: 289–297.

Watson, C.P.N., Deck, J.H., Morshead, C., Van der Kooy, D. and Evans, R.J. (1991) Postherpetic neuralgia: further post-mortem studies of cases with and without pain. Pain, 44: 105–117.

Woolf, C.J. and Thompson, S.W. (1991) The induction and maintenance of central sensitization is dependent on N-methyl-D-aspartic acid receptor activation; implications for the treatment of post-injury pain hypersensitivity states. Pain, 44: 293–299.

Woolf, C.J. and Wall, P.D. (1982) Chronic peripheral nerve section diminishes the primary afferent A-fibre mediated inhibition of rat dorsal horn neurones. Brain Res., 242: 77–85.

Woolf, C.J. and Wall, P.D. (1986) Relative effectiveness of C primary afferent fibers of different origins in evoking a prolonged facilitation of the flexor reflex in the rat. J. Neurosci., 6: 1433–1442.

Woolf, C.J., Shortland, P. and Coggeshall, R.E. (1992) Peripheral nerve injury triggers central sprouting of myelinated afferents. Nature, 355: 75–78.

Wynn-Parry, C.B. (1980) Pain in avulsion lesions of the brachial plexus. Pain, 9: 41–53.

Wynn Parry, C.B. (1984) Brachial plexus injuries. Br. J. Hosp. Med., 32: 130–132, 134–139.

Herpes Zoster and Postherpetic Neuralgia, 2nd Revised and Enlarged Edition
Pain Research and Clinical Management, Vol. 11
Edited by C.P.N. Watson and A.A. Gershon

An essay on the mechanisms which may contribute to the pain of postherpetic neuralgia

Patrick D. Wall [*]

Centre for Neuroscience Research, Hodgkin Building, King's College London, London SE1 1UK, UK

1. Introduction

The chapters in this book preceding this one bring together the remarkable facts about the painful state of postherpetic neuralgia. I take it as my task to examine these facts and to ask how an adequate therapy might be achieved. Fortunately for me, the chapter by Rowbotham, Petersen, Baron and Fields proposes a clear structure which implies causative mechanisms which I can explore. Their scheme defines three subtypes:

(1) Irritable nociceptors, in which there is marked allodynia, thermal sensitivity, prolonged relief from local anaesthetics, a sympathetic component and pain produced by capsaicin.

(2) Deafferentation without allodynia, in which there is a severe sensory deficit, no allodynia, no effect of local anaesthetics, no sympathetic component and no response to capsaicin.

(3) Deafferentation with allodynia, a mixture of subtypes one and two.

In any clinical pain syndrome, there is inevitably a search for a peripheral cause or a central cause or a mixture of both. One interpretation of the first subtype would be that it has a purely peripheral origin in the sensitisation of normal nociceptors by the disease so that the threshold for producing pain is so lowered that normally innocuous stimuli produce pain and allodynia. This has the charm of simplicity and classical plausibility. It would require no central changes since nociceptors with their intact central projections simply become excited by low-level stimuli. This would be primary allodynia and implies a chronic inflammation of normally high threshold nociceptors. Since this is the simplest hypothesis, let us examine the evidence.

1.1. Evidence for irritable nociceptors

The histopathology of PHN cases is necessarily limited. No one doubts that continuous chronic PHN pain may follow acute viral infection of the dorsal root ganglia. The question is what structures change to cause the pain. In the acute phase, we know almost nothing of the significant predictive changes. The severity of acute pain is only very slightly worse in those patients who go on to develop PHN than in those who recover (Baron et al., 1997). They do show a generalised deficit of vibration detection threshold during the acute phase suggesting a large fibre disor-

[*] Correspondence to: Professor Patrick D. Wall, 1 Lake House, South Hill Park, London NW3 2SH, UK. Phone/Fax: +44 (20) 7435-9139; E-mail: patrick.wall@kcl.ac.uk

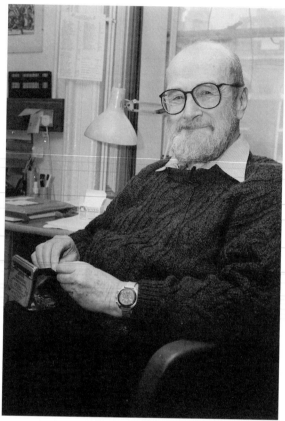

Prof. Patrick D. Wall

der. It is curious that, in the very early painful stages before the appearance of skin signs, one would expect an unmyelinated fibre-evoked triple response of wheal and flare if nociceptors were being excited. It appears to be a disease limited to cutaneous afferents but we do not know which of the many types of cutaneous afferent are involved. There is no evidence for infection of afferents supplying deep tissue such as muscle.

The pathology found in the PHN stage is described in the chapter by Watson, Oaklander and Deck. Widespread scattered destruction of dorsal root ganglion cells and therefore of both peripheral and central axons is clear. However, it is not clear which if any of these changes is crucial to the development of PHN. Signs of ongoing inflammation are reported but with no consistency. Similarly there is no agreement on the fibre spectrum of sur-

viving fibres. Most important, we do not know if some fibres survive with retracted terminal arborisations which have withdrawn from their normal position in skin. Only Noordenbos (1959) biopsied peripheral intercostal nerves in PHN patients and showed a preferential loss of large fibres. This has not been repeated for the very good reason, which Noordenbos later emphasised, that cutting nerves is a hazardous procedure likely to enhance the problems of deafferentation. This is presumably the reason why there are no reports of microneuronographic recording from PHN nerves which would be capable of identifying irritable nociceptors. The quite large needles used in this technique are capable of further damaging a nerve (Wall and McMahon, 1985) and therefore are a potential danger in the presence of an obvious neuropathy. Biopsies of skin in PHN repeatedly show a very marked decrease of nociceptors in PHN (Rowbotham et al., 1996; Oaklander et al., 1998). Similarly functional studies in search of nociceptors such as the histamine flare show a severe deficit of nociceptors (Baron and Saguer, 1993). The only known examples of irritable nociceptors are associated with tissue damage and therefore with the infiltration of inflammatory cells. No such cells have been reported in the skin biopsies of patients in the chronic state of PHN. The dorsal root ganglia do not show consistent signs of inflammation (Smith, 1978) in PHN patients. Therefore there is no histopathological evidence for the presence of long-term irritation of nociceptors.

There have been extensive experiments designed to produce prolonged sensitisation of nociceptors particularly by the school of Ferreira (reviewed in Ferreira et al., 1999 and Poole et al., 1999). They concentrate on the long lasting effects of cytokines and kinins produced by various cells during the course of inflammation. They can induce a delayed and prolonged hyperalgesia by injecting the prostaglandin E2 or the sympathomimetic agonist, dopamine. They produce persistent hyperalgesia by successive daily injections. After 6–9 daily injections, the sensitivity of the nociceptors does not return to its basal level but, instead, reaches a plateau. If this plateau is maintained by a further 7–9 days of daily injections, the hyperalgesia persists in the absence of further injections for up to 30 days. This is the only example I can find in the literature of persistent sensitisation of nociceptors in the absence of frank inflammation of tissue of the type hypothesised by Rowbotham et al. However, the effect does fade in the absence of further injections. This is to be expected with the continuous ongoing generation of replacement receptors and structural proteins continually synthesised in the dorsal root ganglion cells and transported into the axon. Furthermore the long lasting effect is abolished by treatment with dipyrone, diclofenac or flurbiprofen. Unfortunately this is not a characteristic of the pain of PHN attributed to irritable nociceptors by Rowbotham et al. Fibres and cells that survive the initial acute phase of inflammation would be expected to reconstitute their premorbid structure and excitability and therefore would not remain irritable in the absence of ongoing inflammation. It is conceivable that the period of viral duplication during the acute phase might change the nature of the surviving dorsal root ganglion cells' nuclei or of surrounding cells but there is no evidence for such an effect in cells which are not undergoing mitosis.

1.2. Indirect central and peripheral effects of peripheral nerve degeneration

I am assured in a personal communication with Professor Fields that it was not their intention to attribute the tenderness of skin in PHN entirely to the primary irritation of nociceptors. There is certainly growing evidence that the presence of degenerating fibres in a peripheral nerve induces excitatory changes in neighbouring 'intact' fibres. These new results follow the demonstration in rats that section of spinal nerves was followed by a mechanical and cold hyperalgesia in skin innervated by the neighbouring intact spinal roots (Kim and Chung, 1992). This result repeated similar effects seen in monkey (Kirk and Denny-Brown, 1970). These authors attributed the hyperalgesia to the development of ongoing activity in the dorsal root ganglion whose axons had been cut since they claimed that the hyperalgesia disappeared if the

dorsal root was cut or blocked central to the ganglion whose spinal nerve was cut. However, subsequent work has clearly failed to confirm this result. Li et al. (2000) showed that subsequent cutting of the L5 dorsal root after section of the L5 spinal nerve failed to abolish the hyperalgesia. However, they did show that subsequent section of the L4 dorsal root did abolish the hyperalgesia produced by L5 spinal nerve section. Similarly, Eshenfelder et al. (2000) showed that L5 dorsal root section had no effect on the hyperalgesia produced by L5 spinal nerve section. This implies that the hyperalgesia originates not from the cut nerve but from neighbouring intact nerves. Ali et al. (1999) had shown in monkey that uninjured C-fibre nociceptors developed spontaneous activity and α-adrenergic sensitivity when neighbouring axons degenerated. Similarly, Michaelis et al. (2000) have shown that intact muscle but not skin afferents develop ongoing discharge after neighbouring nerves have degenerated. Evidently we must consider the possibility that intact fibres in the neighbourhood of degenerating fibres may generate an afferent barrage which might increase central excitability.

2. Primary versus secondary hyperalgesia

It is conceivable that irritable nociceptors contribute to the pain of PHN which would be primary hyperalgesia. Since there is also the phenomenon of secondary hyperalgesia caused by central changes, we must first examine the properties of these two types of hyperalgesia. Fortunately Raja et al. (1999) have recently summarised the data on this subject to which they have themselves made major contributions. Briefly, primary sensitisation is proven when a nociceptor is found to become more sensitive after an initial noxious stimulus has excited it. There are two types of change observed. In one, the threshold of the unit is found to be unchanged on the second test but, as the stimulus intensity is increased, the rate of discharge of the unit escalates at a higher rate than previously. This would produce primary hyperalgesia where a normally painful stimulus produced more pain on a second application. In the second type, the threshold of the unit drops with the second stimulus and then the discharge rate escalates to higher levels than observed with the first stimulus. This would produce primary allodynia where a normally innocuous stimulus produces pain. In hairy skin but not in glabrous skin, heat hyperalgesia is attributed to small myelinated nociceptors and not to unmyelinated C-fibres. Mechanical stimuli of the light stroking type which are so characteristically painful in PHN are *not* associated with any observed sensitisation of nociceptors. Therefore the proposal that mechanical allodynia is produced by sensitised nociceptors is not supported by extensive physiological studies. For thermal stimuli Rowbotham et al. write, "Surprisingly, the magnitude of the thermal sensory deficit was inversely correlated to both ongoing pain and allodynia severity." It is indeed surprising since Nurmikko et al. (1990) showed that only thermal sensory *loss* during zoster was significantly associated with PHN development.

Secondary hyperalgesia and allodynia differs radically in nature and origin from the primary type. It is caused not by changes in the sensitivity of peripheral sensory axons but by an increased sensitivity of central neurons following peripheral damage. Localised thermal, mechanical or chemical painful stimuli are followed by the appearance of a wide zone of ongoing and easily provoked pain. The central mechanisms for this secondary appearance of pain produced by peripheral stimuli is summarised in Doubell et al. (1999). There are rapid processes in which normal inhibitions fail while excitatory effects are augmented. The effect is exaggerated by the slow transport of new substances from the periphery and there may be morphological changes in the circuitry of dorsal horn neurons. Light touch to the skin becomes painful due to the novel effectiveness of normal low-threshold myelinated afferents and not to changes in the periphery. Raja et al. (1999) and many others describe the details of this mechanical allodynia but they firmly emphasise that there is not an associated hyperalgesia to thermal stimuli in the surrounding zone. We can now summarise the situation which leads to the common problems of PHN: (1) raised thresholds to detec-

tion of mechanical and thermal stimuli, (2) raised painful sensitivity to mechanical stimuli when they are detected. The raised thresholds are the expected consequence of the destruction of afferents and the more afferents destroyed the more the threshold rises with anaesthesia in the extreme. The appearance of mechanical allodynia is entirely the consequence of central sensitisation since there is no evidence for peripheral nociceptor sensitisation. This mechanical allodynia is entirely the result of central changes but requires the activity of peripheral afferents to trigger the painful response. Therefore, as more and more afferents are lost, the patient is likely to move from the allodynic type to the deafferentation type. If sensitised mechanically responsive nociceptors can not explain these states, we are left only with the Rowbotham et al. data on thermal changes to explain. They report a number of interesting interventions which they interpret as evidence for irritable nociceptors with which I will deal later. Here I wish only to comment on the basic observations. They find that small decreases of thermal threshold are associated with high allodynia but that is expected because the allodynia requires an afferent input. They report rare cases of actual thermal hyperalgesia but we are not told if the threshold changed or if there was a coincident tactile component in the thermal stimulus. None of this is diagnostic of a change in peripheral nociceptors. Many groups have observed dorsal horn cells which respond to touch and to damage and to skin temperature since I reported them forty years ago (Wall, 1960). These are candidates to provide a central source of both mechanical and thermal evoked pain.

3. Sprouting in the neighbouring peripheral nervous system

In 1979, Devor et al. (Devor et al., 1979) showed that when the sciatic nerve in the rat was sectioned, the intact fibres of the saphenous nerve sprouted and invaded part of the foot evacuated by the degenerated sciatic nerve fibres. We could observe this phenomenon in man (Inbal et al., 1987). The subject remains of lively interest (Mansikka and Pertovaara, 1997; Ahcan et al., 1998; Pertens et al., 1999). Curiously, I do not know of mention of this topic in PHN in spite of the fact that intact survivors must sprout into the territory lost by the destroyed fibres. The problem may be not just the filling in of denervated gaps by collateral sprouts, but there is the possibility that the new sprouts may contribute to the afferent barrage in an abnormal way. It is very well established that sprouts emitted from the cut end of axons become spontaneously active, mechanosensitive and sensitive to sympathetic activity (reviewed in Devor and Seltzer, 1999). Furthermore these changes spread centrally and appear in the dorsal root ganglion cells whose axons have been cut (Wall and Devor, 1983). These phenomena themselves could be relevant to PHN if there was an intermediate pathology of damaged axons between the extremes of complete destruction and complete escape. While it has not been reported, a likely pathology would be of the dying-back type in which nerve endings would be withdrawn from their normal location in epidermis into deeper tissue. We know that many normal terminals are missing from dermis in PHN as described elsewhere in this book. We do not know if the entire axon and dorsal root ganglion is necessarily destroyed. If there are intermediate forms of destruction in which cutaneous axons retain blind neuritic endings in deeper tissue then it is very likely that these neurites and the dorsal root ganglion cells from which they originate would be the source of a steady ongoing afferent barrage and would be mechanosensitive and would be excited by adrenaline. Such endings could be confused with the irritable nociceptors proposed by Rowbotham et al. but would be a fundamentally different phenomenon.

We do not know if these deep neurites exist but the collateral sprouting of nearly intact afferents is certain. The existence of these sprouts has been known for twenty years but little was known of their physiology. Ali et al. (1999) showed that intact C-fibre nociceptors became active when neighbours degenerated. Now a crucial paper has appeared by Michaelis et al. (2000). They started with an experiment which had been done several times before in

which they cut the sural nerve (SU) and the nerve to gastrocnemius soleus (GS) and recorded the development of ongoing ectopic discharge in dorsal root ganglion cells whose axons had been cut. They found that 20.4% of the myelinated axons in GS became spontaneously active while none of the cutaneous dorsal root ganglion cells became active. This confirmed the surprising finding that the ectopic barrage from a cut nerve is limited to muscle afferents following transection of the axons. In the control situation where the nerves had not been cut, there was almost no ectopic activity (1.1%) in dorsal root ganglion cells supplying GS. Finally they made a new and very crucial observation by leaving the nerve to gastrocnemius intact while cutting the surrounding nerves.

The result was that 18.8% of the dorsal root ganglion cells that supply the intact GS became spontaneously active. This discharge had a high mean frequency (6.1 Hz) with intermittent bursts of even higher frequency. The conduction velocity of these active fibres was 5–30 m/s which places them in the group of small muscle fibres which include nociceptors. This means that the substantial changes of chemistry and activity which have been so well studied in axotomised cells spread to involve intact neighbours in a way which could certainly affect the sensory signs of PHN.

4. Central ipsilateral consequences of peripheral nerve damage

It is evident from the work of Watson and colleagues described in this book and reviewed from a different viewpoint by Gilden et al. (2000) that the varicella-zoster infection itself may spread centrally and involve widespread structures. For the sake of argument, I will propose here that the major troublesome symptoms of PHN may all be the consequence of the destructive lesions of the dorsal root ganglion and peripheral nerve and that it is not necessary to propose direct central destruction to explain the major pain problems of on-going pain, deafferentation and increased sensitivity. While the entire PHN group of syndromes is, of course, unique and diagnostic, individual examples of the troublesome symptoms are apparent after traumatic and surgical lesions which only affect the periphery in the primary lesion. Similarly, the three animal models that imitate some aspects of PHN, all involve only peripheral initial lesions (Devor and Seltzer, 1999). Therefore we will now explore the central secondary consequences of various peripheral lesions.

4.1. The totally deafferented cell

This phase applies to a cell which has suffered such severe destruction of its sensory afferent input that it fails to respond to any peripheral stimuli. It does not mean a cell which is stripped of all synaptic contacts which can never occur in the central nervous system. Every dorsal horn cell receives many inputs other than those arriving over the dorsal roots. These include inputs from nearby cells and from cells in other segments and from descending systems. Furthermore the evacuation of some synaptic sites by the degeneration of afferent fibres provokes local sprouting from nearby intact endings on the same cell which then spread to occupy the empty sites. Cells which have lost their effective peripheral input by experimental section of nearby dorsal roots become steadily more excitable and increase their rate of spontaneous firing (Basbaum and Wall, 1976). As this increases, the cells begin to emit high-frequency bursts of impulses. At a further stage, mutual interaction between the deafferented cells leads to synchronisation of the bursts. Similar but less dramatic changes are observed after extensive peripheral nerve lesions as with lesions of the sciatic and saphenous nerves in cats and rats (Devor and Wall, 1981; Wall and Devor, 1983). A variable component in the induction of this change can be the massive impulse barrage produced by the injury of the axons at the time of their section. However, a slower component is also involved and is due to the change in the delivery of trophic molecules which are normally transported from the periphery over the afferent fibres. The overall change can be seen as a homeostatic mechanism in which the cell having detected a loss of input induces an increase of gain in an attempt to compensate for the decreased input. It is reasonable to assume that this state is seen with brachial plexus avulsions with root damage in which the patient reports an ongoing burning pain in the anaesthetic limb accompanied by unprovoked intermittent stabs of pain.

4.2. The partially deafferented cell

Given the large overlapping areas occupied by the terminal arborisations of entering afferent axons, it is not surprising that partial deafferentation is far more common than complete deafferentation even with quite extensive root or peripheral nerve lesions (Basbaum and Wall, 1976; Devor and Wall, 1981). Here the individual cell may go through a period of complete failure to respond to peripheral stimuli but, as the process of rising excitability proceeds, the cell begins to respond to peripheral stimuli carried to the spinal cord over nearby intact nerves. This amounts to an expansion of the cell's normal receptive field in its intact state. With large lesions, the expansion of the receptive field may be dramatic. In the case of root lesions, cells may begin to respond to inputs arriving many segments away from the cell. This widespread recruitment of distant inputs contrasts with the normal state where cells respond only to afferents present in nearby roots so that the combination of normal receptive fields generates a precise somatotopic map. Not only do the novel responses originate from stimuli in a previously inert region, but the nature of the input–output relations of the novel connections is abnormal. The mechanism by which these changes occur is presumed to be exactly the same as those which were described above as responsible for the increased excitability of completely deafferented cells. Coincident with the rise of excitability, and perhaps its cause, is a collapse of both pre- and postsynaptic inhibitions. This raises a particular therapeutic problem in deafferentation states since most drug therapy for pain depends on boosting existing inhibitory systems. If the disease state has been produced by the destruction of the very inhibitory systems on which the drugs work, it is not surprising that normally analgesic drugs are no longer effective. One mechanism which would seem reasonable to explain the appearance of expanded receptive fields is the central sprouting of the terminal arborisations of intact afferents. This leaves the possibility that there is a functional readjustment of the physiology of normally existing connections. This is an optimistic conclusion since therapy should be able to prevent or reverse such changes of excitability much more easily than would be the case if new anatomical connections had been formed.

An educational clinical example of the consequences of partial deafferentation is seen in the results of a neurological examination of any amputee. Sensory testing on the stump far removed from the area of injury reveals areas of increased sensitivity. Furthermore when the abnormal sensation is provoked, it radiates into the phantom. Here we must assume that stimulation of normal afferents in normal tissue provokes normal responses in the cells which correspond to the stimulated area but the input also spreads to cells with exalted excitability.

4.3. The prolonged central effects of afferent impulses

It was classically assumed that after impulses arrived at a synapse there was a very brief change of excitability after which the cell returned to its rest state until the next impulses arrived. It followed from this that prolonged postsynaptic activity would only be produced by prolonged afferent bombardment. It now becomes evident that many central cells produce very prolonged changes after excitation in addition to the classical rapidly reversible changes (Woolf, 1983, 1991). At least three types of chemical transmitter are now being considered as released by afferents: excitatory amino acids such as glutamate and aspartate, peptides which are the particular speciality of unmyelinated afferents and purines such as ATP. These in turn act on receptors including the two quite different types NMDA and non-NMDA receptors. The latter appear to fulfil the classical requirements of rapid response and rapid restoration. In contrast the NMDA receptors have quite different properties and which are revealed and cre-

ated by prolonged depolarisation and perhaps by the peptides. They appear responsible for the gradually rising excitability of cells, 'wind up', produced by the repeated arrival of volleys of impulses in small-diameter afferent fibres. Furthermore they appear responsible for the very prolonged (hours) increases of excitability which may follow brief (seconds) input barrages over unmyelinated afferents, particularly those originating from deep tissue (Woolf and Wall, 1986).

The crucial issue which faces us here in relation to postherpetic neuralgia is whether these changes can become permanent. The extreme example would be the death of cells produced by calcium entry following NMDA receptor activation (Bennett and Xie, 1988). Artificial application of particularly effective excitatory amino acids such as kainic acid can certainly kill cells. Some believe that pathologically provoked afferent discharges such as that produced by section of nerve fibres which causes an injury discharge is sufficient to kill some cells. Short of frank destruction, brief afferent bombardment can certainly produce prolonged intracellular changes such as the unmasking of the oncogene c-fos which may persist for over a week after only minutes of enhanced afferent input in small fibres (Hunt et al., 1987). It is not even known if these intracellular changes are associated with a prolonged change of excitability. A less dramatic plausible possibility is that the cells become sensitised to overreact to normally innocuous inputs even though, in the absence of input, the cells return to a normal resting state.

These hugely important practical questions are not answered and are not simple to answer. The answers require that physiologists should be able to monitor the excitable state of neurons over long periods of months. It may be that particular combinations of transmitters and modulators and particular states of intracellular chemistry and of membrane receptors co-operate to produce steady-state changes in afferents and in postsynaptic excitability, all triggered by an initial period of enhanced afferent barrage. Certainly such long-term changes can be produced by peripheral nerve or root section but we do not know the relative roles of the initial impulse barrage and of the subsequent changes in trophic chemicals and the chemical environment of the central cells.

4.4. Central effects of changed peripheral tissue

Thanks to the brilliantly incisive experiments of workers such as Sperry and Levi-Montalcini we now know rather exactly how peripheral to central connections are established in the embryo by a combination of programs inherent in differentiating and growing axons of nerve cells and of properties inherent in the target tissue contacted by the growing axons (Levi-Montalcini, 1988). It now becomes apparent that these interactions continue throughout adult life. For example, in the normal adult, the chemistry and physiology and central connectivity of skin nerve such as the sural nerve differs from that of a muscle nerve such as the nerve to gastrocnemius. However, if these nerves are cross-anastomosed in the adult so that the skin nerve is forced to regenerate into muscle and vice versa many of these properties reverse (McMahon and Gibson, 1987). The peripheral unmyelinated C-fibres appear responsible for this ongoing interaction. The C-fibres are literally tasting the tissue which they contact and are signalling to their cell bodies and indirectly to central structures that they should change to the appropriate chemistry, morphology and physiology. One of the chemicals responsible for this signalling has been identified as nerve growth factor, NGF. If a cut nerve is artificially supplied with a substitute source of NGF when it is cut off from its normal peripheral supply (Fitzgerald et al., 1985), many of the changes which follow nerve section do not occur. Furthermore, if muscle which is normally low in NGF production has its NGF concentration artificially raised in the adult, the C-fibres supplying muscle change their chemistry and central connections to those normally associated with a peripheral tissue such as skin which is normally rich in NGF (Lewin and McMahon, 1991). Furthermore we have described above that there are physiological changes in intact fibres in the presence of degeneration of neighbours.

The reason why these phenomena are relevant to the present issue is that the primary acute phase may have permanently changed the nature of the tissue surrounding the primary afferent fibres. These changes could be of three types. In the first, scar tissue may remain in deep or cutaneous tissue and thereby change the excitability of peripheral fibres or of their central connections. Second, there may have been a dying back of some peripheral axons which fail to regenerate. Such fibre terminals would remain along the course of the peripheral nerve and, since they fail to re-establish contact with their normal peripheral target, their cell bodies and central connections would remain in the exalted state. If this were the case, one might expect a distributed tenderness and Tinel sign along the course of affected peripheral nerves. As far as I know, this has not been reported, but I also do not know if it has been investigated either clinically or histologically. Finally we do not know if the surround Schwann cells and glial cells revert to their premorbid state after the acute phase is complete. If they do not, we should investigate the consequence of the changed external environment around the affected afferent fibres.

5. Contralateral and widespread ipsilateral changes

There is now a wide range of examples in the literature in which unilateral interventions produce bilateral effects (Koltzenburg et al., 1999). We quote fourteen papers in which manipulation of sensory nerves on one side produce changes in the contralateral sensory nerves. The first example comes from the work of Lisney and associates (Lisney and Devor, 1987) who found that section and regeneration of the saphenous nerve on one side changed the ability of the contralateral intact saphenous nerve to generate neurogenic inflammatory responses. In PHN, Oaklander et al. (1998) found in 18 patients with chronic pain after shingles that there was a marked drop in the number of cutaneous neurites at the ipsilateral shingles site from 1661 in normal skin to 339 neurites/mm^2 in the shingles site. However, when they biopsied the non-painful skin contralateral to the painful shingles site, they also found a highly significant 50% drop in the number of neurites. When they examined the skin of patients who had had shingles but had not developed the painful late stage there was also some loss of neurites at the old lesion site but no contralateral changes.

We discussed the possible mechanisms for these contralateral effects and dismissed the idea of some humoral mechanism since the changes are precisely localised to the equivalent contralateral locus. Similarly there is no evidence for bilateral central structures as an explanation for these examples which might apply in midline structures such as the bladder. We are forced to conclude that a signal travels into the CNS and ultimately affects contralateral homonymous neurones. We give reasons to doubt that this signal is contained in the pattern of nerve impulses. It is true of course that there are commissural neurones which could provide a pathway over which the signal could be carried. The most likely candidate for the nature of the signal is that it is made by neurotrophin concentrations and there is now much evidence for the power of these transported growth factors (reviewed in McMahon and Bennett, 1999).

In PHN, there are clear signs of a contralateral movement of signs of the disorder even though the painful symptoms do not accompany this spread. If this is occurring contralaterally, it is surely likely that there will also be ipsilateral signs in segments rostal and caudal to the clinical symptom-affected segment. The paper by Oaklander et al. (1998) strongly suggests that signals associated with pain development move from the periphery to the central nervous system since, in the pain-free patients who had recovered from their acute zoster, there were no contralateral effects; I take this to imply no extensive central involvement in the pain-free cases.

6. Summary and conclusions

I wish to propose that the various forms of PHN are the result of the single process of a more and more complete destruction of dorsal root ganglion cells which produces secondary changes in the periphery and centrally. This single process does not require the existence of irritable nociceptors. It is still not known if this dorsal root ganglion cell or trigeminal ganglion cell destruction has to be selective or may simply be randomly scattered. It may be that cells supplying both skin and deep tissue must suffer. Similarly we do not know if the disease must destroy a particular type of axon preferentially, such as large-diameter axons. It is true that cutaneous nerve lesions which eventually destroy all types of fibre as in cutaneous leprosy are not necessarily painful. It is clear that the viral infection may spread centrally from the dorsal root ganglia and may involve glia, but it is not evident that this extension plays a necessary role in typical PHN. I will therefore explore the single hypothesis that the symptoms are explained by a progressive and random destruction of sensory nerve cells.

6.1. Complete sensory recovery after acute herpes zoster

We now know that in the common situation of recovery from zoster there is a substantial loss of fibres in skin biopsies from the previously affected area and yet no change of sensory threshold. This is reminiscent of biopsies of leprous nodules where more than 50% of the fibres must be destroyed before raised sensory thresholds appear. This is not to be explained away by the trivial use of the word 'redundancy'. It means that there is an active dynamic feedback stabilised central homeostatic mechanism which maintains normal sensitivity over a wide range of numbers of input channels. The central mechanism does this by raising its excitability as the number of active input channels drops.

6.2. PHN with allodynia

As the number of input fibres drops below a critical level, the compensatory increased excitability of central structures can no longer successfully compensate for the loss of input and handles the remaining input with excessive amplification but a raised threshold.

This produces a secondary allodynia and hyperalgesia which has two causative components.

(1) Arriving afferent impulses in normal and secondarily sensitised sensory fibres synapse on cells which are in an exalted state of excitability.

(2) The central cell excitability depends on ongoing central activity and on the steady afferent barrage. In PHN, this afferent barrage may be exaggerated by the presence of end neuromas in damaged fibres which have died back and certainly by the presence of collateral sprouting and excitability in neighbouring fibres described above.

We can now examine the list of signs used by Rowbotham et al., whereas I propose a secondary allodynia caused by the input from axons not involved in the primary insult.

(A) The sensory thresholds are characteristic of secondary and not primary allodynia.

(B) Anaesthetic infiltration will affect all fibres both stimulated and spontaneously active. The more active fibres there are, the more will be the effect. Furthermore local anaesthetics in neuralgia have an effect which outlasts the period of nerve block (Arner et al., 1990; Wall, 1998). Even low systemic doses silence ectopic firing of dorsal root ganglion cells (Wall and Devor, 1983).

(C) Capsaicin sensitivity affects a fraction of any sensitive afferents and does not differentiate primary from secondary hyperalgesia.

(D) Epinephrine infiltration will affect any retracted axon neurones and neurites of collateral sprouts from undamaged neurones. I have written on the problems of interpreting this effect (Wall, 1995).

(E) Topical NSAIDS would be interesting if the effect was confirmed but seems to me unlikely given the poor response to high systemic doses. In summary, I do not think it necessary to invent chronically sensitised nociceptors.

6.3. Deafferentation PHN

Here the mechanism is entirely central with no peripheral nerve contributory component as in brachial plexus avulsion where no afferent input persists.

7. Prevention

Time will tell if the new generation of children immunised against chicken pox will ever develop PHN. Similarly, as discussed in my preface to this book, it may be that the explosion of latent virus in older adults can be prevented by reimmunising them in their later years. We may be faced with the appearance of adult chicken pox in people who escaped immunisation and which was so disastrous in isolated communities such as Fiji when colonial invasion brought indigenous people in contact with varicella for the first time as adults. Perhaps HIV positive patients should be immunised if their immune system is sufficiently strong to generate a significant immune response.

It is tempting to consider preventative measures during the long period as acute zoster evolves into PHN. For that we would need to know when, why and where the crucial lesions occur. Before zoster appears on the skin, there is a period of localised pain. Perhaps the triggering damage is already complete in this phase in which case it might be justified to start antiviral treatment during this time even though the diagnosis is speculative. I will be very interested to read in this book if the evidence is good that treatment during the zoster phase with antiviral agents arrests the transition from zoster to PHN. Since the inflammation is suspected as a cause of secondary changes in the periphery, there is good reason but no evidence that vigorous anti-inflammatory treatment during zoster might decrease the long-term evolution. It could also be that the long-term changes are secondary to the painful afferent barrage during acute zoster which changes central excitability. Therefore analgesic procedures during zoster might improve the late outcome as well as comforting the patient during the acute phase. This might justify vigorous acute treatment including analgesics, local anaesthesia and sympathectomy.

8. Treatment

This book would not be written if there was an adequate existing therapy for PHN. An intense search is in progress by pharmacologists for effective drug therapy since narcotics are rarely effective. One target is to discover a practical NMDA antagonist since NMDA is strongly suspected as a factor involved in the hyperexcitability of partially deafferented cells in spinal cord dorsal horn and medulla. Powerful antagonists exist but thus far have such wild psychedelic side effects when leaking systemically that they are quite impractical. Similarly compounds in the 'caine family' have excellent inhibitory effects on hyperexcitable central cells but these sodium channel blockers in therapeutic systemic doses are close to producing fatal cardiac effects. Therefore there is a search for channels characteristic of hyperexcitable neurons for which blockers might be synthesised. Similarly there is a search for drugs which would specifically block impulses in damaged but not intact axons. For that reason, the discussion about whether the pain-provoking impulses from the periphery are carried by damaged axons, or, as I maintain, by intact axons has a powerful bearing on the pharmacological research needed. Finally there is no doubt that partial or complete deafferentation carries a signal to which central cells react. That signal is almost certainly a neurotrophin or mixture of such neuronal factors. The most optimistic contemporary research now concentrates on neurotrophins which might prevent or reverse the effects of afferent nerve damage (Bennett et al., 1996, 1998; Ramer et al., 2000).

References

Ahcan, V., Arnez, Z.M., Bajrovic, F. and Janko, M. (1998) Collateral sprouting in the human palm after peripheral nerve injury. Br. J. Plast. Surg., 51: 436–443.

Ali, Z., Ringkamp, M., Hartke, T.V., Chien, H.F., Flavahan, N.A., Campbell, J.N. and Meyer, R.A. (1999) Uninjured C-fiber nociceptores develop spontaneous activity and alpha-adrenergic sensitivity following L6 spinal nerve ligation in monkey. J. Neurophysiol., 81: 455–466.

Arner, S., Lindblom, V., Meyerson, B.A. and Molander, C. (1990) Prolonged relief of neuralgia after regional anaesthesia blocks. Pain, 43: 287–295.

Baron, R. and Saguer, M. (1993) Are C nociceptors involved in signalling and maintaining tactile allodynia. Brain, 116: 1477–1496.

Baron, R., Haendler, G. and Schulte, H. (1997) Afferent large fibre polyneuropathy predicts the development of postherpetic neuralgia. Pain, 72: 231–238.

Basbaum, A.I. and Wall, P.D. (1976) Chronic changes in the response of cells in adult cat dorsal horn following partial deafferentation. Brain Res., 116: 181–204.

Bennett, D.L.H., French, J., Priestly, J.V.P. and McMahon, S.B. (1996) NGF but not NT-3 or BDNF prevents A fibre sprouting into lamina II. Mol. Cell. Neurosci., 8: 211–220.

Bennett, D.L.H., Michael, G.J., Ramachandran et al. (1998) GDNF is protective for a distinct group of small DRG cells after nerve injury. J. Neurosci., 18: 3059–3072.

Bennett, G.J. and Xie, Y.K. (1988) A peripheral neuropathy in rat. Pain, 33: 87–107.

Devor, M. and Seltzer, Z. (1999) Pathophysiology of damaged nerves in relation to chronic pain. In: P.D. Wall and R. Melzack (Eds.), Textbook of Pain 4E., Churchill-Livingstone, Edinburgh.

Devor, M. and Wall, P.D. (1981) The effect of peripheral nerve injury on receptive fields of cells in cat spinal cord. J. Comp. Neurol., 199: 277–291.

Devor, M., Schonfeld, D., Seltzer, Z. and Wall, P.D. (1979) Two modes of cutaneous reinnervation following peripheral nerve injury. J. Comp. Neurol., 185: 211–220.

Doubell, T.P., Mannion, R.J. and Woolf, C.J. (1999) The dorsal horn: state-dependent sensory processing, plasticity and the generation of pain. In: P.D. Wall and R. Melzack (Eds.), Textbook of Pain 4E. Churchill-Livingstone, Edinburgh.

Eshenfelder, S., Habler, H.-J. and Janig, W. (2000) Dorsal root section elicits signs of neuropathic pain rather than reversing them in rats with L5 spinal nerve injury. Pain, 87: 213–219.

Ferreira, S.H., Sacks, D., Cunka, F.Q. and Lorenzetti, B.B. (1999) Persistent hyperalgesia and cytokin. In: N.E. Saade, A.V. Apkarian and S.J. Jabar (Eds.), Pain and Neuroimmune Interactions. Plenum, New York, pp. 3–8.

Fitzgerald, M., Wall, P.D., Goedert, M. and Emson, P.C. (1985) Nerve growth factor counteracts the neurophysiological and neurochemical effects of chronic nerve section. Brain Res., 332: 131–141.

Gilden, D.H., DeMasters, B.K., Laguardia, J.J., Mahalingam, R. and Cohrs, R.J. (2000). Neurologic complications of the reactivation of varicella-zoster virus. N. Engl. J. Med., 342: 635–645.

Hunt, S.P., Pini, A. and Evan, G. (1987) Induction of c-fos like protein in spinal and neurons following sensory stimulation. Nature, 328: 632–634.

Inbal, R., Rousso, M., Ashur, H., Wall, P.D. and Devor, M. (1987) Collateral sprouting in skin and sensory recovery after nerve injury in man. Pain, 28: 141–154.

Kim, S.H. and Chung, J.M. (1992) An experimental model for peripheral neuropathy produced by segmental spinal nerve ligation in the rat. Pain, 50: 355–363.

Kirk, E.J. and Denny-Brown, D. (1970) Functional variation in dermatomes in the Macaque monkey following dorsal root lesions. J. Comp. Neurol., 139: 307–320.

Koltzenburg, M., Wall, P.D. and McMahon, S.B. (1999) Does the right hand know what the left is doing. Trends Neurosci., 22: 122–127.

Levi-Montalcini, R. (1988) In Praise of Imperfection. Basic Books, New York.

Lewin, G.R. and McMahon, S.B. (1991) Reorganisation of primary afferent connectivity in the adult spinal cord: evidence for tissue-specific neurotrophic influences from the periphery. Eur. J. Neurosci., 3: 1112–1122.

Li, Y., Dorsi, M.J., Meyer, R.A. and Belzberg, A.J. (2000) Mechanical hyperalgesia after an L5 spinal nerve lesion in the rat is not dependent on input from injured nerve fibres. Pain, 85: 493–502.

Lisney, S.J.W. and Devor, M. (1987) After discharge and interactions among fibres in damaged peripheral nerve. Brain Res., 415: 122–136.

Mansikka, H. and Pertovaara, A. (1997) Submodality selective hyperalgesia adjacent to partially injured sciatic nerve in the rat is dependent on capsaicin-sensitive afferents and independent of collateral sprouting or a dorsal root reflex. Brain Res., Bull., 44: 237–245.

McMahon, S.B. and Bennett, D.L.H. (1999) Trophic factors in pain. In: P.D. Wall and R. Melzack (Eds.), Textbook of Pain. Churchill-Livingstone, Edinburgh.

McMahon, S.B. and Gibson, S. (1987) Peptide expression is altered when afferent nerves reinnervate inappropriate tissue. Neurosci. Lett., 73: 9–15.

Michaelis, M., Xiangmo, L. and Jänig, W. (2000) Axotomised and intact muscle afferents but not skin afferents develop ongoing discharges after peripheral nerve lesions. J. Neurosci., 7: 2742–2748.

Noordenbos, W. (1959) Pain. Elsevier, Amsterdam.

Nurmikko, T.J., Rasadnen, A. and Hakkinen, V. (1990) Observations on acute herpes zoster. Clin. J. Pain, 6: 284–290.

Oaklander, A.L., Romans, K., Horasek, S., Stocks, A., Hauer, P. and Meyer, R.A. (1998) Unilateral postherpetic neuralgia is associated with bilateral sensory neuron damage. Ann. Neurol., 44: 789–795.

Pertens, E., Urschel-Gysbes, B.A., Holmes, M., Pal, R., Foester, A., Kril, Y. and Diamond, J. (1999) Intraspinal and behavioural consequences of nerve growth factor-induced sprouting and nerve growth factor-induced hyperalgesia. J. Comp. Neurol., 410: 73–89.

Poole, S., Cunha, F. de Q. and Ferreir, S.H. (1999) Bradykinin, cytokines and inflammatory hyperalgesia. In: N.E. Saade, A.V. Apkarian and S.J. Jabber (Eds.), Pain and Neuroimmune Interactions. Plenum, New York.

Raja, S.N., Meyer, R.A., Ringkamp, M. and Campbell, J.N. (1999) Peripheral neural mechanisms of nociception. In: P.D. Wall and R. Melzack (Eds.), Textbook of Pain 4E. Churchill-Livingstone, Edinburgh.

Ramer, M.S., Priestley, J.V. and McMahon, S.B. (2000) Functional regeneration of sensory axons into the adult spinal cord. Nature, 403: 312–316.

Rowbotham, M.C., Yosipovitch, G., Connolly, M.K., Finlay, D., Forde, G. and Fields, H.L. (1996) Cutaneous innervation density in the allodynic form of postherpetic neuralgia. Neurobiol. Dis., 3: 205–214.

Smith, F.P. (1978) Pathological studies of spinal nerve ganglia in relation to intercostal pain. Surg. Neurol., 10: 50–53.

Wall, P.D. (1960) Cord cells responding to touch, damage and temperature of the skin. J. Neurophysiol., 23: 197–210.

Wall, P.D. (1995) Noradrenaline-evoked pain in neuralgia. Pain, 63: 1–2.

Wall, P.D. (1998) New horizons: an essay. In: M.J Cousins and P.O. Bridenbaugh (Eds.), Neural Blockade 3E. Lippincott-Raven, Philadelphia, PA.

Wall, P.D. and Devor, M. (1983) Sensory afferent impulses from dorsal root ganglia as well as from the periphery in normal and nerve injured rats. Pain, 17: 321–339.

Wall, P.D. and McMahon, S.B. (1985) Microneuronography and its relation to perceived sensation. Pain, 21: 209–229.

Woolf, C.J. (1983) Evidence for a central component in post-injury pain hypersensitivity. Nature, 306: 686–688.

Woolf, C.J. (1991) Generation of pain: central mechanisms. In: C. Wells and C.J. Woolf (Eds.), Pain Mechanisms and Management. Br. Med. Bull., 47: 523 –533.

Woolf, C.J. and Wall, P.D. (1986) Relative effectiveness of C primary afferent fibres of different origins in evoking a prolonged facilitation of the flexor reflex. J. Neurosci., 6: 1433–1442.

Herpes Zoster and Postherpetic Neuralgia, 2nd Revised and Enlarged Edition
Pain Research and Clinical Management, Vol. 11
Edited by C.P.N. Watson and A.A. Gershon
© 2001 Elsevier Science B.V. All rights reserved

CHAPTER 18

Prevention of postherpetic neuralgia by corticosteroids

Barbara T. Post [1], John T. Philbrick [2] and C. Peter N. Watson [3,*]

[1] *University of Virginia School of Medicine, Northridge Internal Medicine, 2955 Ivy Road, Suite 305, Charlottesville, VA 22901, USA,* [2] *University of Virginia School of Medicine, Box 494, Charlottesville, VA 22908, USA and* [3] *Department of Medicine, University of Toronto and 1 Sir Williams Lane, Toronto, ON M9A 1T8, Canada*

1. Introduction

Since the first edition of this book, further studies (Wood et al., 1994; Whitley et al., 1996) have indicated that there is no benefit from corticosteroids in preventing postherpetic neuralgia (PHN).

For many years, ACTH and corticosteroids have been used as standard therapy in patients with herpes zoster to prevent PHN, particularly in patients at high risk for development of the disorder. The first reports of patients treated with ACTH were by Nickel (1951) and Sulzberger et al. (1951). Other case reports followed (Frank and Lysiak, 1953; Gelfand, 1954; Sauer, 1955; Appelman, 1955), most describing success with corticosteroid treatment. Elliott (1964) and colleagues in a cohort study of 15 patients concluded that corticosteroid therapy prevented PHN. Two randomized controlled trials (Eaglstein et al., 1970; Keczkes and Basheer, 1980) reported statistically significant benefits with corticosteroid therapy. These studies led to the general acceptance of this mode of therapy by the medical community. Dermatology textbooks (Habif, 1990) have long recommended prophylactic steroid therapy in immunocompetent patients at risk for development of PHN. A survey of practising dermatologists (Levinson and Shaw, 1983) found that: (1) 81% of respondents routinely used corticosteroids in healthy patients older than 60 years of age; (2) 68% used corticosteroids in patients who were 50–60 years old; (3) in patients under 50, 20% used corticosteroids; and (4) steroids were more frequently prescribed in patients with cranial nerve involvement. Typically, treatment with the equivalent of 40–60 mg of prednisone per day for three to six weeks, starting early in the course of the disease, has been employed.

More recently, others have argued that corticosteroid therapy is ineffective in preventing PHN. Two randomized trials in the 1980s (Clemmensen and Andersen, 1984; Esmann et al., 1987) reported no significant benefit from corticosteroids. Even more recently, two studies (Wood et al., 1994; Whitley et al., 1996) have shown no additional benefit of steroids in preventing PHN when added to acyclovir therapy. In addition, concerns about known complications of corticosteroids have been raised, including a possible risk of dissemination associated with corticosteroid treatment of herpes zoster (Merselis et al., 1964). Other potential concerns raised when considering steroid treatment include: glucose intolerance, hypertension, increased intraocular pressure, cataracts, peptic ulcer disease, exacerbation of congestive heart failure, osteoporosis and avascular necrosis of the femoral head.

---

* Correspondence to: Dr. C.P.N. Watson, Department of Medicine, University of Toronto and 1 Sir Williams Lane, Toronto, ON M9A 1T8, Canada. Phone: +1 (416) 239-3494; Fax: +1 (416) 239-6365; E-mail: peter.watson@utoronto.ca

TABLE I

Summary of study methodologies and compliance with standards[1]

Study	1	2	3	4 Active drug	4 Comparison regime	4 Duration of pretreatment symptoms	5 Regimen	5 E[2]	6 Neuralgia	6 Adverse steroid effects (N)	7
Eaglstein et al. (1970)	−	+	−	Triamcinolone, 48 mg/day × 7 days; 16 mg/day × 7 days	Lactose	Approximately 5 days	Codeine tap water soaks	−	Pain in zoster region	None	+
Keczkes and Basheer (1980)	−	+	+	Prednisolone, 40 mg/day × 10 days; gradual taper to zero × 21 days	Carbamazepine, 100 mg q.i.d. × 28 days	5.3 days (prednisolone); 5.0 days (carbamazepine)	Topical neomycin/Gramicidin; talcum powder	+	Presence or absence of pain	None	−
Clemmensen and Andersen (1984)	+	+	−	Prednisone, 45 mg/day × 7 days; 30 mg/day × 7 days; 15 mg/day tapered to zero over 7 days	Placebo	4.1 days (prednisone); 4.0 days (placebo)	Topical chlorhexidine lidocaine; aspirin/codeine; potassium chloride	−	Four-point pain scale; daily consumption of analgesics	Dizziness (2); periorbital oedema (1); elevated blood sugar (1)	+
Esmann et al. (1987)	−	+	+	Prednisolone, 40 mg/day × 7 days; 30 mg/day × 3 days; 20 mg/day × 3 days; 10 mg/day × 4 days; 5 mg/day × 3 days; acyclovir 800 mg 5 × daily × 7 days	Calcium lactate; acyclovir 800 mg 5 × daily × 7 days	2.2 days (prednisolone); 2.3 days (placebo)	Analgesics as needed; carbowax with 0.2% chlorhexidine/10%; lignocaine 3%; acyclovir cream (ocular lesions)	−	Detailed pain flow chart to type and grade pain; analgesic consumption	−	+
Wood et al. (1994)	+	+	+	Acyclovir, 7 days or 21 days and prednisolone, 40 mg × 3 weeks or placebo	4 groups: acyclovir 21 days + prednisolone versus acyclovir, 7 days + prednisolone	Prodrome = 96 h. Rash 24–72 h.	Other antivirals and steroids excluded	+	Pain severity, quality, duration, 'zoster-associated pain'	Higher with steroids (19% vs. 13%)	+
Whitley et al. (1996)	+	+	+	Acyclovir, prednisone, placebo	4 groups: acyclovir + placebo, acyclovir + prednisone × 21 days, prednisone + placebo × 21 days, placebo × 21 days	Most rash < 2 days (141 versus 44 > 2 days)	Other antivirals and immune globulin excluded	+	Pain, quality of life, sleep, rash healing	No difference in 4 groups	+

[1] Standards: 1 = diagnostic criteria; 2 = random allocation of treatment; 3 = description of patients; 4 = treatments; 5 = supplemental treatments; 6 = outcome measures; 7 = blinded ascertainment and outcomes: (+), compliance with standard; (−), failure to comply with standard.

[2] E = equal allocation of supplemental treatments.

Because of these conflicting views, a systematic analysis of the literature on this subject (Post and Philbrick, 1988) was performed to evaluate the evidence behind this therapy and address the question of corticosteroid efficacy and risk. In this chapter we have extended and updated this analysis to include all relevant publications through June 2000.

2. Methods

All studies involving the use of corticosteroids for the treatment of herpes zoster, published in the English language, were sought for review. This search included a review of *Cumulated Index Medicus* from January 1965 through June 2000, a Medline search through 2000, and all citations from the reference lists of relevant publications. We identified 14 studies, published between 1951 and 2000, that met our selection criteria. Seven were case reports or short series of cases (Nickel, 1951; Sulzberger et al., 1951; Frank and Lysiak, 1953; Gelfand, 1954; Appelman, 1955; Sauer, 1955; Sutton, 1984), one was a cohort study (Elliott, 1964) and six were randomized controlled trials (Eaglstein et al., 1970; Keczkes and Basheer, 1980; Clemmensen and Andersen, 1984; Esmann et al., 1987; Wood et al., 1994; Whitley et al., 1996). Because of the potential for bias causing distortion of the results of uncontrolled, non-randomized trials, we have selected for further review only the six studies conducted as randomized controlled trials. To help in judging the methodological strength of these trials, we applied to them seven standards used in evaluating clinical trials for the purpose of reducing the chance of bias and distortion. These standards were the same used in an earlier review (Post and Philbrick, 1988) which was adapted from Gifford and Feinstein (1969).

3. Compliance with methodologic standards

The seven standards used to evaluate study methodology are described in the paragraphs that follow.

We provide the ratings of the six randomized trials below and in Table I.

3.1. Standard 1: establishment of diagnostic criteria

To investigate the success of any therapy in the treatment of a disease, it is necessary to include a precise statement of diagnostic criteria for that disease. Since the diagnosis of herpes zoster is made primarily on clinical grounds, for a study to satisfy this standard we required a statement of criteria for the diagnosis of herpes zoster including at least: (1) presence of an acute vesicular eruption; and (2) dermatomal distribution of the rash. Three (Clemmensen and Andersen, 1984; Wood et al., 1994; Whitley et al., 1996) of the six trials met this standard.

3.2. Standard 2: random allocation of treatment

The purpose of randomization is to ensure that every subject in a study has the same chance of being assigned to the treatment or comparison groups. Randomization prevents conscious or unconscious decisions of investigators creating groups that are unequal in important factors that could affect outcomes, such as disease severity or age. To satisfy this standard, we required only a simple statement that treatment was assigned by a random method. All six studies (Eaglstein et al., 1970; Keczkes and Basheer, 1980; Clemmensen and Andersen, 1984; Esmann et al., 1987; Wood et al., 1994; Whitley et al., 1996) met this standard.

3.3. Standard 3: adequate description of patients

The standard of adequate description of patients required that the authors provide: (1) basic patient demographic data (at least age and sex according to treatment group); (2) dermatomal location of the rash; and (3) presence of other co-morbid illnesses that could be adversely affected by corticosteroid therapy, such as diabetes, tuberculosis, or human immunodeficiency virus infection. This information is important for appropriate generalization of the results of a study. In addition, it is important to use this information in small studies to compare the treatment groups in order to demonstrate that randomization succeeded in creating similar groups. Five studies (Keczkes and Basheer, 1980; Clemmensen and Andersen, 1984; Esmann et al., 1987; Wood et al., 1994; Whitley et al., 1996) provided the required simple demographic information. Four (Keczkes and Basheer, 1980; Esmann et al., 1987; Wood et al., 1994; Whitley et al., 1996) provided information on dermatomal distribution. All six studies satisfied the third part of this standard by excluding patients who might have diseases adversely affected by steroid therapy. Four (Keczkes and Basheer, 1980; Esmann et al., 1987; Wood et al., 1994; Whitley et al., 1996) satisfied all three parts of this standard.

3.4. Standard 4: adequacy of treatment

An effective and timely treatment regimen is essential to a well-designed study evaluating that treatment. In all six studies (Eaglstein et al., 1970; Keczkes and Basheer, 1980; Clemmensen and Andersen, 1984; Esmann et al., 1987; Wood et al., 1994; Whitley et al., 1996) approximately equivalent doses of corticosteroids were used, and treatment was begun 2.2–5.3 days after the onset of symptoms (see Table I for the exact regimens). The duration of treatment lasted from 10 to 21 days. The treatment regimes were similar to those generally recommended (Habif, 1990).

3.5. Standard 5: equality of supplemental treatment

When supplemental therapy is provided to patients in addition to the primary treatment modality being investigated for efficacy, it is essential that these supplemental regimes be provided equally to all treatment arms of the study. If this is not done, then it is possible that any treatment effect could be due to supplemental therapy rather than the primary treatment. All six studies (Eaglstein et al., 1970; Keczkes and Basheer, 1980; Clemmensen and Andersen, 1984; Esmann et al., 1987; Wood et al., 1994; Whitley et al., 1996) noted supplemental treatments when used (see Table I for those used). One

of the six studies (Keczkes and Basheer, 1980) noted that these treatments were applied equally; in five (Eaglstein et al., 1970; Clemmensen and Andersen, 1984; Esmann et al., 1987; Wood et al., 1994; Whitley et al., 1996) some or all supplemental treatments were used according to patients' needs.

3.6. Standard 6: appropriate outcome measures

Because treatment with corticosteroids has potential for harm as well as benefit, this standard has two parts: one dealing with ascertainment of pain and the other with observed adverse effects of corticosteroids.

Since accurate reports of pain levels are notoriously difficult to measure, we required for the first part of this standard that researchers utilize techniques to 'harden' subjective data to improve the validity of their measures of pain. Two studies (Eaglstein et al., 1970; Keczkes and Basheer, 1980) failed to meet this standard because only the presence or absence of pain was noted. Four studies (Clemmensen and Andersen, 1984; Esmann et al., 1987; Wood et al., 1994; Whitley et al., 1996) met the first part of standard. Clemmensen and Andersen (1984) utilized a four-point 'pain score' as well as keeping a record of supplemental analgesics used. Esmann et al. (1987) used a detailed pain flow chart to obtain a description of the type and grade of pain. This study did not find that the number of analgesics correlated well with severity of pain, and so did not use this analysis as part of the results. Wood et al. (1994) used the measure zoster-associated pain. Whitley et al. (1996) used a category scale for pain and follow-up for pain duration.

For the second part of this standard, we required at a minimum that each study report the number and nature of side effects attributable to corticosteroids. Only one of the six studies failed to provide this information (Esmann et al., 1987). Only four patients were reported to have suffered side effects and all were reported in the same study (Clemmensen and Andersen, 1984). Two patients reported dizziness, one patient reported periorbital oedema and one patient developed elevated blood sugar. Wood et al.

TABLE II

Reported results of studies

Study	Weeks after start of treatment	Persistent pain		P [1]	$N_{s.e.}$ [2]
		corticosteroid	control		
Eaglstein et al. (1970)	>8	3/15 (20) [3]	11/19 (58) [3]	0.03	0
	>52	1/15 (6.6)	1/19 (5.3)	NS	0
Keczkes and Basheer (1980)	>8	3/20 (15)	13/20 (65)	0.002	0
	>52	0/20 (0)	2/20 (10)	NS	0
Clemmensen and Andersen (1984)	>6	4/19 (21)	1/19 (5.2)	NS	4
Esmann et al. (1987)	2	13/41 (35)	21/37 (50)	0.02	0
	26	9/41 (23)	9/37 (24)	NS	0
Wood et al. (1994)	>20	no difference	no difference	NS	38 (vs. 26 on acyclovir alone $P > 0.1$)
Whitley et al. (1996)	24 weeks	no difference	no difference	0.10	No difference ($P > 0.05$)

[1] Fisher's exact test; NS = not significant.
[2] Number of patients with corticosteroid side effects.
[3] Number of patients with persistent pain/total number of patients × 100 (percentage with persistent pain).

(1994) reported more side effects in the steroid group and those were chiefly gastrointestinal. Whitley et al. (1996) reported no difference in adverse effects between the steroid and other groups. All of these side effects readily reversed when the steroid therapy was stopped. No episodes of dissemination of herpes zoster or life-threatening side effects were reported as a result of corticosteroid therapy.

3.7. Standard 7: blinded ascertainment of outcomes

In order to avoid patient or investigator bias in the assessment of the effectiveness of treatment, it is crucial in clinical trials that neither the patient nor the investigator know what treatment is being given. Five (Eaglstein et al., 1970; Clemmensen and Andersen, 1984; Esmann et al., 1987; Wood et al., 1994; Whitley et al., 1996) of the six studies were truly 'double-blind' with treatment appearing the same to both the patient and the investigator. In the fourth study, (Keczkes and Basheer, 1980) there was no such effort at blinding.

3.8. Compliance results

Eaglstein et al. (1970) satisfied three of the seven standards; Keczkes and Basheer (1980) and Esmann et al. (1987) satisfied four of the standards;

and Clemmensen and Andersen (1984) satisfied five. Wood et al. (1994) and Whitley et al. (1996) satisfied all seven standards.

4. Results of reviewed studies and critique

Table II presents the results of the six studies. The studies varied in size from 34 to 400 patients. Two studies were performed in Denmark (Clemmensen and Andersen, 1984; Esmann et al., 1987) and two each in Great Britain (Keczkes and Basheer, 1980; Wood et al., 1994) and the USA (Eaglstein et al., 1970; Whitley et al., 1996). Three studies (Eaglstein et al., 1970; Keczkes and Basheer, 1980; Esmann et al., 1987) treated patients initially as inpatients and three (Clemmensen and Andersen, 1984; Wood et al., 1994; Whitley et al., 1996) treated patients solely as outpatients. Esmann et al. (1987) found decreased pain in the steroid group during the first two weeks, and that there was no difference at the end of the six month study. Both Eaglstein et al. (1970) and Keczkes and Basheer (1980) reported significantly less pain in patients treated with corticosteroids at eight weeks but no difference at one year. Clemmensen and Andersen (1984) reported no difference at six weeks between the corticosteroid and placebo groups. Wood et al.

(1994) found no significant differences between any of the four treatment groups in the time to either first or complete pain resolution. Whitley et al. (1996) found that zoster-associated pain was not significantly reduced in the acyclovir plus prednisone group compared with the acyclovir plus placebo group ($P = 0.10$). There are several probable explanations for the contradictory conclusions of these six studies. They are described in the following sections.

4.1. Differences in patient characteristics between studies

There are marked differences in the rates of pain after several months among these studies. High rates of persistent pain at six to eight weeks in the placebo groups were reported in the three studies finding an early positive effect of corticosteroid therapy. These rates ranged from about 50% (Esmann et al., 1987) to 65% (Keczkes and Basheer, 1980). On the other hand, the negative study of Clemmensen and Andersen (1984) reported only a 5.2% rate of pain at 6 weeks in the placebo-treated patients. In the three positive studies the placebo groups differed from placebo groups of the negative study in other ways. The subjects were all initially treated as inpatients in the positive studies while they were outpatients in the negative study. Also, Keczkes and Basheer's (1980) patients averaged 68.5 years of age, Esmann et al.'s (1987) averaged 72 years of age, and 79% of Eaglstein et al.'s (1970) patients were over the age of 60. In contrast, Clemmensen and Andersen's (1984) patients averaged only 56 years of age. These data suggest that the three studies which report a higher incidence of PHN enrolled patients who were older, more severely ill, and at high risk for PHN. This difference in patient characteristics may account for differences in response to corticosteroid treatment. Unfortunately, the small size of the studies and the lack of detailed clinical information limit our ability to investigate this hypothesis further. There was no difference in the patient groups in the studies of Wood et al. (1994) or Whitley et al. (1996).

4.2. Differing treatment regimes

The relative doses of corticosteroids in the six studies varied somewhat, but there was no trend toward a lower dose in the Clemmensen and Andersen (1984) study to explain inefficacy of treatment. In the study by Keczkes and Basheer (1980), an active placebo, carbamazepine, was compared to prednisone therapy. However, there has been some suggestion that carbamazepine may be helpful in treating PHN (Price, 1982), and we would expect this design to decrease the difference between the study groups. In the Esmann et al. (1987) study, acyclovir was given to all patients. While this design could change the natural history of herpes zoster infections, it should not invalidate the comparison between the corticosteroid and placebo arms of the study. In addition, acyclovir did not appear to reduce the incidence of the reporting of persistent pain compared to the other two studies with high rates of persistent pain at six to eight weeks (Eaglstein et al., 1970; Keczkes and Basheer, 1980). Supplemental treatments were not provided equally in three studies (Eaglstein et al., 1970; Clemmensen and Andersen, 1984; Esmann et al., 1987), but it seems unlikely that these topical treatments and pain medications could have led to differences in PHN after the skin lesions had healed.

4.3. Bias and ascertainment of pain

Pain was chosen as the major measure of outcome in all six randomized controlled trials. The presence of pain is an inherently subjective symptom and therefore difficult to quantify. Even with attempts to quantify or 'harden' pain levels, its presence or absence is highly subject to bias. It is particularly difficult in PHN since this pain typically is episodic, is influenced by external stimuli, and does not have a readily identifiable end point. In all but one of the studies (Keczkes and Basheer, 1980) attempts were made to blind both the patients and investigators to the treatment being given. However, because high-dose prednisone therapy has predictable side effects, including fluid retention, glucose intolerance, and psychological effects including mood swings and euphoria, it is unlikely that efforts at maintaining blinding of patients and physicians were entirely successful. Failure of blinding could explain the results of the positive studies. For example, patients taking corticosteroids may report less pain than those in the control group, due to steroid-induced 'euphoria' or just from placebo effect. Efforts to more objectively measure pain by creating a scale with which to rate pain and looking at analgesic consumption rate could not prevent this bias from occurring. None of the studies investigated the success of the blinding procedures by asking the patients and investigators to guess in which treatment arm the patient was enrolled. In three studies reporting a beneficial effect of steroid treatment (Eaglstein et al., 1970; Keczkes and Basheer, 1980; Esmann et al., 1987) the benefit was seen early in the study and was not apparent later on. This is consistent with the above-described bias, since attenuation of the steroid-induced 'euphoria' or the placebo effect is likely to have occurred after the drugs were discontinued. The use of the term zoster-associated pain as an outcome is a useful one in this type of study (Wood et al., 1994). This is the continuum of pain from study enrollment to final resolution and does not require a discrimination between acute zoster pain and PHN.

4.4. Type II error

In a negative study, before the conclusion that a therapy is ineffective can be reached, an analysis for Type II error, or beta error, must be made. Type II error is measure of the likelihood of failing to discover a therapeutic effect that actually exists. The ability to detect an effective therapy in a study is dependent on the frequency of the outcome under study (greater ability with mid-range frequencies, lesser with low and high frequencies), the efficacy of the treatment (greater ability with more efficacious treatments), and the number of patients in each study group (greater ability with larger study groups). For example, if the expected incidence of PHN found in the treatment group in the Clemmensen and Andersen (1984) study (21%, Table II) were to be reduced

by treatment by 50%, 117 patients would be needed in both the treatment and control groups to have even a 50% chance of detecting this effect at the 5% level of significance. Because this study had only 19 patients per treatment arm, it is quite possible that an actual therapeutic effect was missed. The three studies (Eaglstein et al., 1970; Keczkes and Basheer, 1980; Esmann et al., 1987), although reporting an early beneficial effect from corticosteroid therapy, found no statistically significant benefit at six or twelve months. Although they included more patients than Clemmensen and Andersen (1984), they also had insufficient numbers to exclude an effect of treatment of the size in the above illustration. Lycka (1990) pooled the results of the four randomized trials in order to create larger study groups and achieve greater statistical power to detect a difference between groups. Although Lycka's statistical analysis is carefully performed and in some circumstances such pooling is proper, Post and Philbrick (1989) and others (Schmader and Studenski, 1989) have concluded that such pooling should not be done because of the methodologic weaknesses of and differences between the studies. We are concerned that when studies are too different and flawed methodologically, combining results of the studies will only result in magnifying the distortions that may be present and give false confidence in the results. Guidelines have been published for determining when arithmetic pooling of results may be appropriate (Goldman and Feinstein, 1979; Gerbarg and Horwitz, 1988).

5. Discussion

In this review we have carefully analyzed all the published randomized controlled trials investigating the effect of a short course of corticosteroids on the prevention of PHN. Although some of the studies have a number of methodologic strengths, weaknesses include limited clinical information describing the patients treated, potential failure of blinding to treatment group resulting in biased ascertainment of outcomes, and the potential for missing a therapeutic effect that actually existed because of inadequate statistical power of the studies.

It is now possible to state with increasing confidence that prophylactic corticosteroid treatment as currently given is not beneficial in preventing PHN. For long-term pain (that lasting six months or more), none of the six studies suggested benefit. We have skepticism about any conclusions concerning long-term pain relief that is based on our concern about inadequate statistical power in some of the trials to detect clinically important differences between treatment groups. There was no consistent trend in the studies toward corticosteroid efficacy. Since prevention of long-term pain is the primary concern of clinicians in management of herpes zoster, our review does not support the use of corticosteroids for that purpose.

Three (Eaglstein et al., 1970; Keczkes and Basheer, 1980; Esmann et al., 1987) of the six randomized trials reported improvement in pain at six to eight weeks after initiation of the two or three week course of corticosteroids. These were the three trials reporting high rates of pain in the control groups, presumably because the studies enrolled patients at high risk to develop PHN. The results can be interpreted in two ways. The first possible explanation is that corticosteroids are effective in reducing the early pain of herpes zoster, but not the long-term and permanently debilitating neuralgia. The second explanation is that there is no effect of corticosteroids on PHN; but rather, reported differences were due to an unavoidable failure of blinding from the effects of high-dose corticosteroids and the subjective nature of pain reporting. We cannot say which is the true explanation.

Any decision as to whether to use corticosteroids in this situation should be made based on weighing the potential for harm as well as the potential benefits. Only four of the patients given corticosteroids in these series required discontinuation of steroid therapy for readily reversible side effects. None of the six studies (Eaglstein et al., 1970; Keczkes and Basheer, 1980; Clemmensen and Andersen, 1984; Esmann et al., 1987; Wood et al., 1994; Whitley et al., 1996) reported dissemination of herpes zoster while on steroid therapy, nor any other life-threatening complications. It seems, therefore, that the 3–6 weeks course of steroid therapy suggested for use in herpes zoster appears to be quite safe. Although the concern of dissemination of herpes zoster with steroid therapy was raised by Merselis et al. (1964), we have found no further episodes of dissemination reported since that initial series. The risks of dissemination appear to be primarily associated with individuals with impaired immunologic response, who may be at risk for dissemination because of their underlying disease.

Corticosteroids have no discernible effect on the disabling chronic neuralgia of herpes zoster. However, they may have some efficacy in reducing pain in a proportion of patients at high risk for pain in the first several weeks and months after initiating the drug. However, this temporary benefit must be weighted against the potential for side-effects and complications of short-term corticosteroid use.

6. Summary

Short courses of corticosteroid therapy have been used for many years in the treatment of acute herpes zoster infections with the hope of preventing the chronic pain of PHN. This practice has been based on experience reported in case reports and clinical trials. When the evidence for this mode of therapy is evaluated critically, it appears that this practice has not been supported by methodologically sound studies of adequate size. A review of the six randomized trials evaluating the effect of corticosteroids suggests that corticosteroids may reduce pain six to eight weeks after the onset of the rash but have no effect on the presence of pain at six to twelve months.

References

Appelman, D.H. (1955) Treatment of herpes zoster with ACTH. N. Engl. J. Med., 253: 693–695.

Clemmensen, O.J. and Andersen, K.E. (1984) ACTH versus prednisone and placebo in herpes zoster treatment. Clin. Exp. Dermatol., 9: 557–563.

Eaglstein, W.H., Katz, R. and Brown, J.A. (1970) The effects of early corticosteroid therapy on the skin eruption and pain of herpes zoster. JAMA, 211: 1681–1683.

Elliott, F.A. (1964) Treatment of herpes zoster with high doses of prednisone. Lancet, 2: 610–611.

Esmann, V., Geil, J.P., Kroon, S. et al. (1987) Prednisolone does not prevent postherpetic neuralgia. Lancet, 2: 126–129.

Frank, L. and Lysiak, R. (1953) Herpetic and postherpetic pain treated with cortisone and ACTH. N.Y. J. Med., 53: 2379.

Gelfand, J.L. (1954) Treatment of herpes zoster with cortisone. JAMA, 154: 911–912.

Gerbarg, Z.B. and Horwitz, R.I. (1988) Resolving conflicting clinical trials: Guidelines for meta-analysis. J. Clin. Epidemiol., 41: 503–509.

Gifford, R.H. and Feinstein, A.R. (1969) A critique of methodology in studies of anticoagulant therapy for acute myocardial infarction. N. Engl. J. Med., 280: 351–357.

Goldman, L. and Feinstein, A.R. (1979) Anticoagulants and myocardial infarction: The problems of pooling, drowning and floating. Ann. Intern. Med., 90: 92–94.

Habif, T.P. (1990) Clinical Dermatology. CV Hosby Co., St. Louis, p. 295.

Keczkes, K. and Basheer, A.M. (1980) Do corticosteroids prevent postherpetic neuralgia? Br. J. Dermatol., 102: 551–555.

Levinson, W. and Shaw, J.C. (1983) Survey of all active members of the Oregon Dermatological Society.

Lycka, B.A.S. (1990) Postherpetic neuralgia and systemic corticosteroid therapy. Int. J. Dermatol., 29: 523–527.

Merselis, J.G., Jr., Kaye, D. and Hook, E.W. (1964) Disseminated herpes zoster, a report of 17 cases. Arch. Intern. Med., 113: 679–686.

Nickel, W.R. (1951) Herpes zoster treated with ACTH. Arch. Dermatol. Syph., 64: 372.

Post, B.T. and Philbrick, J.T. (1988) Do corticosteroids prevent postherpetic neuralgia? J. Am. Acad. Dermatol., 3: 605–610.

Post, B.T. and Philbrick, J.T. (1989) Corticosteroids and postherpetic neuralgia. J. Am. Acad. Dermatol., 3: 524.

Price, R.W. (1982) Herpes zoster: An approach to systemic therapy. Med. Clin. North Am., 66: 1106–1118.

Sauer, G.C. (1955) Herpes zoster: Treatment of postherpetic neuralgia with cortisone, corticotropin and placebo. Arch. Dermatol., 71: 488–491.

Schmader, I.E. and Studenski, S. (1989) Are current therapies useful for the prevention of postherpetic neuralgia? J. Gen. Int. Med., 4: 83–89.

Sulzberger, M.B., Sauer, G.C., Hermann, F. et al. (1951) Effects of ACTH and cortisone on certain diseases and physiologic functions of the skin: I. Effects of ACTH. J. Invest. Dermatol., 16: 323–337.

Sutton, G. (1984) Steroid stoss therapy in the treatment of herpes zoster. Br. J. Clin. Pract., 38: 21–24.

Whitley, R.J., Weiss, H., Gnann, J.W. et al. (1996) Acyclovir with and without prednisone for the treatment of herpes zoster, a randomized placebo-controlled trial. Ann. Int. Med., 125: 376–383.

Wood, M.J., Johnson, R.W. and McKendrick, M.W. (1994) A randomized trial of acyclovir for 7 days or 21 days with and without prednisolone for treatment of acute herpes zoster. N. Engl. J. Med., 330: 896–890.

Herpes Zoster and Postherpetic Neuralgia, 2nd Revised and Enlarged Edition
Pain Research and Clinical Management, Vol. 11
Edited by C.P.N. Watson and A.A. Gershon

CHAPTER 19

The prevention of postherpetic neuralgia

C. Peter N. Watson [*]

Department of Medicine, University of Toronto and 1 Sir Williams Lane, Toronto, ON M9A 1T8, Canada

For it happens in this, as the physicians say it happens in hectic fever, that in the beginning of the malady it is easy to cure but difficult to detect, but in the course of time, not having been either detected or treated in the beginning, it becomes easy to detect but difficult to cure.

Niccolò Machiavelli, *The Prince*

Postherpetic neuralgia (PHN) and severe ocular involvement are the two most feared complications of herpes zoster. PHN may reasonably be compared with other end-stage disorders in which damage to an organ occurs and that structure is unable or not fully able to repair itself and respond to treatment. Evidence for this position lies with epidemiologic, clinical, and pathologic information, which will be reviewed here. As many as half of the patients with established PHN are incompletely relieved or totally refractory to the best therapies available (Table I). Because of this and of the possibility of preventing this disorder, we must consider early, vigorous treatment even though the effect of this is unproven. Optimally, this approach to treatment should be studied in a scientific fashion, but pending the results from such a study, it appears reasonable to proceed with early multi-modal intervention with herpes zoster and to also consider the possibility of prevention or attenuation of the disease by vaccination of older adults.

1. Epidemiology

Herpes zoster is the most common neurologic disease (Kurtzke, 1984). PHN is a painful disorder that occurs 1 month after herpes zoster infection in about 10% (overall incidence) of those with the infection (Burgoon et al., 1957; Hope-Simpson, 1975; Ragozzino et al., 1982). The incidence of PHN, however, increases with age, affecting 50% of herpes zoster patients by age 60, and the incidence rises steadily with increasing age (De Moragas and Kierland, 1957). The number of those affected will likely increase in the future with the shift of demographics to an increase in the aged population. The prognosis for patients with established PHN is poor, since at least half continue to suffer for many years — some even until death (Watson et al., 1991a). Of the 50% who seem to do reasonably well, many require continual pharmacotherapy, often with unpleasant side effects. These data are from a clinic that specializes in the treatment of PHN; patient outcome may be worse elsewhere.

2. Clinical findings

Clinical findings indicate that the nervous system is altered by this disease such that there are areas of sensory loss and widespread areas of sensitive skin,

---

* Correspondence to: Professor C.P.N. Watson, Department of Medicine, University of Toronto and 1 Sir Williams Lane, Toronto, ON M9A 1T8, Canada. Phone: +1 (416) 239-3494; Fax: +1 (416) 239-6365; E-mail: peter.watson@utoronto.ca

TABLE I

Number of postherpetic neuralgia patients responding poorly or not at all to treatment with antidepressants or opioids in controlled trials

Study/year	Agent	% of subjects not responding to treatment with	
		Opioid or antidepressant [1]	Placebo
Watson et al., 1982	Amitriptyline	8/24, 33%	100%
Max et al., 1988	Amitriptyline	21/41, 53%	84%
Kishore-Kumar et al., 1990	Desipramine	14/26, 54%	89%
Watson et al., 1992	Amitriptyline and/or maprotiline	17/32, 53%	No placebo
Watson et al., 1998	Amitriptyline and/or nortriptyline	10/31, 32%	No placebo
Watson and Babul, 1998	Oxycodone	17/38, 42%	82%

[1] Data are No_1 responding/No_1 treated, %.

which respond to the lightest touch with severe pain (Fig. 1). There are three types of pain associated with PHN: steady, often burning pain; lancinating, shock-like pain; and pain on non-painful stimulation of the skin (allodynia). These are often all present in a single case. The allodynia suggests that central neurones have expanded their receptive fields and have lowered thresholds to sensory stimulation. There is no evidence that the sensory changes are reversible.

Table I summarizes controlled trials of antidepressant and opioid therapies in PHN. These data indicate that 30%–50% of the patients responded poorly or not at all to some antidepressants and to an opioid (Watson and Babul, 1998). Even with these drugs, responses are usually incomplete, with total relief unusual. Side effects occur in nearly all treated patients. Newer treatments such as gabapentin and topical lidocaine also leave many patients with no or unsatisfactory relief. For most, other treatments are ineffective and include a variety of trial-and-error approaches, which may benefit an occasional patient with differing pain mechanisms (Watson, 1995).

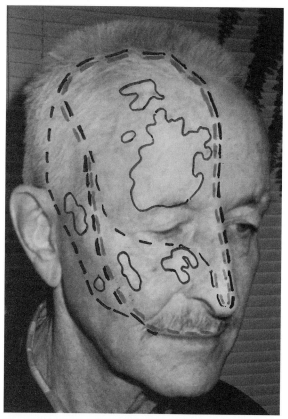

Fig. 1. Ophthalmic zoster with postherpetic neuralgia and loss of right eye. Solid line outlines scarring; dashed lines outline area of sensory loss and sensitive skin (allodynia).

3. Pathology

The few pathologic studies of PHN cases indicate that there is extensive damage to the peripheral and central nervous system (Watson et al., 1988, 1991b). The peripheral nerve, ganglion, and sensory root are extensively scarred, leading to the loss of normal structures (see Chapter 15). Surviving nerve fibers appear to shift to the smaller fiber population, which may be predominantly excitatory and may fire spontaneously or in response to the lightest of tactile stimulation. Further, there is evidence of central nervous system damage in that the dorsal horn of the spinal cord is infiltrated by inflammatory cells and later becomes atrophic because of the destruction of nerve fibers and neurones (see Chapter 15). There is no evidence that any of these pathologic changes are reversible.

4. Discussion

It is not known whether vaccination of older adults will attenuate or prevent herpes zoster; however, on the basis of current concepts of the pathogenesis of the disorder (i.e., it is thought that declining cell-mediated immunity is an important factor in the eruption of zoster), it would seem reasonable to study this approach. Clinical trials are currently underway, but the results will not be known for some years.

The other preventive avenue is to treat herpes zoster early and aggressively. This would require education of the general population so that patients would recognize the symptoms of zoster, contact a physician, and make arrangements to be seen promptly. Physicians' secretaries, nurses, and physicians also need to realize the importance of scheduling the patient on the day of the call. Educational material regarding herpes zoster is available from the Varicella Zoster Research Foundation [1] (Chapter 2). It is important that antiviral therapy with valacyclovir or famciclovir be initiated within 72 h of the onset of pain or rash in order to inhibit viral replication. It appears that there is a modest reduction in zoster-associated pain with this approach (Beutner et al., 1995; Tyring et al., 1995).

Another measure that should be considered is the early, aggressive use of analgesics to prevent the development of sensitization of the nervous system.

Opioids may be required, in which case, infectious disease specialists may wish to consult a pain management expert. There is some evidence that regional anesthesia of the painful area (by an anesthesiologist expert in these techniques) may help to resolve acute pain, and although not scientifically proven (the studies not having been done) to prevent PHN, this treatment may do so, particularly in conjunction with other approaches.

Antidepressants have been repeatedly shown to have an analgesic action in PHN that is independent of an antidepressant effect (Watson et al., 1982, 1992, 1998; Max et al., 1988; Kishore-Kumar et al., 1990). It is suggested that this action is via inhibition of re-uptake of serotonin and noradrenaline in the central nervous system. These are inhibitory neurotransmitters for pain pathways. Only amitriptyline, nortriptyline, desipramine, and maprotiline have been shown to relieve established PHN (Watson et al., 1982, 1992, 1998; Max et al., 1988; Kishore-Kumar et al., 1990). It has been suggested that early antidepressant therapy at the stage of herpes zoster may help to prevent persistent pain (Bowsher, 1996). Treatment may be instituted with low doses (10–25 mg, depending on the patient's age) of amitriptyline. This dose can be titrated every few days by similar increments until relief occurs or side effects supervene, and then the dose can be slightly reduced and held steady (Watson, 1995).

These preventive measures need to be studied scientifically to see if they alter the long-term natural course of PHN (Burgoon et al., 1957; De Moragas and Kierland, 1957; Hope-Simpson, 1975; Ragozzino et al., 1982; Watson et al., 1991b). However, used by experienced practitioners, these approaches have minimal untoward effects; thus, it seems reasonable to make them part of the management of herpes zoster until such studies are completed.

References

Beutner, K.R., Friedman, D.J., Forszpaniak, C., Andersen, P.L. and Wood M.J. (1995) Valacyclovir compared with acyclovir for improved therapy for herpes zoster in immunocompetent

---

[1] VZV Research Foundation, 40 East 72nd Street, New York, NY 10021; Phone, +1 (212) 472-7148; Fax: +1 (212) 861-7033.

adults. Antimicrob. Agents Chemother., 39: 1546–1553.

Bowsher, D. (1996) Postherpetic neuralgia and its treatment: A retrospective survey of 191 patients. J. Pain Symptom Manage., 12: 327–331.

Burgoon, C.F., Burgoon, J.S. and Haldridge, G.D. (1957) The natural history of herpes zoster. JAMA, 164: 265–269.

De Moragas, J.M. and Kierland, R.R. (1957) The outcome of patients with herpes zoster. Arch. Dermatol., 75: 193–196.

Hope-Simpson, R.E. (1975) Postherpetic neuralgia. J. R. Coll. Gen. Pract., 25: 571–575.

Kishore-Kumar, R., Max, M.B. and Schafer, S.C. et al. (1990) Desipramine relieves postherpetic neuralgia. Clin. Pharmacol. Ther., 47: 305–312.

Kurtzke, J.F. (1984) Neuroepidemiology. Ann. Neurol., 16: 265–277.

Max, M.B., Schafer, S.C., Culnane, M., Smoller, B., Dubner, R. and Gracely, R. (1988) Amitriptyline but not lorazepam relieves postherpetic neuralgia. Neurology, 38: 1427–1432.

Ragozzino, M.W., Melton, I.J., Kurland, L.T. et al. (1982) Population based study of herpes zoster and it sequelae. Medicine, 21: 310–316.

Tyring, S., Barbarash, R.A., Nahlek, J.E. et al. (1995) Famciclovir for the treatment of acute herpes zoster: Effects on acute disease and postherpetic neuralgia. Ann. Intern. Med., 123: 89–96.

Watson, C.P.N., Evans, R.J., Reed, K., Merskey, H., Goldsmith, I. and Warsh, J. (1982) Amitriptyline versus placebo in postherpetic neuralgia. Neurology, 32: 671–673.

Watson, C.P.N., Morshead, C., Van der Kooy, D., Deck, J. and Evans, R.J. (1988) Postherpetic neuralgia: Post-mortem analysis of a case. Pain, 34: 129–138.

Watson, C.P.N., Deck, J.H., Morshead, C., Van der Kooy, D. and Evans, R.J. (1991a) Postherpetic neuralgia: Further post-mortem studies of cases with and without pain. Pain, 44: 105–117.

Watson, C.P.N., Watt, V.R., Chipman, M., Birkett, N. and Evans, R.J. (1991b) The prognosis with postherpetic neuralgia. Pain, 46: 195–199.

Watson, C.P.N., Chipman, M., Reed, K., Evans, R.J. and Birkett, N. (1992) Amitriptyline versus maprotiline in postherpetic neuralgia; A randomized, double-blind, crossover trial. Pain, 48: 29–36.

Watson, C.P.N. (1995) The treatment of postherpetic neuralgia. Neurology, 45: 58–59.

Watson, C.P.N. and Babul, N. (1998) Oxycodone relieves neuropathic pain: A randomized trial in postherpetic neuralgia. Neurology, 50: 1837–1841.

Watson, C.P.N., Chipman, M. and Reed, K. (1998) Amitriptyline versus nortriptyline in postherpetic neuralgia. Neurology, 51: 1166–1171.

Herpes Zoster and Postherpetic Neuralgia, 2nd Revised and Enlarged Edition
Pain Research and Clinical Management, Vol. 11
Edited by C.P.N. Watson and A.A. Gershon

CHAPTER 20

Nerve blocks, herpes zoster, and postherpetic neuralgia

Perry G. Fine [*]

Department of Anesthesiology and Pain Management Center, University of Utah Health Sciences Center,
Salt Lake City, UT 84108, USA

1. Introduction

The role of nerve block therapy in the management of pain due to acute herpes zoster eruption and the prevention or control of postherpetic neuralgia (PHN) continues to be unclear. There has been very little done in the way of methodologically sound studies to clarify the role or value of this type of intervention over the last several years, although many pain management anesthesiologists continue to prescribe nerve block therapies as preventative or therapeutic adjuncts. The controversy over the timing (when and how often), type (what block with what drug(s)), and other variables which might help define the indications for nerve blocks is compounded by the potential risks and economic costs of such therapies. This latter but timely issue is not addressed in the medical literature dealing with the prevention and management of zoster pain, so there is little to draw upon in the way of references. Nevertheless, upon considering the literature which focuses on nerve block therapies, it is important to keep this issue in mind. Balancing the potential risks versus benefits of such therapies in this light may help direct us toward reasonable therapeutic dispositions. For instance, due to the extremely debilitating

nature of intractable postherpetic neuralgia, and the economic costs of chronic treatment, nerve block therapy which is *possibly* effective but has some potential risk and is somewhat costly in the short run may be worth pursuing. This chapter explores these issues in depth and concludes with suggestions for dealing with the present controversies raised by this unresolved subject.

2. General considerations

In all branches of medicine, mythology and science are entwined. The lore of nerve block therapy as a useful tool in the management, prevention or treatment of pain due to herpes zoster is a richly laden case in point. Documentation of this form of therapy as a useful tool for this problem dates back to the beginning of this century (Loeser, 1986).

In view of the terribly demoralizing nature of this pain producing disorder, it is easy to see, through the eyes of the sanguine, albeit, frustrated clinician, how hope and wishful thinking might promote inordinately positive claims and unproven conclusions. And, after all, who would be so cruel as to cast shadows with the skeptical lamp of empirical sci-

[*] Correspondence to: Dr. Perry G. Fine, Pain Management Center Administrative Offices, Suite 2000, 546 Chipeta Drive, Salt Lake City, UT 84108, USA. Phone: +1 (801) 585-7690; Fax: +1 (801) 585-7694; E-mail: fine@aros.net

ence, when there might be some chance, however remote, of benefit to the sufferer. It is within this quite understandable emotional context coupled with the difficulties inherent in carrying out prospective controlled clinical studies for this type of problem that, almost a century and many reports later, we have not moved beyond the limits of our impressions in this particular field.

Although unintended at its inception, in its evolution this chapter may now appear to be a study in disillusionment for those who believe there is an empiric basis and well-defined role for the prescription of nerve block therapies in those with herpes zoster. Rigorous review and honest evaluation of the existing literature in its entirety challenges such notions. The art of medicine may be served by adhering to such beliefs and practices, but the science is not. And so, with sincere apologies to those firm believers, this chapter will serve more as a critique of inadequate study design and a plea for correcting this deficiency in future studies, than as a clinical guide of what to do and how, when, and where to do it.

3. Timing of interventions

There are three time periods or phases during the presentation of the herpes zoster syndrome when useful treatment information regarding pain can be derived. These include treatment of pain during the acute infectious/inflammatory period, preemptive treatments during the acute period to prevent chronicity, and treatment of protracted neuralgic pain. Nerve block therapies have been applied with a view toward each of these.

3.1. Acute pain control

Rosenak (1938) reported the results of treating 22 patients with symptoms of herpes zoster for two to fourteen days. He performed somatic or sympathetic nerve blocks with procaine and described 90% success in achieving pain relief and vesicular healing after 48 hours. No long-term follow-up is provided. Street (1943) and Findley and Patzer (1945) report

a total of 7 cases who obtained marked pain relief and rapid healing from sympathetic block using procaine. Similarly, Ferris and Martin (1950) used stellate ganglion and lumbar sympathetic blocks in 22 patients with acute zoster. Of the twenty patients seen within 5 days of symptoms, complete pain relief and crusting over of lesions after one or two blocks is reported. One of the two patients who were treated 4 weeks into their disease had similar results, but the other did not respond to nerve blocks. Again, no long-term follow-up is provided.

Using steroid infiltration around the painful lesions in lieu of local anesthetic, Lefkovits (1961) described complete or marked relief in 4 patients with symptoms for less than 3 months. No follow-up information is provided.

Colding has submitted two reports in the English language literature investigating the efficacy of sympathetic blocks in controlling pain during the acute phase of zoster. In the first (Colding, 1969), 243 patients were treated with regional sympathetic blocks and results were analyzed according to the duration of precedent symptoms. In 204 patients with zoster for less than 14 days, 15% experienced no relief compared to 30% in the 38 patients who had had symptoms longer than 14 days. Incomplete relief in these two groups was 23% and 26%, respectively. In his subsequent report (Colding, 1973) he reviews the results of sympathetic blocks in 483 patients with acute zoster pain. He found that 10% of patients with symptoms less than 2 weeks old fail to obtain pain relief compared with a 60% non-response rate in those treated who had symptoms longer than 2 weeks. Similar results were reported by LaFlamme et al. (1979). These investigators used sympathetic blocks to treat acute zoster pain of the trigeminal distribution. Three of five patients studied had complete relief after 5–12 blocks, applied at two-day intervals.

Riopelle et al. (1984) studied the effects of different types of nerve blocks (epidural, stellate ganglion, peripheral nerve) in 72 patients with symptoms of herpes zoster for 30 days or less. Pain relief was described as prompt with all these techniques and relief lasted for hours to days. Patients could return as often as desired for repeat blocks. Patients' clinical courses were followed for 6 months. Bonica and Buckley (1990) give a testimonial of complete relief of pain during the acute phase of zoster in 126 patients treated with several nerve blocks daily followed by intermittent blocks thereafter. Unfortunately, this is an unpublished account without extensive details.

Perkins and Hanlon (1978) describe the use of serial epidural injections of local anesthetic with steroid in 7 patients with acute zoster pain. They report virtually complete relief of pain with this method.

Using a rather novel technique at the time, Marmer (1965) provided a single case report of continuous epidural analgesia in a 70 year old man for the control of acute zoster pain. This treatment lasted 11 days with reportedly excellent pain control, but no follow-up information was provided. Using a different continuous technique, Reiestad et al. (1989) report the efficacy of local anesthetic mediated analgesia using pleural catheters in 18 patients with acute zoster. Catheters remained in place for 2–3 weeks during the acute eruptive phase. No significant complications arose.

What can be concluded from these reports? Most evident is the fact that none of these represent controlled clinical trials. A variety of techniques are described with varying degrees of efficacy reported, but there are no controls against which one can attribute specificity to the technique in question. Similarly, the nerve blocking or infiltrating methods described are not compared to other conventional treatment modalities such as peripheral or central acting analgesics, either by efficacy, cost, or risk. Nevertheless, in severe cases where the risk of other treatments or their lack of efficacy exceeds that of nerve blocking, it may be quite reasonable to proceed with these more invasive means.

Contrary to the frequently encountered yet unsubstantiated statements which appear in the literature, there is no well-demonstrated 'technique of choice' for this indication. Based upon the known and hypothetical mechanisms by which acute zoster produces pain, the location and severity of symptoms, the underlying health status of the patient,

the experience of the treating physician, and the resources available, a rational plan can be determined. In these cases, the best measure of 'success' will be the subjective response of the patient and objective functional changes that are pertinent and measurable. Placebo-controlled randomized clinical trials in clinically similar populations or in blinded 'double-dummy' cross-over trials will be the only means of discerning the relative merits of any technique.

3.2. Preemptive nerve blocks to prevent postherpetic neuralgia

Two essential criteria which need to be met in order to assess the efficacy of nerve block therapy as a prophylaxis against persistent neuralgia following herpes zoster infection are: 1) the performance of nerve block(s) during the acute phase of the disease, and 2) follow-up for a period of time long enough to determine whether postherpetic neuralgia has developed. Unfortunately, there are few studies in the literature which meet even these minimal criteria.

Colding's reports (see Colding, 1969 and 1973) are the earliest which set out to answer this question. Combining results, in those patients who provided information 5–6 months after onset of zoster symptoms and treatment with sympathetic blocks, 10–20% had continued pain. Follow-up information from less than one third of the initial study population was obtainable, and this sample was not selected at random. This introduces an insurmountable source of bias. In addition, stratification by age is not reported. Since it is well-established that advancing age is a significant factor in persistent pain after zoster, lumping results without regard to age is not illuminating. Thus, these data cannot be critically compared to other studies evaluating the 'natural history' of the disease process. Without concurrent controls, conclusions regarding treatment specificity, even under better sampling conditions, are not valid.

The non-randomized, uncontrolled studies from Perkins and Hanlon (1978) using epidural anesthetics with steroids, Riopelle et al. (1984) using sympathetic, epidural and peripheral nerve blocks, Milligan and Nash (1985) using stellate ganglion blocks, Dan et al. (1985) using various nerve block techniques, Reiestad et al. (1989) using continuous pleural analgesia, and the unpublished accounts of Bonica (see Bonica and Buckley, 1990) suffer from the same limitations.

Yanagida et al. (1987) retrospectively analyzed the incidence of postherpetic neuralgia in two groups of patients receiving stellate ganglion, epidural, or caudal blocks, depending upon the location of their acute zoster pain. One group received blocks prior to eruption of the typical zoster rash and the other received treatment immediately after the rash appeared. Surveys were completed after one year by 91.8% and 83.2% of these two groups, respectively. There was no difference in the incidence of persistent pain between groups. The authors conclude that preemptive blocks early in the course of the disease do not prevent the syndrome of postherpetic neuralgia. Although this statement would appear to be an honest appraisal, the study is flawed in its design. Without concurrent controls, any difference in outcome compared with the natural history as it might unfold in these patients is impossible to assess.

This study was criticized by Bauman (1987). He takes issue with the conclusion that preemptive blocks do not contribute significantly to a reduction in the incidence of postherpetic neuralgia, citing his own experience to the contrary. His criticism is based mostly upon technical questions surrounding the performance of the nerve blocks. Although these points are debatable, this type of attack is misplaced, distracting from the real issue of drawing conclusions from non-controlled, non-randomized, retrospective data. Yanagida's conclusions may or may not be true. However, technical disqualifications and the refutation of a study do not serve as proof of equally unsubstantiated opinions.

Tenicela et al. (1985) published a study which may shine some light on this question. In a randomized, double-blind, placebo-controlled, cross-over trial, the investigators studied 20 patients over the age of 50 with herpes zoster for less than 6 weeks. Subjects were treated with sympathetic blocks or placebo blocks during four consecutive days. All patients with continued pain went on to have another series of blocks with known active drug (bupivacaine). There was no other therapy with the exception of prn weak oral analgesics. Follow-up was via questionnaire every two months for one year and then at six month intervals. The groups were demographically similar and there was one subject from the placebo group who, although there was no substantial relief of pain, refused further blocks.

Ninety per cent of subjects from the sympathetic block group had long-term pain relief, whereas only 20% from the placebo group had initial pain relief. About 55% of the remaining control group went on to have long-term resolution of pain after sympathetic blocks. This left 30% from the initial control group who continued to have long-term pain. Again, the only difference in this group was the use of placebo blocks for four days prior to sympathetic blocks. This translates into a 25% postherpetic neuralgia incidence overall. The limitation of this study is in the numbers of subjects, especially when stratified by age. Were the differences in numbers of subjects from each group who went on to have postherpetic neuralgia a function of the interventions, or a function of coincidental uneven distribution of predisposed patients in the two groups, in spite of randomization? When the differences boil down to 1 patient versus 3 patients, as was the case in this study, larger numbers are required in order to be conclusive.

3.3. Treatment of postherpetic neuralgia with nerve blocks

Published accounts of injection therapy for postherpetic pain date back to Russell et al. (1957). These authors describe the use of various techniques, including 'injection therapy', in 100 patients with postherpetic neuralgia and present a few descriptive cases. There are no data given and no formal study invoked. Lefkovits (1961) used local infiltration of steroid in three patients with symptoms of 5 months, 2 years, and 5 years duration. The shorter-term patients are reported to have had either complete or partial relief, with indeterminate results in the patient with symptoms for 5 years. There is no information given regarding long-term results and there were no controls.

Colding (1969) studied the effect of sympathetic blocks in 34 patients with PHN for an average of two years. Thirteen patients were available for follow-up 5–6 months later, and none had complete pain relief, although three reported less pain than pre-block. Four years later, the same author reported on the results of treating 67 patients with postherpetic pain (2 months to 11 years duration) with up to 10 sympathetic blocks (see Colding, 1973). He reports that 50% of patients experienced short-term pain relief. He presented follow-up information on 34 of these patients, 6–12 months after treatment. Half of this follow-up group experienced no pain relief with block therapy but two patients from this group experienced spontaneous remission of pain. Of the group who had experienced some pain relief (17 patients), about 30% had maintained complete relief of painful symptoms while 50% had gone back to their previous pain levels and the remainder reported some improvement compared to pre-block levels. Putting this all together reveals 10 patients out of the follow-up group of 34 with some perceived long-term pain reduction (2 spontaneous, 8 attributed to blocks), or a figure of 29% improvement. It needs to be recalled that this figure is generated from a non-random follow-up sample of a non-randomized, non-controlled treatment group.

Perkins et al. (1978) treated 5 patients with PHN with 1–3 epidural injections consisting of local anesthetic and steroid. One patient reported 50% pain reduction several months later, and the others reported 0–25% reduction in pain. The authors conclude that this form of therapy is ineffective in treating postherpetic neuralgia. Forrest (1980) also tested epidural steroids for the control of PHN, but came to a different conclusion. Thirty-seven patients with pain for more than six months were enrolled after screening with psychometric tests, drug detoxification, and an appropriate response to a graduated epidural analgesia test. Subjects received weekly epidural injections of methylprednisolone acetate for three weeks. Follow-up occurred for twelve months. Eighty-nine per cent were reported being pain-free at the end of the follow-up period. Although this is an intriguing finding, missing is the use of concurrent controls assigned with randomization. This is needed in order to attribute this result specifically to the therapeutic intervention with statistical analysis.

Other case reports using techniques such as gasserian ganglion block with steroid (see Yamashiro et al., 1990), cryoanalgesia (see Barnard et al., 1981 and Jones and Murrin, 1987), stellate ganglion block (see LaFlamme et al., 1979 and Milligan and Nash, 1985) have either failed to prove efficacy or have been inconclusive. Although they suggest potentially useful ideas, they universally fail to follow a randomized controlled methodology.

As well, anecdotal reports of techniques such as stellate ganglion phenol neurolysis (see Racz and Holubec, 1989) or epidural phenol injections (see Racz et al., 1989) for this indication are suspect. Without data being provided in well controlled studies, and without publication of such trials in peer review journals, it is not possible, no less responsible, to assign any scientific merit to such suggestions. Fair evaluation by clinicians and the patients they serve is simply not possible under these circumstances.

In one case of seemingly intractable postherpetic pain, the use of local anesthetic with the opioid, fentanyl, in a stellate ganglion block led to protracted relief of several week's duration (see Fine and Ashburn, 1988). Although only a single case study, the study design (double-blind, cross-over, placebo-controlled) adds credibility to the findings. The use of an opioid to supplement the effects of local anesthetic is a novel approach. This is predicated upon the finding of opioid receptors within ganglionic tissue, and the notion that some degree of sympathetically maintained pain may be involved in the pathophysiology of pain in some patients with PHN. Arias et al. (1989) have demonstrated a similar result, using sufentanil, in the treatment of refractory reflex sympathetic dystrophy. In the case of the individual referenced above, the use of opioid stellate ganglion blocks has not been a panacea. He is still burdened by the slow recurrence of pain for which he elects to undergo a block almost every month.

4. Conclusions

Given that the randomized controlled trial is the gold standard for clinical studies, a certain form of analytical alchemy would be required to infer a well-defined role for nerve block therapy in the management of pain due to zoster, based upon the available literature. This rather bleak summary notwithstanding, certain conclusions are possible. Clearly, during the acute phase of zoster infection, nerve blocks can be used to provide acute pain relief. Weighing risks and benefits, costs, availability of resources and patient acceptance, nerve blocks may provide a viable alternative to other medical therapies. This places herpes zoster in the same domain as many other acutely painful conditions (infectious, traumatic, postoperative, and so forth) which might be palliated by this treatment modality. And, in a similar vein to acute pain management for other conditions, the circumstances which would point to a specific type of nerve block as the *best* choice have not been clearly defined in the literature. Until the time that this is the case, such decisions would appear to be a matter of personal choice between patient and physician.

Scientifically based data regarding the efficacy of nerve blocks for either prevention or long-term treatment of postherpetic neuralgia are not available. Regrettably, some conclusions which are drawn in the existing literature can be misleading. Statements such as "instant relief from pain and rapid healing of lesions" (see Findley and Patzer, 1945), "Epidural injection of bupivacaine with or without methylprednisolone acetate is the treatment of choice for the pain of cutaneous herpes zoster" (see Perkins and Hanlon, 1978) or "the use of sympathetic block, alone or combined with somatic nerve blocks, if begun early after the onset of pain or the eruption of acute herpes zoster, results in a high incidence of prompt pain relief, appears to decrease the severity and duration of the eruption, and accelerates healing" (see Bonica and Buckley, 1990) are unsubstantiated. From an academic viewpoint, these must be regarded with healthy skepticism and held up to scientific scrutiny. These hopeful and tempting, but unproven, messages can not yet serve as standards for routine clinical practice.

From a practical standpoint, is there nonetheless a justification for performing nerve blocks in an effort to prevent or treat the horrible after-effects of zoster infection? Might this be especially reasonable in the susceptible elderly? Should the anecdotal experiences and impressions of many clinicians be discounted simply because of a non-compelling literature? These are important questions, and they can only be answered within the context of one's own ethical deliberations. Without a solid scientific literature to back clinical decisions, we must rely on practicality mounted upon a foundation of ethical reasoning and judgement.

In this situation, the principles which must be balanced are those of *nonmaleficence* (doing no harm), *beneficence* (doing good) and *autonomy* (served by the provision of informed consent). This would necessarily include a disclosure of the unproven value of this form of therapy as well as the financial costs, risks, alternatives, and probabilities of outcome in the event of non-treatment. Patients with this problem are desperate and ingenuous physicians are compelled to do what they can to help. Within the limits of our present knowledge and capabilities, the irreducible processes of caring for patients and maintaining the integrity of medicine are best served by this approach.

References

Arias, L.M., Schwartzman, R.J., Bartkowski, R., Tom, C.M. and Grossman, K.L. (1989) Sufentanil stellate ganglion injection in the treatment of refractory reflex sympathetic dystrophy. Reg. Anesth., 14: 90–92.

Barnard, D., Lloyd, J. and Evans, J. (1981) Cryoanalgesia in the management of chronic facial pain. J. Max.-Fac. Surg., 9: 101–102.

Bauman, J. (1987) Prevention of postherpetic neuralgia. Anesthesiology, 67: 441–442.

Bonica, J.J. and Buckley, F.P. (1990) Regional analgesia with local anesthetics. In: J.J. Bonica (Ed.), The Management of Pain, Vol. 2. Lea and Febiger, Philadelphia, PA, 2nd ed., pp. 1938–1939.

Colding, A. (1969) The effect of regional sympathetic blocks in the treatment of herpes zoster. Acta Anaesthesiol. Scand., 13: 133–141.

Colding, A. (1973) Treatment of pain: organization of a pain clinic: treatment of acute Herpes zoster. Proc. R. Soc. Med., 66: 541–543.

Dan, K., Higa, K. and Noda, B. (1985) Nerve block for herpetic pain. In: H.L. Fields (Ed.), Advances in Pain Research and Therapy, Vol. 9. Raven Press, New York, pp. 831–838.

Ferris, L.M. and Martin, G.H. (1950) The use of sympathetic nerve block in the ambulatory patient with special reference to its use in Herpes Zoster. Ann. Intern. Med., 32: 257–260.

Findley, T. and Patzer, R. (1945) Treatment of herpes zoster by paravertebral procaine block. JAMA, 128: 1217–1219.

Fine, P.G. and Ashburn, M.A. (1988) Effect of stellate ganglion block with fentanyl on postherpetic neuralgia with a sympathetic component. Anesth. Analg., 67: 897–899.

Forrest, J.B. (1980) The response to epidural steroid injections in chronic dorsal root pain. Can. Anaesth. Soc. J., 27: 40–46.

Jones, M.J.T. and Murrin, K.R. (1987) Intercostal block with cryotherapy. Ann. R. Coll. Surg. Engl., 69: 261–262.

LaFlamme, M.Y., LaBreque, B. and Mignault, G. (1979) Zona ophtalmique: traitement de la névralgie zonateuse par infiltrations stellaires répétées. Can. J. Ophthalmol., 14: 99–101.

Lefkovits, A.M. (1961) Postherpetic neuralgia. Neurology, 11: 170–171.

Loeser, J.D. (1986) Herpes zoster and postherpetic neuralgia. Pain, 25: 149–164.

Marmer, M.J. (1965). Acute Herpes zoster: successful treatment by continuous epidural analgesia. Calif. Med., 103: 277–279.

Milligan, N.S. and Nash, T.P. (1985) Treatment of post-herpetic neuralgia. A review of 77 consecutive cases. Pain, 23: 381–386.

Perkins, H.M. and Hanlon, P.R. (1978) Epidural injection of local anesthetic and steroids for relief of pain secondary to Herpes zoster. Arch. Surg., 113: 253–254.

Racz, G.B. and Holubec, J.T. (1989) Stellate ganglion phenol neurolysis. In: G.B. Racz (Ed.), Techniques of Neurolysis. Kluwer Academic Publishers, Boston, MA, p. 140.

Racz, G.B., Heavner, J. and Haynworth, R. (1989) Repeat epidural phenol injections in chronic pain and spasticity. In: G.B. Racz (Ed.), Techniques of Neurolysis. Kluwer Academic Publishers, Boston, MA, pp. 205–206.

Reiestad, F., Kvalheim, L. and McIlvaine, W.B. (1989) Pleural analgesia for the treatment of acute severe thoracic herpes zoster. Reg. Anesth., 14: 244–246.

Riopelle, J.M., Naraghi, M. and Grush, K.P. (1984) Chronic neuralgia incidence following local anesthetic therapy for herpes zoster. Arch. Dermatol., 120: 747–750.

Rosenak, S. (1938) Procaine injection treatment of Herpes Zoster. Lancet, Nov. 5: 1056–1058.

Russell, W.R., Espir, M.L.E. and Morganstern, F.S. (1957) Treatment of post-herpetic neuralgia. Lancet, Feb. 2: 242–245.

Street, A. (1943) Use of sympathetic nerve block in herpes zoster, Bell's palsy. Mississippi Doctor, 20: 480–481.

Tenicela, R., Lovasik, D. and Eaglstein, W. (1985) Treatment of Herpes zoster with sympathetic blocks. Clin. J. Pain, 1: 63–67.

Yamashiro, H., Hara, K. and Gotoh, Y. (1990) Relief of intractable postherpetic neuralgia with gasserian ganglion block using methyl prednisolone. Masui, 39: 1239–1244.

Yanagida, H., Suwa, K., and Corssen, G. (1987) No prophylactic effect of early sympathetic blockade on postherpetic neuralgia. Anesthesiology, 66: 73–76.

Herpes Zoster and Postherpetic Neuralgia, 2nd Revised and Enlarged Edition
Pain Research and Clinical Management, Vol. 11
Edited by C.P.N. Watson and A.A. Gershon

CHAPTER 21

Topical agents for post-herpetic neuralgia

Michael C. Rowbotham [1,*] and C. Peter N. Watson [2]

[1] *Departments of Neurology and Anaesthesia, University of California, San Francisco, and UCSF Pain Clinical Research Centre, Francisco, CA, USA and* [2] *Department of Medicine, University of Toronto, Toronto, ON, Canada*

1. Introduction

Since the previous edition of this volume, good science supports the use of a topical lidocaine patch in post-herpetic neuralgia (PHN). This chapter provides an update on this data. PHN would appear to be the ideal chronic pain syndrome to treat with topical agents. The disease begins with a cutaneous rash and the chronic state is notable for skin scarring and painfully sensitive skin. Although the initial outbreak may be widespread, occasionally appearing to cover more than the area of skin innervated by a single dorsal root ganglion, most PHN patients are able to localize a limited area of skin as the source of their pain (Rowbotham and Fields, 1989a,b). An effective topical agent could be applied directly by the patient, obviating the need for repetitive physician-administered invasive therapies like nerve blocks. The topical agents studied to date are essentially free of systemic side effects.

The available alternatives to topical therapy have significant drawbacks (Loeser, 1986; Portenoy et al., 1986; Watson and Evans, 1986). The primarily elderly patients with PHN frequently cannot be treated with tricyclic antidepressants because of pre-existing cognitive impairment, cardiac disease, or systemic illness. Side effects like constipation, dry mouth and sedation may prove so bothersome that compliance becomes a major problem in therapy. Anticonvulsants other than gabapentin (Rowbotham et al., 1998) are of uncertain efficacy, non-narcotic analgesics are rarely effective, and benzodiazepines have been proven ineffective. Opioids are effective, but have numerous side effects (Rowbotham et al., 1991; Watson and Babul, 1998). Few PHN patients are willing to undertake invasive neurosurgical procedures with limited evidence for efficacy, such as dorsal column stimulation and deep brain stimulation, and destructive procedures, like dorsal root entry zone (DREZ) lesions. Nerve sectioning, neurolytic nerve blocks, cordotomy and rhizotomy have no proof of efficacy.

Topical therapies for PHN fall into three categories: capsaicin preparations, aspirin/nonsteroidal, anti-inflammatory preparations and local anaesthetics. In the USA, the capsaicin preparations are commercially available (as Zostrix® 0.025% capsaicin and Axsain® 0.075% capsaicin). The lidocaine patch (Lidoderm®) has been recently approved in the USA. Outside the USA, EMLA® (Eutectic Mixture of Local Anaesthetics) is available, but not widely promoted as therapy for PHN.

PHN patients nearly always have a sensory abnormality in the region of pain (Noordenbos, 1959;

* Correspondence to: Dr. M.C. Rowbotham, UCSF Pain Clinical Research Center, 1701 Divisadero Street, Suite 480, San Francisco, CA 94115, USA. Phone: +1 (415) 885-7899; Fax: +1 (415) 885-7855; E-mail: mcrwind@itsa.ucsf.edu

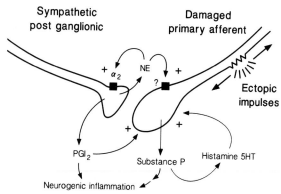

Fig. 1. Targets for topical analgesics. Sympathetic post-ganglionic fibres and damaged primary afferents have multiple sites for interaction. Capsaicin may target C-fibres, substance P, other neuropeptides and the process of neurogenic inflammation. Topical aspirin and nonsteroidal anti-inflammatories may target prostaglandins and other inflammatory mediators, C-fibres and the process of neurogenic inflammation. Local anaesthetics target primary afferents directly, including sites of ectopic impulse generation, and possibly all other interaction sites shown. (Redrawn by permission of Howard Fields.)

Rowbotham and Fields, 1989b; Bjerring et al., 1990; Nurmikko and Bowsher, 1990; Nurmikko, 1991). The intent of all three categories of topical remedies for PHN is to further alter sensory function in the skin to reduce the ability of mediators of inflammation to activate nociceptors. The interactions of potential targets for topical analgesics are shown in Fig. 1. Both local anaesthetics and capsaicin preparations will subtly increase the sensory deficit already present.

2. Capsaicin preparations

Capsaicin is a natural product extracted from pungent red chili peppers. Hot peppers have been used since ancient times as food additives and preservatives, as ingredients in certain social rituals, and as herbal medicines for itch, pain, constipation and other maladies. Beginning in the 1940s, the Hungarian pharmacologist Nicholas Jancso began his extensive characterization of the pharmacological properties of capsaicin and congeners on sensory processes (Jancso et al., 1977). Interest in capsai-

cin has remained intense since it was discovered that, depending on the concentration used, capsaicin can selectively activate, inactivate and even destroy small-diameter primary afferents (Buck and Burks, 1986; Lynn, 1990). Given systemically to neonatal rats, capsaicin destroys most unmyelinated primary afferents, but leaves larger diameter primary afferents and the central nervous system intact. These animals have an enduring deficit in pain sensitivity and a loss of substance P, a peptide thought to be a neurotransmitter involved in pain transmission, in the spinal cord dorsal horn. Capsaicin is not selective for substance P; levels of other peptides in small-diameter primary afferent neurons such as calcitonin gene-related peptide (CGRP), somatostatin, and vasoactive intestinal polypeptide (VIP) are reduced by capsaicin treatment.

The activation of primary afferents by capsaicin is due to an increase in cation permeability (Dray et al., 1990). There is selectivity for capsaicin; large-diameter primary afferents and non-nociceptive C-fibres are not activated. Application of high concentrations produces conduction block in C-polymodal nociceptor fibres (C-PMNs), but not in C-cold thermoceptor axons (Petsche et al., 1983). Acute exposure to high concentrations of capsaicin leads to immediate toxic reactions in C-fibres and their cell bodies in the dorsal root ganglion with an eventual reduction in the number of dorsal root ganglion cells (Jancso et al., 1985). At 2 months after exposure, the overall reduction in C-fibres in peripheral nerve may still be 40%, with up to 80% of the C-PMN fibres absent (Lynn et al., 1987; Pini et al., 1990).

When stimulated by capsaicin, unmyelinated primary afferent C-fibres release substance P at their peripheral terminals. Release of substance P in the periphery produces neurogenic inflammation marked by swelling, vasodilatation and hyperalgesia. In man, a single treatment with capsaicin produces a burning sensation followed by hyperalgesia to heat or skin pressure that may last for up to 24 h (Simone et al., 1987, 1989). Repeat application on normal skin within 24 h led to diminished effects, with pain reduced or absent and less vasodilation. After multiple applications, capsaicin no longer produces a sensa-

TABLE I

Trials of capsaicin for post-herpetic neuralgia

Reference	Strength (%)	Location	n[1]	t (weeks)[2]	Controlled?[3]	Outcome
Bernstein et al. (1987)	0.025	Variable	14	4	No	12/14 completed; 9/12 improved
Watson et al. (1988)	0.025	Variable	33	4	No	23/33 completed; 13/33 severe burning; 3/23 completers good/excellent relief
Bernstein et al. (1989)	0.075	Variable	32	6	Yes	29/32 completed; significant relief and VAS decrease
Drake et al. (1990)	0.025	Variable	30	3	Yes	No difference from vehicle in VAS or verbal ratings
Bjerring et al. (1990)	0.10	Variable	8	5	No	Could not blind study. VAS decreased 25 and 62% moderate/better relief. 0/8 used drug long-term
Peikert et al. (1991)	0.025	Non-trigeminal	39	8	No	19/39 improved; 5/39 intolerable burning; 13/39 no benefit. At follow-up only 33 still used drug
Watson et al. (1993)	0.075	Variable	143	6	Yes	'Significant' relief

[1] n, number of patients.

[2] t, duration in weeks.

[3] Controlled?, was it a controlled trial?

tion. At this time, the axon reflex flare is absent, whether provoked by skin heating, electrical stimulation, allergic response or irritant chemicals (Anand et al., 1983). Hyperalgesia to skin heating disappears after about 24 h, replaced by hypalgesia and possibly a diminution in warm sensitivity. Sensitivity to innocuous cooling or mechanical stimuli remains normal. When treatment is stopped, normal sensitivity and axon reflex flare return over 1–2 weeks time (Lynn, 1990). Re-innervation of the epidermis takes place over many weeks (Nolano et al., 1999).

It has been suggested that the therapeutic effects of capsaicin in treatment of pain are largely due to depleting substance P in C-fibres, both peripherally and centrally. From two different approaches in animal studies, it appears that capsaicin mostly reduces substance P by causing C-fibre degeneration, not depletion in otherwise intact cell processes (Lynn, 1990; Dickenson, 1991). The contribution to pain relief from capsaicin from the reduction in other neuropeptides may be major (Stewart et al., 1976). Any therapeutic rationale must remain firmly based on evidence of efficacy in clinical trials.

Capsaicin-containing preparations for PHN pain have received much attention in recent years. Con-

troversy has surrounded clinical trials of capsaicin because of the difficulty of blinding such studies (Cotton, 1990). On normal skin, capsaicin reliably evokes warmth or a burning sensation. In patients with PHN, a substantial proportion report burning, sometimes of intolerable intensity, which cannot be innocuously mimicked by any placebo (Watson et al., 1988; Peikert et al., 1991). Patients who do not experience burning when applying it to the affected skin may still become unblinded because of burning sensations in the hand they use to apply the cream, or if they are unfortunate enough to have come in contact with the eye or other mucosal surface. A recent study has shown that many PHN patients are exquisitely sensitive to capsaicin application (Petersen et al., 2000; see Chapter 21). The severe pain evoked has implications for the underlying pain mechanisms in this group.

The results of controlled and uncontrolled trials of capsaicin in concentrations varying from 0.025% to 0.10% are summarized in Table I (Bernstein et al., 1987, 1989; Watson et al., 1988; Bjerring et al., 1990; Drake et al., 1990; Peikert et al., 1991). Not included are anecdotal reports of benefit with differing concentrations in individual patients. Several uncontrolled studies have been reported, with variable results. In a study of 14 patients, Bernstein and colleagues reported partial relief in 6 and complete relief in 3 of the 12 patients completing the study (Bernstein et al., 1987). Only one patient reported burning.

Watson and coworkers used 0.025% capsaicin in an open label study of 33 patients with established PHN (Watson et al., 1988). Burning was reported by 26 of the 33 patients (79%). Eleven dropped out due to intolerable burning after using capsaicin from 1 day to 3 weeks, although one of these dropouts was able to resume the trial by applying capsaicin to a smaller area, using oral analgesics, and pretreating the area with 5% Xylocaine ointment. Using a conservative definition of success, Watson reported a good result in 11 patients, and excellent results in two patients, for an overall rate of 39%. In an interview study of 156 patients followed for up to 11 years, Watson and coworkers found both topical capsaicin and antidepressants useful (Watson et al., 1991).

In an elegant study of the effects of capsaicin in a 0.1% concentration, Bjerring and colleagues demonstrated increased thresholds to warmth and pain induced by argon laser stimulation at baseline in the area affected by PHN (Bjerring et al., 1990). After only 1 week of treatment, thresholds increased further and remained stable and elevated for the remainder of the 5-week study with application 5 times daily. The study was initially intended to be blinded and placebo-controlled, but all eight subjects experienced warmth and burning with capsaicin and could recognize the active drug. Five of the eight subjects reported pain relief, which occurred during the first week of treatment and thereafter remained stable. For the entire group, a 24% decrease in pain VAS was recorded. However, although five subjects achieved relief, only three desired to continue treatment after the study ended, and they all discontinued treatment within 1 month post-study.

The longest duration trial of capsaicin is 8 weeks in the open label study of 39 patients with PHN reported by Peikert et al. (1991). Using the 0.025% concentration, five patients dropped out due to intolerable burning, and another five reported severe burning, but remained in the study. Overall, 66% of subjects reported capsaicin-induced burning. Seven patients tried applying 5% lidocaine cream 15 min before capsaicin, but this was successful in only two patients. Of the total group, 15 were classed as nonresponders. Fourteen subjects achieved good or excellent relief of pain, with another five achieving moderate relief (the next lower category rating was 'unchanged'); all 19 were classified as responders (49%). In the 'excellent' and 'good' responders, the decline in VAS scores was an impressive 75% and five patients had completely discontinued all analgesics, including antidepressants. Perhaps due to the lower concentration of capsaicin used, onset of relief was much slower than in Bjerring's patients; only 7 of the 19 responders achieved substantial relief after 1 week of therapy. Interestingly, at long-term follow-up of these 19 responders 10–12 months later, only six continued to use capsaicin even irregularly. However, 72% of the responders remained improved.

At least four double-blind, placebo-controlled studies have been carried out, with mixed results. Drake reported no benefit of 0.025% capsaicin compared to placebo in a randomized, double-blind study, but results have not yet been published in a full length paper (Drake et al., 1990). Thirty patients, all over the age of 60, applied 0.025% capsaicin or placebo five times a day for 3 weeks. No differences were found in pain scores overall, including components of background pain, shooting pains, and hyperaesthesia.

Another multicentre placebo-controlled study of the 0.075% concentration in 143 patients treated for 6 weeks with open label follow-up was completed in 1990. In the 59 patients comprising two of the arms of that study and analysed separately, no benefit of capsaicin was found (Watson, 1991). An efficacy analysis of those completing the study showed a significant effect in favour of capsaicin although usually this did not translate into complete or satisfactory relief for most patients and burning remained an important and unresolved problem (Watson et al., 1993).

Although studies using 0.025, 0.075 and 0.10% capsaicin have been carried out, it is not clear what concentration should be recommended. From human and animal studies, it appears that the higher concentrations produce changes in sensory function more rapidly and perhaps are associated with an earlier onset of pain relief. Despite this, there does not appear to be any clear relationship of burning to capsaicin concentration in the damaged, painfully sensitive skin so characteristic of PHN. Even with the 0.025% concentration, 66% of Peikert's patients and 79% of Watson's patients reported burning. Using lidocaine cream or ointment prior to applying capsaicin does not appear particularly effective in preventing burning. In addition, burning is not always transient, and significantly limits treatment in many patients. Until an effective method for preventing or treating capsaicin-induced burning is developed, the use of capsaicin for therapy of PHN will not reach its full potential. If it is true that the severity of burning is not reliably related to concentration, then the highest concentration available should be tried first in order to provide relief as quickly as possible.

Despite the large number of basic and clinical studies of capsaicin, only limited conclusions can be drawn. First, it has been thoroughly established using laser stimulation and other techniques that capsaicin application alters unmyelinated primary afferent function in both normals and PHN patients (Arendt-Nielsen and Bjerring, 1989). Second, at least some patients achieve definite pain relief with all of the capsaicin concentrations tested so far. It is not possible to reliably estimate the percentage because of the possibility that a truly blind study cannot be carried out with capsaicin. It is clear that capsaicin is not a panacea for treatment of PHN (Watson, 1994), and the clinical literature is notable for divergent results and a lack of full reporting of the placebo-controlled clinical trials carried out to date.

3. Topical anti-inflammatory agents

Using a variety of drugs and application modes, several studies of topical inhibitors of prostaglandin synthesis have appeared since Alexander's first report in 1985 (Alexander, 1985). Results have been mixed. King (1988) has reported on powdered aspirin in chloroform; DeBenedittis et al. (1992) have reported on aspirin in ethyl ether; Morimoto et al. (1990) have reported on indomethacin, and McQuay et al. (1990) have reported on benzydamine cream. A pilot placebo-controlled trial showed aspirin superior to placebo, but longer-term use comparisons of the different compounds in this category have not been reported (DeBenedittis et al., 1992).

The proposed mechanism of action for this approach is still uncertain. Presumably, all agents tried to date in this category share common mechanisms of altering the immediate tissue environment of cutaneous nociceptors (King, 1988; Levine et al., 1988). In pain associated with tissue trauma and inflammation, increased levels of tissue prostaglandins occur. This is likely the case during the active and early post-herpetic phase. Tissue samples from a few cases of post-herpetic neuralgia have shown inflammatory cell infiltrates persisting more than 3 months after the onset of zoster. In normal skin, prostaglandin injection produces hyperalgesia that is associated with a lowering of the threshold of C-PMNs. Subdermal infusions of prostaglandin E-1, bradykinin and histamine do not produce pain when they are administered singly. Prostaglandin E-1 added to either histamine or bradykinin produces severe pain (Flower, 1974; Kuehl and Egan, 1980). The aspirin-like drugs inhibit biosynthesis of prostaglandins, but have little effect upon the release of histamine, 5-HT, bradykinin, lytic enzymes, and many other byproducts of arachidonic acid. The direct effect of aspirin at the tissue level may be desensitization of nerve terminals altered by the inflammatory process, which may involve a combination of blockade of receptors of inflammatory mediators, stabilization of neuronal membranes, and inhibition of prostaglandin synthesis (Ziel and Krupp, 1976; Neto, 1980). Interestingly, in only a subset of C-PMNs does aspirin prevent injury-induced sensitization. In other C-PMNs, not responsive to aspirin, indomethacin prevents sensitization (King, 1988).

Once PHN is well-established, it is likely that active tissue inflammation is no longer present. In theory, abnormal activity in damaged or sensitized primary afferents may produce neurogenic inflammation by release of substance P and other peptides into the skin. The peptides might then further sensitize primary afferents by evoking the local synthesis of prostaglandins and other mediators of inflammation. The cycle could continue indefinitely because of ongoing abnormal activity in damaged nerve (Levine et al., 1988). Antiprostaglandin drugs applied topically could inhibit the cycle by blocking the link between abnormal neural activity and continuing sensitization of primary afferents.

Benzydamine is a pyrazole inhibitor of prostaglandin synthetase. Applied on skin and mucous membranes in cream form, it is marketed as a topical analgesic and anti-inflammatory. The initial uncontrolled studies by Alexander and by Coniam and Hunton suggested benefit in PHN patients (Alexander, 1985; Coniam and Hunton, 1988). However, this was not confirmed in a multiple-dose, placebo-controlled, crossover study using 3% benzydamine cream by McQuay and coworkers at the Oxford Regional Pain Relief Unit in the UK. There were 23 patients with PHN of more than 5 months duration in the 6-week study. Patients received 2 weeks of active and placebo cream with a 1-week run-in period and one cream-free week during the crossover period. Patients were allowed to continue their regular analgesics and were instructed to apply the cream up to 6 times per day as needed for pain relief. The results were entirely negative on outcome measures of category pain relief scores, category pain intensity scores, analgesic use, sleep duration, and patient drug preference.

In 1988, King reported his experience with a time-honoured remedy he had learned from a local physician in Booneville, NY (King, 1988). Although King had used the technique for years, his paper recounted the effects in his most recent 12 patients with acute zoster or PHN. The technique consists of crushing two 350 mg aspirin tablets and mixing with 15–30 ml of chloroform. The cloudy suspension is then daubed onto the painful skin with a cotton ball, leaving behind a powdery residue when the chloroform evaporates. The chloroform acts as a solvent that removes desquamated skin, cutaneous

fats, waxes and oils. The suspension typically produced relief within 20 min and lasted 4–12 h. Most patients repeated the application 2–3 times per day as needed. Chloroform alone was pleasantly cooling, but gave no lasting relief. Special care was needed with lesions near the eye because of potentially damaging effects from chloroform. Kassirer reported good results in a few cases treated with crushed aspirin mixed in an over-the-counter skin cream, indicating that the vehicle may not need to be a powerful solvent, like chloroform (Kassirer, 1988).

Following King's lead, DeBenedittis et al. (1992) have reported their uncontrolled experience with 750–1500 mg of crushed acetylsalicylic acid mixed with 20–30 ml of ethyl ether in patients with acute herpetic neuralgia and PHN, and also compared this mixture with two other nonsteroidal anti-inflammatory drugs (NSAIDs) in a pilot-controlled study. In 28 patients with acute herpetic neuralgia, aspirin treatment appeared to accelerate healing and prevent development of PHN. Patients with PHN also responded. Only aspirin was superior to placebo in the 11-subject blinded comparison of aspirin, indomethacin, and diclofenac in topical form. No side effects or adverse reactions were observed. Whether or not long-term treatment was required and the frequency of dosing recommended for best results were not reported.

Using an application mode popular in Japan, Higa and colleagues reported in abstract form on the effects of indomethacin in the form of an adherent medicated cloth (stupe) (Morimoto et al., 1990). Eighteen patients with PHN were treated in this way, but the protocol details were not specified other than stating single-use evaluations and repeated-use evaluations were carried out. The authors reported that compared to aspirin in chloroform, indomethacin stupes provided equivalent analgesia and were much easier to use.

In summary, topical aspirin and nonsteroidal anti-inflammatory agents have promise. Additional research, both basic and clinical, is clearly justified in this area. Aspirin in chloroform, ethyl ether, or other vehicles have the advantage of being readily available, but the applications are messy to use and some solvents can be very irritating to mucous membranes. Indomethacin in stupe form is a more convenient way to treat PHN affecting the torso and limbs. However, if a large enough area of skin surface is treated on a continuous basis with this method, transdermal absorption of indomethacin in amounts sufficient to cause gastrointestinal upset or ulceration is possible.

4. Topical local anaesthetics

The use of local anaesthetics to control the pain of herpes zoster and PHN has a history dating back to the report by Wood (1929) of complete relief of ophthalmic PHN from injection of procaine into the supraorbital nerve. Since that time, local anaesthetics have been given to millions of patients by the epidural route, intravenously, as stellate ganglion blocks, as peripheral nerve and intercostal nerve blocks, and by nearly every other conceivable route to control the pain of acute zoster and PHN (Colding, 1971; Riopelle et al., 1984; Dan et al., 1985; Loeser, 1986; Portenoy et al., 1986; Watson and Evans, 1986; Yanagida et al., 1987). Once PHN is well established, local anaesthetic peripheral nerve, epidural or sympathetic blocks are unlikely to provide relief that is any more than temporary. For such a chronic condition, it is difficult to justify highly invasive procedures with substantial risks to gain hours or days of relief. Following the lead of the report by Secunda et al. (1941) of relief of PHN pain with subcutaneous local anaesthetic infiltration, Rowbotham and Fields (1989b) reported their experience with lidocaine infiltration in 12 patients with PHN. Nine of 12 achieved at least 50% relief, with seven achieving over 90% relief that lasted from hours to weeks from a single subcutaneous infiltration into the area of maximum pain.

The stratum corneum of intact skin presents a formidable barrier for drug delivery. Anecdotal experience in PHN patients using commercially available local anaesthetic sprays and ointments has been disappointing. Comparing a large number of available preparations in blocking pain from experimentally-induced sunburn and painful electrical stimulation, Dalili and Adriani found in 1971 that the only topically effective preparations contained the base form of the drug in relatively high concentration (Dalili and Adriani, 1971). However, most available preparations contain the drug in the hydrochloride form, which cannot pass through cell membranes, instead of the base form of the lipophilic local anaesthetics, which can. Not surprisingly, Russo et al. (1980) found that topical application of 4% lidocaine hydrochloride was ineffective in producing analgesia in intact skin, but subcutaneous infiltration and iontophoresis did affect sensation. By contrast, Niamtu et al. (1984) reported that lidocaine base 30% in cream form produced sufficient effect to allow minor skin operations.

Beginning in the early 1980s, new formulations of local anaesthetics designed specifically to penetrate intact skin and produce analgesia have appeared. EMLA® (Eutectic Mixture of Local Anesthetics), a 2.5% lidocaine base and 2.5% prilocaine base combination in emulsion cream form, has been extensively studied (Ehrenstrom and Reiz, 1982; Evers et al., 1985). EMLA application under occlusion produces sufficient sensory change to significantly reduce the pain of venipuncture, lumbar puncture, minor skin operations and harvesting skin for split-thickness skin grafts (Hallén et al., 1984, 1985; Young et al., 1987; Lahteenmaki et al., 1988). EMLA application to the forearm under occlusion for 90 min or longer produces analgesia to needle insertion for a depth of up to 5 mm (Arendt-Nielsen and Bjerring, 1988; Bjerring and Arendt-Nielsen, 1990).

Gesztes and Mezei (1988) formulated tetracaine into liposomes and compared it with tetracaine hydrochloride 1% cream in 24 normal adult volunteers. Liposomes are vesicles consisting of phospholipid membranes that can be used to encapsulate a variety of drugs, and can function as drug carriers through the stratum corneum. Using the pinprick method to assess anaesthesia of the skin, liposomal tetracaine, but not tetracaine cream, produced anaesthesia. After 1-h application under occlusion on the forearm, liposomal tetracaine made 80–95% of pinpricks painless for the 4 h of testing. By contrast, tetracaine cream made less than 10% of the pinpricks painless.

Using high-energy heat stimulation of the skin with an argon laser, Arendt-Nielsen and Bjerring have elegantly demonstrated the influence of skin thickness and vascularity in determining the time of onset and duration of analgesia with EMLA (Arendt-Nielsen et al., 1990). They compared hand dorsum, cheek, forehead, antecubital fossa and low back, using EMLA under Tegaderm® plastic occlusion. Areas with thick stratum corneum, such as the hand and antecubital fossa, had a slower onset of analgesia than the back, which has a thinner epidermis, but similar blood flow. Areas of high vascularity, such as the forehead, had a rapid onset of analgesia, but a reduced efficacy and short duration. This finding can be explained by the location of the main portion of the cutaneous free nerve endings at the dermal–epidermal junction close to the papillary capillaries. If the vascular uptake of local anaesthetic is high, the dose in the microenvironment around the nerve endings will remain low and will produce inadequate analgesia. Vascularity is an important determinant of the duration of analgesic effect. In areas of relatively low blood flow, analgesia continues for a time after the drug is wiped off the skin surface because the skin acts as a drug reservoir. In areas of high vascularity, the rate of vascular uptake may be comparable to influx of drug through the skin and no reservoir is formed. In these areas, as soon as the drug is wiped off the skin, analgesic efficacy begins to decline.

The specific analgesic mechanism of action of local anaesthetics applied topically for the pain of PHN remains unknown. Damaged, abnormally functioning or sensitized cutaneous nerve endings sending increased nociceptive signals to the spinal dorsal horn may be the main source of pain in some PHN patients. Using an isolated, perfused rabbit cornea model, which is innervated only by A-δ and C-fibres, Tanelian and MacIver (1991) have shown that local anaesthetics suppress tonic nerve fibre discharges produced by acute injury. The concentration required in the nerve environment is only 1–20 µg/ml. Damaged and regenerating nerve endings express changes in number and location of sodium channels, the tar-

get of local anaesthetic drugs. There is evidence that damaged peripheral nerve is particularly susceptible to local anaesthetics, so that abnormal tonic, evoked and ectopic activity in neuromas is suppressed by local anaesthetic concentrations far below that required to block nerve impulse conduction (Chabal et al., 1989). It therefore may not be necessary to produce the type of dermal anaesthesia required for skin operations to relieve the pain of PHN. In addition, effects of local anaesthetics in the microenvironment of damaged skin on release of peptides, mediators of inflammation and sensitization of primary afferents has been little studied and could contribute significantly to the quality and duration of pain relief achieved.

Numerous studies of topical local anaesthetics for PHN have been carried out. Rowbotham and Fields (1989a) reported success in an uncontrolled study of 11 patients using 10% lidocaine base in a gel vehicle formulated to penetrate intact skin. Kissin et al. (1989) mixed lidocaine in glycerin and reported their clinical experience that relief of varying duration, sometimes prolonged, was the norm. Stow et al. (1989) reported significant pain reduction in an uncontrolled study of 12 patients with PHN treated with EMLA cream under an occlusive dressing for 24 h. For the entire group, pain intensity scores were lowest at 6 h after application, but the subset with trigeminal PHN had reduced pain intensity beginning at 2 h and lasting until 10 h after application.

Rowbotham and coworkers have reported a randomized, double-blind, vehicle-controlled study of 5% lidocaine in gel form (Rowbotham et al., 1995). A total of 39 patients completed the three-session study. The 16 patients with facial or upper cervical PHN had gel applied without an occlusive dressing during the 8-h sessions, and the 23 patients with torso or limb PHN had gel applied under Tegaderm® occlusion for 24 h. In order to obtain data on gel effects and systemic absorption of lidocaine through normal and post-herpetic skin, both the painful area and the matching contralateral area of skin were treated with gel during each session. One session was a double-placebo session, one session consisted of lidocaine gel application to the painful area and vehicle to contralateral normal skin, and one session consisted of lidocaine gel application to the matching contralateral normal skin and vehicle on the painful area. A significant decrease in pain intensity VAS and a significant increase in pain relief scores were found with lidocaine gel compared to vehicle at 8 and 24 h in the torso/limb group. In the facial/upper cervical group, there were no significant differences between active drug and vehicle in pain intensity VAS scores, but pain relief scores significantly favoured active drug at nearly all time points. Thirteen of the 16 patients in the facial/upper cervical group of the study described above requested open label treatment with lidocaine gel. Follow-up for up to 14 months duration indicated that 10 of the 13 continued to use it as needed. For many patients with PHN affecting the torso and limbs, Tegaderm or plastic food wrap as occlusive dressings over EMLA cream or lidocaine gel have proven cumbersome to use long term.

Lidocaine has been formulated into adhesive patches (Lidoderm®) with a soft, woven, stretchy backing that can be applied to cover the area of pain. A randomized, placebo-controlled trial (Rowbotham et al., 1996) demonstrated benefit of Lidoderm patches. Thirty-five subjects with PHN affecting the torso or extremities completed a four-session, random-order, double-blind, vehicle-controlled study of the analgesic effects of this patch. Lidoderm patches were applied in two of the four 12-h-long sessions. In one session, vehicle patches were applied and one session was a no-treatment observation session. Lidocaine-containing patches significantly reduced pain intensity at all time points from 20 min to 12 h compared to no treatment observation and at all time points at 4–12 h compared to vehicle patches. Lidoderm patches were superior to both no-treatment observations and vehicle patches in averaged category pain relief scores. Minimal systemic absorption was documented. No systemic side effects occurred and patches were well tolerated on allodynic skin for 12 h. The majority of subjects reported partial pain relief with 10 of 35 noting moderate or better relief.

A randomized, vehicle-controlled trial (Galer et al., 1999) addressed the issue of the contribution of the patch alone versus the Lidoderm patch in providing relief in PHN since the patch itself appeared to offer some relief. This study utilized an enriched enrollment design since all subjects had been successfully treated with topical lidocaine patches on a regular basis for 1 month prior to study enrollment. The Lidoderm patch was found to provide significantly more pain relief for PHN than did the vehicle patch. The US Food and Drug Administration has approved Lidoderm for the specific indication of PHN pain.

In summary, topical local anaesthetics hold significant promise for the treatment of PHN pain. Side effects are minor, and blood levels of lidocaine have been very low (Evers et al., 1985; Rowbotham and Fields, 1989a; Stow et al., 1989; Rowbotham et al., 1996). More longer-term use data is needed. The relationship between change in sensation produced by the drug and pain relief needs further exploration.

5. Conclusions

Three categories of topical agents for PHN pain have now received substantial study. Capsaicin remains the most controversial of the topical agents. Several hundred patients have now participated in controlled and uncontrolled clinical trials, and two concentrations have been commercially available and in widespread use for several years. Yet, even in larger-scale studies, there is a wide divergence in reported results, with some investigators reporting no benefit in well-designed, controlled studies. Others have reported success rates for capsaicin that seem extraordinarily high for a condition long thought to be among the most intractable of chronic pain syndromes, and substantially higher than shown in controlled studies of antidepressants, the 'gold standard' for treatment of PHN. Crushed aspirin in either chloroform or ethyl ether is internationally available and the topical lidocaine patch (Lidoderm®) has been approved in the USA. EMLA® is available outside the USA.

Patient selection for use of all topical agents is an important, but often overlooked issue. In the study of EMLA® for PHN pain carried out by Stow et al. (1989), only patients who had obtained pain relief from subcutaneous injection of a local anaesthetic–steroid combination were invited to participate. In the controlled studies by Rowbotham et al. (1995, 1996), only patients with a component of superficial pain and areas of painfully sensitive skin on examination were allowed to participate. It is not known to what degree this could be a factor in trials of other topical agents for PHN.

At least with the local anaesthetics, it seems logical that subcutaneous infiltration prior to initiating topical treatment would have some predictive value. At the present time, there are no practical and accepted ways of doing this with the anti-inflammatories and capsaicin compounds. Although PHN may seem a homogenous disorder due to its aetiology and ease of diagnosis, experience from seeing hundreds of patients with this disorder is that symptomatology is quite variable. A subset, though undoubtedly the majority, have pain that seems potentially treatable with topical agents. Until factors predicting success with the topical drugs reviewed here (and the proven systemic therapies, such as antidepressants) are clearly identified, how to choose the best treatment modality for individual PHN patients will remain uncertain.

Acknowledgements

Dr. Rowbotham is supported by Grants RO-1 NS39521, P50 NS21445, and K-24 NS02164 from the National Institute of Neurological Disorders and Stroke. Dr. Rowbotham has received educational support, consulting fees, and other income from Endo Pharmaceuticals (the North American licensee for Lidoderm®).

References

Alexander, J. (1985) Post-herpetic neuralgia. Anaesthesia, 40: 1133–1134.

Anand, P., Bloom, S.R. and McGregor, G.P. (1983) Topical capsaicin pretreatment inhibits axon reflex vasodilatation caused by somatostatin and vasoactive intestinal polypeptide in human skin. Br. J. Pharmacol., 78: 665–669.

Arendt-Nielsen, L. and Bjerring, P. (1988) Laser-induced pain for evaluation of local analgesia: a comparison of topical application (EMLA) and local injection (lidocaine). Anesth. Analg., 67: 115–123.

Arendt-Nielsen, L. and Bjerring P. (1989) Use of a new argon laser technique to evaluate changes in sensory and pain thresholds in human skin following topical capsaicin treatment. Skin. Pharmacol., 2: 162–167.

Arendt-Nielsen, L., Bjerring, P. and Nielsen, J. (1990) Regional variations in analgesic efficacy of EMLA cream. Acta. Dermatol. Venereol. (Stockholm), 70: 314–318.

Bernstein, J.E. (1988) Capsaicin in postherpetic neuralgia, Resid. Staff Physician, October.

Bernstein, J.E., Bickers, D.R., Dahl, M.V. and Roshal, J.Y. (1987) Treatment of chronic postherpetic neuralgia with topical capsaicin. J. Am. Acad. Dermatol., 17: 93–96.

Bernstein, J.E., Korman, N.J., Bickers, D.R., Dahl, M.V. and Millikan, L.E. (1989) Topical capsaicin treatment of chronic postherpetic neuralgia. J. Am. Acad. Dermatol., 21: 265–270.

Bjerring, P. and Arendt-Nielsen, L. (1990) Depth and duration of skin analgesia to needle insertion after topical application of EMLA cream. Br. J. Anaesth., 64: 173–177.

Bjerring, P., Arendt-Nielsen, L. and Soderberg, U. (1990) Argon laser induced cutaneous sensory and pain thresholds in postherpetic neuralgia: quantitative modulation by topical capsaicin. Acta Dermatol. Venereol., 70: 121–125.

Buck, S.H. and Burks, T.F. (1986) The neuropharmacology of capsaicin: Review of some recent observations. Pharmacol. Rev., 38: 179–226.

Chabal, C., Russell, L.C. and Burchiel, K.J. (1989) The effect of intravenous lidocaine, tocainide and mexiletine on spontaneously active fibers originating in rat sciatic neuromas. Pain, 38: 333–338.

Colding, A. (1971) Treatment of pain: Organization of a pain clinic: treatment of acute herpes zoster. Proc. R. Soc. Med., 66: 541–543.

Coniam, S.W. and Hunton, J.J. (1988) A study of benzydamine cream in post-herpetic neuralgia. Res. Clin. Forums, 10: 65–66.

Cotton, P. (1990) Compliance problems, placebo effect cloud trials of topical analgesic. J. Am. Med. Assoc., 264: 13–14.

Dalili, H. and Adriani, J. (1971) The efficacy of local anesthetics in blocking the sensations of itch, burning, and pain in normal and 'sunburned' skin. Clin. Pharmacol. Ther., 12: 913–919.

Dan, K., Higa, K. and Noda, B. (1985) Nerve block for herpetic pain. In: H. Fields, R. Dubner and F. Cervero (Eds.), Advances in Pain Research and Therapy, Vol. 9. Raven Press, New York, pp. 831–838.

DeBenedittis, G., Besana, F. and Lorenzetti, A. (1992) A new topical treatment for acute herpetic neuralgia and postherpetic neuralgia: the aspirin/diethyl ether mixture. An open label study plus a double-blind controlled clinical trial. Pain, 48: 383–390.

Dickenson, A.H. (1991) Capsaicin: gaps in our knowledge start to be filled. Trends Neurosci., 14: 265–266.

Drake, H.F., Harries, A.J., Gamester, G.E. et al. (1990) Randomised double-blind study of topical capsaicin for treatment of post-herpetic neuralgia. Pain, 5 (Suppl.): S58 (abstract).

Dray, A., Bettaney, J. and Forster, P. (1990) Actions of capsaicin on peripheral nociceptors of the neonatal rat spinal cord-tail in vitro: dependence of extracellular ions and independence of second messengers. Br. J. Pharmacol., 101: 727–733.

Ehrenstrom, G.M.E. and Reiz, S.L.A. (1982) EMLA — a eutectic mixture of local anesthetics for topical anesthesia. Acta Anaesthesiol. Scand., 26: 596–598.

Evers, H., VonDardel, O., Johlin, L., Ohlsen L. and Vinnars, E. (1985) Dermal effects of compositions based on the eutectic mixture of lignocaine and prilocaine (EMLA). Br. J. Anaesth., 57: 997–1000.

Flower, R.I. (1974) Drugs which inhibit prostaglandin biosynthesis. Pharmacol. Rev., 62: 33–67.

Galer, B.S., Rowbotham, M.C., Perander, J. and Friedman, E. (1999) Topical lidocaine patch relieves postherpetic neuralgia more effectively than a vehicle topical patch: results of an enriched enrollment study. Pain, 80: 533–538.

Gesztes, A. and Mezei, M. (1988) Topical anesthesia of the skin by liposome-encapsulated tetracaine. Anesth. Analg., 67: 1079–1081.

Hallén, B., Olsson, G.L. and Uppfeldt, A. (1984) Pain-free venipuncture. Anaesthesia, 39: 969–972.

Hallén, B., Carlsson, P. and Uppfeldt, A. (1985) Clinical study of a lignocaine–prilocaine cream to relieve the pain of venepuncture. Br. J. Anaesth., 57: 326–328.

Jancso, G., Kiraly, E. and Jancso-Gabor, A. (1977) Pharmacologically induced selective degeneration of chemosensitive primary sensory neurons. Nature (London), 270: 741–742.

Jancso, G., Kiraly, E., Joo, F., Such, G. and Nagy, A. (1985) Selective degeneration by capsaicin of a subpopulation of primary sensory neurons in the adult rat. Neurosci. Lett., 59: 209–214.

Kassirer, M.R. (1988) King and Robert: Concerning the management of pain associated with herpes zoster and of post-herpetic neuralgia [Pain 33 (1988) 73–78]. Pain, 35: 368–369.

King, R.B. (1988) Concerning the management of pain associated with herpes zoster and of postherpetic neuralgia. Pain, 33: 73–78.

Kissin, I., McDanal, J. and Xavier, A.V. (1989) Topical lidocaine for relief of superficial pain in postherpetic neuralgia. Neurology, 39: 1132–1133.

Kuehl, F.A. and Egan, R.W. (1980) Prostaglandins, arachidonic acid and inflammation. Science, 210: 978–984.

Lahteenmaki, T., Lillieborg, M., Ohlsen, L., Olenius M. and Strombek, J.O. (1988) Topical analgesia for the cutting of split-skin grafts: a multicenter comparison of two doses of a lidocaine/prilocaine cream. Plast. Reconstr. Surg., 82: 458–462.

Levine, J.D., Coderre, T.J. and Basbaum, A.I. (1988) The peripheral nervous system and the inflammatory process. In: R. Dubner, G.F. Gebhart and M.R. Bonds (Eds.), Proc. Vth World Congress on Pain. Elsevier, Amsterdam, pp. 33–43.

Loeser, J.D. (1986) Herpes zoster and postherpetic neuralgia. Pain, 25: 149–164.

Lynn, B. (1990) Capsaicin: actions on nociceptive C-fibres and therapeutic potential. Pain, 41: 61–69.

Lynn, B., Pini, A. and Baranowski, R. (1987) Injury of somatosensory afferents by capsaicin: selectivity and failure to regenerate. In: L.M. Pubols and B.J. Sessle (Eds.), Effects of Injury on Trigeminal and Spinal Somatosensory Systems. Alan R. Liss, New York, pp: 115–124.

McQuay, H.J., Carroll, D., Moxon, A., Glynn, C.J. and Moore, R.A. (1990) Benzydamine cream for the treatment of post-herpetic neuralgia: minimum duration of treatment periods in a cross-over trial. Pain, 40: 131–135.

Morimoto, M., Inamori, K. and Hyodo, M. (1990) The effect of indomethacin stupe for post-herpetic neuralgia — particularly in comparison with chloroform–aspirin solution. Pain, 5 (Suppl.): S59 (abstract).

Neto, F.R. (1980) Further studies on the action of salicylates on nerve membranes. Eur. J. Pharmacol., 68: 155–162.

Niamtu, J. III, Campbell, R.L. and Garrett, M.S. (1984) The anesthetic skin patch for topical anesthesia. J Oral Maxillofac. Surg., 42: 839–840.

Nolano, M., Simone, D.A., Wendelschafer-Crabb, G., Johnson, T., Hazen, E. and Kennedy, W.R. (1999) Topical capsaicin in humans: parallel loss of epidermal nerve fibers and pain sensation. Pain, 81: 135–145.

Noordenbos, W. (1959) Pain. Elsevier, Amsterdam, 185 pp.

Nurmikko, T. (1991) Neuropathic pain. Academic dissertation. University of Tampere, Finland, 95 pp.

Nurmikko, T. and Bowsher, D. (1990) Somatosensory findings in postherpetic neuralgia. J. Neurol. Neurosurg. Psychiatry, 53: 135–141.

Peikert, A., Hentrich, M. and Ochs, G. (1991) Topical 0.025 and percent; capsaicin in chronic post-herpetic neuralgia: efficacy, predictors of response and long-term course. J. Neurol., 238: 452–456.

Petersen, K.L., Fields, H.L., Brennum, J., Sandroni, P. and Rowbotham, M.C. (2000) Capsaicin activation of 'irritable' nociceptors in post-herpetic neuralgia. Pain, 88: 125–133.

Petsche, U., Fleischer, E., Lembeck, F. and Handwerker, H.O. (1983) The effect of capsaicin application to a peripheral nerve on impulse conduction in functionally identified afferent nerve fibres. Brain Res., 265: 233–240.

Pini, A., Baranowski, R. and Lynn, B. (1990) Long term reduction in the number of C-fibre nociceptors following capsaicin treatment of a cutaneous nerve in adult rats. Eur. J. Neurosci., 2: 89–97.

Portenoy, R.K. and Foley, K.M. (1986) Chronic use of opioid

analgesics in non-malignant pain: Report of 38 cases. Pain, 25: 171–186.

Portenoy, R.K., Duma, C. and Foley, K.M. (1986) Acute herpetic and postherpetic neuralgia: clinical review and current management. Ann. Neurol., 20: 651–664.

Riopelle, J.M., Naraghi, M. and Grush, K.P. (1984) Chronic neuralgia incidence following local anesthetic therapy for herpes zoster. Arch. Dermatol., 120: 747–750.

Rowbotham, M.C. and Fields, H.L. (1989a) Topical lidocaine reduces pain in post-herpetic neuralgia. Pain, 38: 297–302.

Rowbotham, M.C. and Fields, H.L. (1989b) Post-herpetic neuralgia: the relation of pain complaint, sensory disturbance, and skin temperature. Pain, 39: 129–144.

Rowbotham, M.C., Reisner, L.A. and Fields, H.L. (1991) Both intravenous lidocaine and morphine reduce the pain of postherpetic neuralgia. Neurology, 41: 1024–1028.

Rowbotham, M.C., Davies, P.S. and Fields, H.L. (1995) Topical lidocaine gel relieves postherpetic neuralgia. Ann. Neurol., 37: 246–253.

Rowbotham, M.C., Davies, P.S., Verkernpinck, C. and Galer, B.S. (1996) Lidocaine patch: double-blind controlled study of a new treatment method for postherpetic neuralgia. Pain, 65: 39–44.

Rowbotham, M.C., Harden, N., Stacey, B., Bernstein, P. and Magnus-Miller, L. (1998) Gabapentin for the treatment of postherpetic neuralgia. JAMA 280: 1837–1842.

Russo, J., Lipman, A.G., Comstock, T.J., Page, B.C. and Stephen, R.L. (1980) Lidocaine anesthesia: comparison of iontophoresis, injection, and swabbing. Am. J. Hosp. Pharm., 37: 843–847.

Secunda, L., Wolf, W. and Price, J. (1941) Herpes zoster: local anesthesia in the treatment of pain. New Engl. J. Med., 224: 501–503.

Simone, D.A., Ngeow, J.Y.F., Putterman, G.J. and LaMotte, R.H. (1987) Hyperalgesia to heat after intradermal injection of capsaicin. Brain Res., 418: 201–203.

Simone, D.A., Baumann, T.K. and LaMotte, R.H. (1989) Dose-dependent pain and mechanical hyperalgesia in humans after intradermal injection of capsaicin. Pain, 38: 99–107.

Stewart, J.M., Getto, C.J., Neldner, K., Reeve, E.B., Kirvoy, W.A. and Zimmerman, E. (1976) Substance P and analgesia. Nature, 262: 784–785.

Stow, P.J., Glynn, C.J. and Minor, B. (1989) EMLA cream in the treatment of post-herpetic neuralgia: efficacy and pharmacokinetic profile. Pain, 39: 301–305.

Tanelian, D.L. and MacIver, M.B. (1991) Analgesic concentrations of lidocaine suppress tonic A-delta and C fiber discharge produced by acute injury. Anesthesiology, 74: 934–936.

Watson, C.P.N. (1991) Presentation at 10th annual scientific meeting of American Pain Society, November.

Watson, C.P.N. (1994) Topical capsaicin as an adjuvant analgesic. J. Pain Symptom Manage., 9: 425–433.

Watson, C.P.N. and Babul, N. (1998) Efficacy of oxycodone in neuropathic pain: a randomized trial in postherpetic neuralgia. Neurology, 50: 1837–1841.

Watson, C.P.N. and Evans, R.J. (1986) Postherpetic neuralgia: A review. Arch. Neurol., 43: 836–840.

Watson, C.P.N., Evans, R.J. and Watt, V.R. (1988) Postherpetic neuralgia and topical capsaicin. Pain, 33: 333–340.

Watson, C.P.N., Watt, V.R., Chipman, M., Birkett, N. and Evans, R.J. (1991) The prognosis with postherpetic neuralgia. Pain, 46: 195–199.

Watson, C.P.N., Tyler, K.L., Bickers, D.R., Millikan, L.E. (1993) A randomized, vehicle-controlled, trial of topical capsaicin in the treatment of postherpetic neuralgia. Clin. Ther., 15: 510–526.

Wood, H. (1929) Herpes zoster ophthalmicus complicated by persistent neuritis. Am. J. Ophthalmol., 12: 759–760.

Yanagida, H., Suwa, K. and Corssen, G. (1987) No prophylactic effect of early sympathetic blockade on postherpetic neuralgia. Anesthesiology, 66: 73–76.

Young, A.C., Shorthall, A., Haynes, W. and Young, G. (1987) Lignocaine–prilocaine cream for lumbar puncture. Lancet, 2: 1533.

Ziel, R. and Krupp, P. (1976) Significance of the membrane stabilizing effect of non-narcotic analgesics. In: J.J. Bonica and D. Albe-Fessard (Eds.), Advances in Pain Research and Therapy, Vol. 1. Raven Press, New York, pp. 517–521.

Herpes Zoster and Postherpetic Neuralgia, 2nd Revised and Enlarged Edition
Pain Research and Clinical Management, Vol. 11
Edited by C.P.N. Watson and A.A. Gershon

The medical treatment of postherpetic neuralgia: antidepressants, anticonvulsants, opioids and practical guidelines for management

C. Peter N. Watson [*]

Department of Medicine, University of Toronto and 1 Sir Williams Lane, Toronto, ON M9A 1T8, Canada

1. Overview

The efficient physician is the man that successfully amuses his patients while nature effects a cure.

Philosophical dictionary, Voltaire (1694–1778)

Of the terrible doubt of appearances. Of the uncertainty after all — that we may be deluded.

Leaves of Grass, Walt Whitman (1819–1882)

It is possible that Voltaire has described much of what has passed for therapy in herpes zoster (HZ) and postherpetic neuralgia (PHN) over the years, since most patients improve with time especially in the first month after the onset of HZ. Walt Whitman further expresses what may be the apparently favourable results of uncontrolled trials in these conditions because of this. This chapter will review both randomized controlled trials and less rigorously studied preventive approaches and treatments for PHN. My bias from clinical experience, research and the literature is that antidepressants, although seriously limited by side effects and incomplete, or in some cases lack of efficacy, are the most consistently use-

ful approaches. The anticonvulsant gabapentin is an alternative, has been proven useful by a single controlled trial and may be attractive because of its side effect profile. Opioids are an option in refractory cases. Topical agents are fully discussed in Chapter 21. Other therapies may have benefit in occasional patients with specific, differing pain mechanisms and so trials of these in refractory patients may be justified both because of this and to mark time, perhaps obtaining placebo relief with the hope for the natural resolution with time that may occur even with PHN of long duration (Watson et al., 1991). Despite all these measures, at least 30% of patients with PHN remain either completely refractory or unsatisfactorily relieved by the best we have to offer, and new approaches to this vexing problem are sorely needed.

2. The prevention of postherpetic neuralgia

One may separate management into the prevention of PHN, by treatment at the stage of HZ, and the treatment of established PHN (that which persists for

---

* Correspondence to: Dr. C.P.N. Watson, Department of Medicine, University of Toronto and 1 Sir Williams Lane, Toronto, ON M9A 1T8, Canada. E-mail: peter.watson@utoronto.ca

TABLE I

Agents used to prevent postherpetic neuralgia

Agent	Source	Study population [1]	Effective?	N/N [1]	C	R	D
Levodopa and benserazide	Kernbaum and Hauchecorne (1981)	HZ	Yes, at 23 days; No, at 60 days	25/47	Y	Y	Y
Vidarabine	Whitley et al. (1982)	HZ, I−	Reduced duration but not incidence	63/121	Y	Y	Y
Interferon-α	Merigan et al. (1978)	HZ, cancer	Reduced severity and duration	45/90	Y	Y	Y
Acyclovir	Peterslund et al. (1981)	HZ, I+	N	Low dose, 27/56	Y	Y	Y
				High dose, 19/29	Y	Y	Y
	Bean et al. (1982)	HZ, I+	N	19/29	Y	Y	Y
	Balfour et al. (1983)	HZ, I±	N	94	Y	Y	Y
Valacyclovir	Beutner et al. (1995)	HZ	Y	?	Y	Y	Y
Famciclovir	Tyring et al. (1995)	HZ	Y	?	Y	Y	Y
Acyclovir vs. vidarabine	Shepp et al. (1986)	HZ, I±	No difference	22	Y	N	N
Adenosine monophosphate	Sklar et al. (1985)	HZ	Y	17/32	Y	Y	Y
Steroids							
Triamcinolone	Eaglstein et al. (1970)	HZ	Y	15/35	Y	Y	Y
Prednisolone	Keczkes and Basheer (1980)	HZ	Y	20/40	Y	Y	N
ACTH, prednisone	Clemmensen and Anderson (1984)	HZ	N	36/60	Y	Y	Y
Prednisolone	Esmann et al. (1987)	HZ	N	39/78	Y	Y	Y
	Wood ct al. (1994)	HZ	N	349/400	Y	Y	Y
Prednisone	Whitley et al. (1996)	HZ	N	201/208	Y	Y	Y
Sympathetic block							
1% Lidocaine hydrochloride with norepinephrine bitartrate	Colding (1969)	HZ	Y	71/303	N		
	Colding (1973)	HZ	Y	155/483	N		
Bupivacaine	Riopelle et al. (1984)	HZ	N	72	N		
Mepivacaine	Dan et al. (1983)	HZ	Y	470	N		
	Dan et al. (1985)	HZ	Y	529	N		
	Yanagida et al. (1987)	HZ	N	49	N		
Amantadine	Galbraith (1983)	HZ	Y	33/67	Y	Y	Y

[1] HZ, herpes zoster; I+, immunocompetent; I±, immunocompromised; I−, immunosuppressed; *N/N*, number of patients treated/total number of patients. Trials: C, controlled; R, randomized; D, double blind.

longer than 1 month). The approaches to prophylactic therapy are summarized in Table I. The efficacy of antiviral agents is dealt with by Richard Whitley in Chapter 6 and by Anne Gershon in Chapter 10. Both uncontrolled and controlled trials have claimed a preventive effect by the use of corticosteroids. This very controversial subject has been addressed by Drs. Barbara Post and John Philbrick in Chapter 18. There have been conflicting reports of the effectiveness of sympathetic blocks employed at the stage of HZ to prevent the development of PHN. Dr. Perry Fine discusses this approach in Chapter 20.

Galbraith (1983) reported a randomized, double-blind, placebo-controlled trial of amantadine hydrochloride for the acute illness in a population with a mean age of 70 years. He found a reduction by half in the time taken to achieve total pain relief with this agent. A double-blind, placebo-controlled study of levodopa and benserazide (Kernbaum and Hauchecorne, 1981) claimed a reduction in PHN in patients 65 years of age and older. Although a difference was detected at 31 days, no such effect was present at 60 days after the onset of the rash. A randomized, placebo-controlled, double-blind trial of intramuscular adenosine monophosphate (AMP) has been reported to markedly reduce PHN (Sklar et al., 1985). The number of patients in this trial was small and concern has been raised that the groups were not comparable as to severity of disease and also about the toxicity of AMP in humans (Sherlock and Corey, 1985). Bowsher has suggested that early treatment with amitriptyline may prevent PHN (Bowsher, 1996). Although unproven, early aggressive acute pain management with opioids if necessary may prevent central sensitization and PHN.

3. The treatment of established postherpetic neuralgia

A summary of various treatments reported to be effective for PHN is presented in Table II.

3.1. Antidepressants

A large number of studies support the utility of antidepressants in a variety of chronic pain problems (Feinmann, 1985; Getto et al., 1987; Goodkin and Gullion, 1989; McQuay et al., 1996; Sindrup and Jensen, 1999). An important part of this literature concerns favourable, well-designed trials of the use of these agents in neuropathic pain, particularly PHN. PHN is a particularly good model of neuropathic pain for drug trials because, if patients are chosen carefully, the pain is fairly chronically stable over time and sufficient numbers of cases can be readily obtained. Antidepressant therapy as opposed to many other putative therapies of this difficult problem, has come to have a sound, scientific basis. Further research in this direction may shed light on this therapy, of at least some of the broader range of less-common neuropathic pain problems which are therefore more difficult to study. These disorders, however, may have heterogeneous mechanisms both between disorders and within a particular dis-

ease entity. This section will review the evolution of investigation into the antidepressant therapy of PHN.

Woodforde et al. (1965) were the first to recognize that amitriptyline could afford relief in truly chronic postherpetic pain problems. They thought that all 14 of their patients were depressed and that was their rationale for using the drug. Their uncontrolled study used an initial dose of 10 mg 4 times a day gradually increasing to 25 mg 4 times a day, achieving good pain relief in 11 patients from 1 to 11 months. Taub (1973) reported successfully treating five subjects with PHN of greater than 3 months' duration with amitriptyline combined with a phenothiazine (fluphenazine, perphenazine or thioridazine). In a later publication, Taub and Collins (1974) used amitriptyline 75 mg with fluphenazine 1 mg 3 times a day in 17 patients with pain of longer than 1 year's duration. Their patients had good relief in both studies, with some mild residual pain at 3–6 years of follow-up. The authors commented on their belief in the lack of efficacy of amitriptyline alone and said that they used it mainly to combat the depressant action of the other drug.

Based on empirical experience, we became convinced that amitriptyline by itself resulted in pain relief in PHN and also thought that phenothiazines alone were ineffective. We also observed that most patients did not seem very depressed except in some cases as a secondary response to pain. We therefore conducted a double-blind, placebo-controlled crossover trial of amitriptyline in 24 patients with this disorder (Watson et al., 1982). All patients had PHN of more than 3 months' duration and good results were achieved in 16 of 24 (67%). Most patients were not depressed, and pain relief occurred without a change in depression ratings in most patients, indicating that the drug appeared to result in pain relief independently of its antidepressant effect. This analgesia occurred at lower doses than usually used to treat depression (median 75 mg). Follow-up was a median 12 months with good results maintained in 12 of 22 (55%). By using small doses (10–25 mg) to start and small increments in this study significant side effects were few. A subsequent trial by Max et al. (1988b) has corroborated these results.

TABLE II

Treatment of postherpetic neuralgia (PHN)

Source	Agent	PHN[1]	Effect?	N	Trial was[1]			
					C	X/P	R	D
Antidepressants and neuroleptics								
Farber and Burks (1974)	Chlorprothixene	Some	Y	30	N			
Nathan (1978)	Chlorprothixene	Y	N	13	Y	X	Y	Y
Nathan (1978)	Chlorprothixene	Y	N	19	N			
Woodforde et al. (1965)	Amitriptyline	Y	Y	14	N			
Taub (1973)	Amitriptyline and perphenazine or fluphenazine or thioridazine	Y	Y	5	N			
Taub and Collins (1974)	Amitriptyline plus fluphenazine	Y	Y	17	N			
Watson et al. (1982)	Amitriptyline	Y	Y	24	Y	X	Y	Y
Max et al. (1988b)	Amitriptyline	Y	Y	58	Y	X	Y	Y
Watson et al. (1985)	Zimelidine	Y	N	15	Y	X	N	N
Watson et al. (1988)	Amitriptyline, nortriptyline	Y	Y	123	N	X	N	N
Kishore-Kumar et al. (1989)	Desipramine	Y	Y	26	Y	X	Y	Y
Watson et al. (1998)	Amitriptyline, nortriptyline	Y	Y	31	Y	X	Y	Y
Opioids								
Watson and Babul (1998)	Oxycodone	Y	Y	50	Y	X	Y	Y
Anticonvulsants								
Killian and Fromm (1968)	Carbamazepine	L	N	6	Y	X	Y	Y
Hatangdi et al. (1976)	Carbamazepine or phenytoin plus nortriptyline	Y	Y	34	N			
Gerson et al. (1977)	Carbamazepine plus clomipramine	Y	Y	16	Y[2]	X	Y	N
Raftery (1979)	Valproic acid plus amitriptyline	Y	Y	20	N			
Rowbotham (1998)	Gabapentin	Y	Y	229	Y	P	Y	Y
Local anesthetic spray and/or vibration								
Russell et al. (1957)	Vibration	?	Y	100	N			
Taverner (1950)	Ethyl chloride	Y	Y	16	N			
Todd et al. (1965)	Ethyl chloride and vibration	Y	Y	86	N			
Sympathetic block								
Colding (1969)	1% Lidocaine with noradrenaline	Y	N	34	N			
Colding (1973)	1% Lidocaine with noradrenaline	Y	N	67	N			
Transcutaneous nerve stimulation (TENS)								
Nathan and Wall (1974)	Continuous TENS	Y	Y	30	N			
Gerson et al. (1977)	Intermittent TENS	Y	N	17	N			
Haas (1977)	TENS	Y	Y	11	N			
Acupuncture								
Lewith et al. (1983)	Acupuncture	Y	N	30/62	Y[3]	N	Y	N
Epidural steroids								
Forrest (1980)	Methyl-prednisolone	Y	Y	37	N			
Intrathecal steroids								
Kotani et al. (2000)	Methyl-prednisolone	Y	Y	82/89	Y	P	Y	Y

Y = yes; N = no; *N* = number.

[1] PHN Y_1 >1 month; L, long-standing. Trials: C, controlled; X, crossover; P, parallel; R, randomized; D, double blind.

[2] Versus TENS.   [3] Versus mock TENS.

Amitriptyline has severe limitations in the long term because of intolerable side effects and the fact that relief is rarely complete and occurs in only about two-thirds of patients. One action of this drug is to potentiate both serotonin and noradrenaline which are thought to be inhibitory neurotransmitters in systems descending from the brainstem on to the dorsal horn of the spinal cord. Subsequent research has explored whether selective serotonergic or noradrenergic agents might be more effective and have fewer untoward effects.

Experience with serotonergic agents (clomipramine, trasodone, nefasodone, fluoxetine and zimelidine) in PHN has been disappointing (Watson and Evans, 1985; Watson et al., 1988; Kishore-Kumar et al., 1989). The evidence supporting the use of noradrenergic agents is more compelling (Watson et al., 1988, 1992, 1998; Max et al., 1988a,b; Kishore-Kumar et al., 1990).

Desipramine, a selective norepinephrine re-uptake inhibitor, has been shown to be more effective than placebo in this disease and pain relief with that drug as well was not mediated by mood elevation (Kishore-Kumar et al., 1990). Although reported to have few side effects, we do not know how it compares to amitriptyline.

A randomized, double-blind trial was conducted comparing maprotiline (noradrenergic) with amitriptyline, attempting to answer the question as to whether such an agent possesses greater analgesia and effectiveness for PHN (Watson et al., 1992). Although we found amitriptyline to be more effective, nine patients responded equally well to both drugs and seven responded only to maprotiline. Thus, 16 of 32 patients (50%) completing the trial may have had predominantly noradrenergic pain-inhibiting systems, whereas eight other responders required an agent with an effect on serotonin and noradrenaline (amitriptyline). All three aspects to the pain of PHN responded to treatment, that is, steady pain, brief (jabbing) pain and pain on tactile skin contact. We found side effects troublesome with both agents, therefore limiting effectiveness. Again, most patients were not depressed and pain relief occurred in most without change in depression-rating scales.

A blinded, randomized trial compared amitriptyline with nortriptyline (more noradrenergic) and found equal efficacy, but less intolerable side effects with nortriptyline (Watson et al., 1998). Based on this information, we believe the initial antidepressant of choice is amitriptyline or nortriptyline. If these fail we would then try selective noradrenergic agents such as desipramine or maprotiline.

Despite the negative results with serotonergic agents in large numbers of patients, occasional patients appear to respond to serotonergic drugs. This may, however, be due to other factors than a true pharmacological action.

The dosing guidelines are similar for amitriptyline, nortriptyline, and maprotiline. In those patients 65 years of age or under, we suggest, depending on body weight, starting with 25 mg at bedtime, and in the age group over 65, we suggest 10 mg. The dose may be increased every 1–2 weeks by 25 or 10 mg until pain relief occurs or side effects supervene. Despite careful follow-up and dosage titration, complete pain relief is unusual. About one-third of patients will not respond well and the side effects of the drugs may be troublesome so that the search for more effective, better tolerated agents of this sort must continue.

3.2. Neuroleptics

Farber and Burks (1974) used high doses of chlorprothixene in patients with postherpetic pain for a duration of 2 days to 8 weeks. In an uncontrolled study of 30 subjects of unstated age, they found total relief of pain within 72 h in all save one. Nathan (1978) attempted to duplicate this work in established PHN (median duration 1 year) by the same method and also by a lower dose, double-blind, placebo-controlled study. He concluded that dosages under 100 mg/24 h were ineffective. He thought that the high-dose regimen helped about one-third of patients, but only in the short term and with a high incidence of side effects. An initial dose of 10 mg 4 times a day was used, achieving at least good relief in 11 patients for 1–11 months. Taub (1973) reported treating five subjects with PHN of over 3 months' duration with amitriptyline and a phenothiazine (perphenazine, fluphenazine, or thioridazine). In a later publication, Taub and Collins (1974) used amitriptyline hydrochloride, 75 mg every night with fluphenazine, 1 mg 3 times a day, in 17 patients with pain of duration longer than 1 year. The subjects in both studies had good relief with some mild residual pain at 6 months to 3 years follow-up. Taub commented on his impression of the ineffectiveness of amitriptyline alone, using it mainly to combat the depressive potential of the phenothiazine. There has been no placebo-controlled trial of a phenothiazine alone in PHN. I believe that beneficial effects seen with the combination of an antidepressant and phenothiazine are due to the antidepressant, the efficacy of which has been proven by controlled trials. I have seen occasional patients improve on different phenothiazines, but have never been certain that the effect was due to the drug or a placebo effect of a result of the natural history of pain resolution.

3.3. Anticonvulsants

Early studies utilizing the anticonvulsants carbamazepine, phenytoin and valproic acid for PHN have been neither unimpressive (Killian and Fromm, 1968) or difficult to interpret because of the concomitant use of antidepressants (Killian and Fromm, 1968; Hatangdi et al., 1976; Gerson et al., 1977; Raftery, 1979). Although carbamazepine is a popular agent for the paroxysmal lancinating pain that commonly occurs, there is no conclusive evidence to justify its use in this fashion. More recently, gabapentin has been proven superior to placebo in PHN with 43% of patients reporting at least moderate improvement (versus 12% with placebo) (Rowbotham et al., 1998). Because it appears to have fewer side effects than antidepressants, it has been suggested as a first-line treatment for this condition. A dose of 3500 mg/day was aimed for in the trial above and many patients achieved that.

3.4. Opioids

For a long time there has been a bias against using opioids for non-malignant pain. There is now increas-

ing support for the view that they are helpful and justifiable in these conditions (Taub, 1982; Tennant and Uelmen, 1983; France et al., 1984; Urban et al., 1986; Wan Lu et al., 1988; Portenoy, 1990; Zenz et al., 1992). Some of these reports were of neuropathic pain (Urban et al., 1986; Portenoy, 1990; Zenz et al., 1992). One report has suggested that opioids do not relieve neuropathic pain (Arner and Meyerson, 1988). However, this study did not include patients with PHN and its conclusions were challenged (Fields, 1988).

Our experience with PHN (Watson et al., 1988) has indicated that opioids are useful for some patients with PHN. We were able to document that 25 of 90 otherwise intractable patients achieved good to excellent results and 50 others had 25–50% relief. Rowbotham et al. (1991) have shown that intravenous morphine was more effective than placebo in relieving PHN in a single session trial. A controlled trial of sustained release oxycodone has shown that 58% of patients experienced at least moderate improvement in pain versus 18% on placebo (Watson and Babul, 1998). I continue to follow many posterpetic patients otherwise refractory to all the usual approaches for whom we regularly renew prescriptions for opioids. I find that these patients do not develop significant problems with tolerance or physical and psychological dependency. There appears to be a ceiling effect with PHN. Below this, some relief occurs and usually complete pain relief does not occur, which is similar to the effect of antidepressant therapy. Opioid analgesics may take the extreme severity of the pain away, but frequently do not result in complete or satisfactory improvement. The relief is enough, however, that patients choose to continue using the drug. Above this apparent ceiling, no further pain relief occurs, but side effects supervene to the point that further dose escalation is refused. Because patients may prefer a particular opioid, we have used a variety, including morphine, hydromorphone, anileridine, levorphanol, codeine and oxycodone. A variety of sustained release oral preparations are now available and may be of advantage, including codeine, morphine, oxycodone, hydromorphone as well as a transdermal preparation of fentanyl.

TABLE III

Number needed to treat (NNT) values for drugs studied by randomized controlled trials in postherpetic neuralgia

Agent	Studies included	Authors calculating NNT	NNT (95% confidence limits)
Antidepressants/ Tricyclics	Watson et al. (1982) Max et al. (1988b) Kishore-Kumar et al. (1990)	McQuay et al. (1996)	2.3 (1.7–3.3)
Gabapentin	Rowbotham et al. (1998)	Sindrup and Jensen (1999)	3.2 (2.4–5.0)
Oxycodone	Watson and Babul (1998)	Sindrup and Jensen (1999)	2.5 (1.6–5.1)

3.5. How effective are these approaches in clinical practice?

The important question for clinicians is how satisfactory these drugs are for patients in terms of relief of pain and disability, tolerability of side effects and long-term benefit. Clinical trials which demonstrate a statistically significant difference in rating scales may not clearly convey effectiveness. The best clinical trial is unlikely to duplicate clinical practice because of such factors as the selection of subjects even if the analysis reports data on all patients entering the study (the intent to treat analysis). The number needed to treat (NNT) has been suggested to convey the meaningful clinical significance for a trial (Laupacis et al., 1988; Cook and Sackett, 1995). This evaluation is a description of an arbitrary therapeutic effect for a desired outcome of 50% improvement or more. It describes the difference between an intervention, such as a drug and a control treatment. It is expressed as the number of patients required to be treated for a favourable response. A comparison of NNT values for antidepressants, gabapentin, and oxycodone is given in Table III. Although the latter two drugs have only been subjected to one randomized controlled trial each, antidepressants and oxycodone may have an advantage in relieving pain; however, their side-effect profile may make them less satisfactory to patients.

Another way of determining a satisfactory response is to report a combined outcome rating of good or better defined as mild or no pain and disability, tolerable side effects, and an expression of satisfaction with the treatment. Antidepressant trials (Watson et al., 1982, 1992, 1998) indicate that between 47 and 60% of patients have a good response when so defined.

3.6. Miscellaneous therapies

Russell et al. (1957) advocated repeated nerve blocks, interspinal ligament injection of hypertonic saline solution, or skin infiltration with procaine hydrochloride for relief of hyperesthesia and spontaneous pain in PHN. They also discussed the use of a hand vibrator over the injured skin. Of 100 patients they provided details for only five. No duration of antecedent pain was stated. Taverner (1950) reported 16 cases treated with ethyl chloride spray to the scarred area. Symptoms for 12 of these were relieved for 3–21 months, with their pain duration being 10 months to 13 years. The spray was applied daily to twice a week. The author commented on the failure of vibration in his experience, cautioning about the risk of skin injury. Todd et al. (1965) reported on 86 patients with PHN of at least 3 months: 58 (67%) obtained relief with a combination of ethyl chloride spray followed by the applications of a hand vibrator, follow-up was 6 months to 6 years. Colding (1969, 1973) concluded that sympathetic blocks for established PHN were of no value. Forrest (1980) treated 37 patients with postherpetic pain of longer than 6 months' duration with three epidural injections of methylprednisolone acetate at weekly intervals. At 1 year, he thought that 90% of the patients were free of pain, with "some patients" followed up for more than 3 years. Forrest postulated that the steroid, local anaesthetic or preservative might have been the effective component. In view of the pathologic findings of fibrosis and lack of inflammation, in most cases, it is difficult to explain how local steroids might be effective. Another study (Perkins and Hanlon, 1978) of five patients with true PHN, treated with epidural bupivacine hydrochloride and methylprednisolone, concluded that no patient had more than 50% relief at 1 and 5 months.

Kotani et al. (2000) reported the results of a randomized, controlled trial of an intrathecal corticosteroid (methylprednisolone), given with lidocaine, in patients with PHN. The authors of this study wisely chose a population of patients with PHN of at least one year's duration that had been unresponsive to conventional treatments. They used a parallel design with two comparison groups (one receiving lidocaine only and one receiving no treatment); this was a useful approach since the control (no treatment) group did not receive a sham injection. Only seven patients were lost to follow-up during the two years of the trial. Patients with involvement of the trigeminal nerve were excluded. This region (usually the forehead) and the thoracic area are the two most common sites of PHN.

Although the treating physician administered the four weekly injections and was aware of the assigned interventions, the investigators assessing the outcomes were unaware of the treatment assignments, as were the patients presumably, except those in the control group, who received no injection. This lack of blinding does not appear to have been an important problem in view of the poor outcomes in the lidocaine-only group. More than 90% of the patients who received methylprednisolone and lidocaine reported excellent or good pain relief at four weeks and at one and two years, as compared with only approximately 6% of those who received only lidocaine and approximately 4% of those who received no treatment. Furthermore, the areas of allodynia were reduced by more than 70% in the methylprednisolone-lidocaine group and by less than 25% in the lidocaine-only group. Allodynic pain from light tactile stimulation, such as that from clothing, hair, or even a breeze, can be one of the most debilitating problems faced by patients with PHN. These results appear remarkable and it will be interesting to see whether further clinical trials and clinical prac-

tice can replicate the efficacy and the safety of this approach used.

During the two years of this trial, no critical adverse effects, such as arachnoiditis or neurotoxic effects from the methylprednisolone, were noted. Adhesive arachnoiditis with chronic inflammation and scarring in the arachnoidea mater around the spinal cord and nerves is one of the most worrisome complications of intrathecal injections. This condition may result in nerve injury and may itself be a cause of intractable neuropathic pain. Use of this technique in larger numbers of patients and observation during longer follow-up periods will be important to identify any occurrences of these potentially severe side effects. Significant ethical and medicolegal issues arise because current preparations of methylprednisolone are not approved for intrathecal use by the manufacturer and a preservative-free preparation is not currently available.

The authors argue that an anti-inflammatory action is the basis of this treatment of PHN. The study by Kotani et al. does not address the important problem of PHN involving the trigeminal nerve, which is one of the most common sites of this condition. Perhaps future studies in patients with intractable PHN should assess the use of injections of corticosteroids into Meckel's cave, which is the area of the subarachnoid space around the trigeminal ganglion.

Nathan and Wall (1974) used prolonged transcutaneous electrical nerve stimulation (TENS) and found good results in 11 of 30 patients with established PHN. Voltage, pulse width, frequency, site of application, and duration were all controlled by the patient. Generally, the subjective sensation of the input was non-painful and tingling. Pain relief often outlasted stimulation by hours. Follow-up duration was not clearly stated in all. Gerson et al. (1977) found the intermittent use of TENS was unsuccessful in 17 patients with chronic PHN. Haas (1977) concluded that TENS was helpful in 9 of 11 patients, with follow-up over 1–18 months. Lewith et al. (1983) thought that acupuncture was of little value in PHN when compared with placebo (mock TENS) in 62 patients. Claims have been made for a variety of other therapies, but these studies suffer from small numbers of patients, lack of controls, inadequate data about the patient population, and/or lack of adequate follow-up.

4. A summary of practical guidelines for prevention and treatment of postherpetic neuralgia

Most of the putative preventive approaches (except antivirals) to PHN can be regarded as not conclusively established by more than one controlled trial with adequate numbers of patients. Pending final proof, it is reasonable to treat patients aggressively to relieve the pain of HZ and to try to prevent PHN if the therapy is safe and well-tolerated (see Chapter 19). Earlier chapters have discussed dermatological approaches to the acute skin lesions (Chapter 9), ophthalmic complications (Chapter 11), and the special problem of the immunosuppressed patient (Chapter 10). It is important to recognize that the population at highest risk for PHN is the age group 60 years and over, who may have a risk of 50% or more of developing this complication. There is no good evidence supporting the use of corticosteroids to prevent PHN (Chapter 18). Valacyclovir and famciclovir should be given within the first 72 h and exert a modest effect at preventing PHN (Beutner et al., 1995; Tyring et al., 1995). Amitriptyline, if used early, may also help to prevent ongoing pain (Bowsher, 1996). Although no controlled trial has ever been done of nerve blocks to treat HZ pain or prevent PHN, they are reasonable and safe in experienced hands and may be repeated, if effective, as symptoms dictate. The use of nonsteroidal inflammatory drugs, and, in the author's view, opioids, are justified to relieve severe pain with the acute illness. Whether better control of acute pain will reduce the occurrence of PHN is unknown, but possible.

For established PHN (neuropathic pain persisting more than 1 month after HZ) the most consistently effective agents appear to be the older antidepressant drugs and several controlled trials in PHN support this approach. These indicate that pain may be taken from moderate or severe to mild in about one-half

to two-thirds of patients. I tend to commence with amitriptyline or nortriptyline in a dose of 10 mg before bed in those over 65 years and with 25 mg in those 65 or under. The dose is increased by similar increments in a single bedtime dose every 7–10 days until relief is obtained or side effects supervene. If these fail, we then usually try a noradrenergic agent, such as desipramine or maprotiline. Occasional patients failing these may benefit from a serotonergic drug, such as trasodone, clomipramine, fluoxetine or other SSRIs, but no controlled trial has been done and we have not been impressed with these agents for most individuals. It is also possible that the addition of a neuroleptic, such as fluphenazine 1 mg up to three times daily, may give added benefit in some. An alternative approach which may also be regarded as first-line is gabapentin increased to as much as 3500 mg/day (Rowbotham et al., 1998). A trial-and-error approach in refractory patients may also include the anticonvulsants carbamazepine, phenytoin, clonazepam or valproate. It is our common practice with resistant cases to prescribe analgesics including opioids on an as needed and/or round the clock basis. A variety of long-acting opioids are available. The dose can be increased to satisfactory relief or unacceptable side effects. The use of topical agents is attractive as it is simple and free of systemic effects. These can be used as sole therapy or as adjuvant agents. These have been discussed in Chapter 21 and include capsaicin, acetylsalicylic acid and local anaesthetic agents, such as lidocaine. Although an unpublished controlled trial showed no difference between capsaicin and vehicle (placebo) ointment, it remains possible that occasional patients with differing pain mechanisms may benefit from this agent. A lidocaine patch has been shown to be useful by randomized controlled trials. TENS may be worth trying. Electrode placement, frequency, intensity and duration of stimulation are a matter of trial and error. Some patients may benefit from nerve blocks which, if efficacious, may be repeated at appropriate intervals. At least 30% of our patients remain totally refractory or unsatisfactorily relieved and our approach with those is to see them regularly, and try any new or older approach that seems reasonable and safe, hoping that with time, as Voltaire said, "nature will effect a cure." Approximately 50% of patients, even those with long duration pain, will improve over the years with one-half of these on no treatment (Watson et al., 1991).

References

Arner, A. and Meyerson, B.A. (1988) Lack of analgesic effect of opioids on neuropathic and idiopathic forms of pain. Pain, 33: 11–24.

Balfour, H.H., Bean, B. and Laskin, O.L. et al. (1983) Acyclovir halts progression of herpes zoster in immunocompromised patients. New Engl. J. Med., 380: 1453.

Bean, B., Braun, C. and Balfour, H.H. (1982) Acyclovir therapy for acute herpes zoster. Lancet, 2: 118–121.

Beutner, K.R., Friedman, D.J. and Forszpaniak, C. et al. (1995) Valacyclovir compared with acyclovir for improved therapy for herpes zoster in immunocompetent adults. Antimicrob. Agents Chemother., 39: 1546–1553.

Bowsher, D. (1996) Postherpetic neuralgia and its treatment: a retrospective survey of 191 patients. J. Pain Symptom Manage., 12: 327–331.

Clemmensen, O.I. and Anderson, K.E. (1984) ACTH versus prednisone and placebo in herpes zoster treatment. Clin. Exp. Dermatol., 9: 557–563.

Colding, A. (1969) The effect of sympathetic blocks on herpes zoster. Acta Anaesthesiol. Scand., 13: 113–141.

Colding, A. (1973) Treatment of pain: organization of a pain clinic, treatment of herpes zoster. Proc. R. Soc. Med., 66: 541–543.

Cook, R.J. and Sackett, D.L. (1995) The number needed to treat: a clinically useful measure of treatment effect. Br. Med. J., 310: 452–454.

Dan, K., Higa, K., Tanaka, K. and Mori, R. (1983) Herpetic pain and cellular immunity. In: T. Yokota and R. Dubner (Eds.), Current Topics in Pain Research and Therapy. Int. Congr. Soc., Vol. 6–12, Excerpta Medica, Amsterdam, pp. 293–295.

Dan, K., Higa, K. and Noda, B. (1985) Nerve block for herpetic pain. In: H.L. Fields, R. Dubner and F. Cerrero (Eds.), Advances in Pain Research and Therapy, Vol. 9. Raven Press, New York, pp. 831–838.

Eaglstein, W.H., Katz, R. and Brown, J.A. (1970) The effects of corticosteroid therapy on the skin eruption and pain of herpes zoster. J. Am. Med. Assoc., 211: 1681–1683.

Esmann, V., Kroon, S. and Peterslund N.A. (1987) Prednisolone does not prevent postherpetic neuralgia. Lancet, 2: 126–129.

Farber, G.A. and Burks, J.W. (1974) Chlorprothixene therapy for herpes zoster neuralgia. South. Med. J., 67: 808–812.

Feinmann, C. (1985) Pain relief by antidepressants: possible modes of action. Pain, 23: 1–8.

Fields, H.L. (1988) Can opiates relieve neuropathic pain?. Pain, 35: 365.

Forrest, J.B. (1980) The response to epidural steroid injections in chronic dorsal root pain. Can. Anaesth. Soc., 27: 40–46.

France, R.D., Urban, B.J. and Keefe, F.J. (1984) Long-term use of narcotic analgesics in chronic pain. Soc. Sci. Med., 19: 1379–1382.

Galbraith, A.W. (1983) Treatment of acute herpes zoster with amantadine hydrochloride (Symmetrel). Br. Med. J., 4: 693–695.

Gerson, G.R., Jones, R.B. and Luscombe, D.K. (1977) Studies on the concomitant use of carbamazepine and clomipramine for the relief of postherpetic neuralgia. Postgrad. Med. J., 54(Suppl. 4): 104–109.

Getto, C.J., Sorkness, C.A. and Howell, T. (1987) Antidepressants and chronic non-malignant pain: a review. J. Pain Symptom Manage., 2: 8–18.

Goodkin, K. and Gullion, C.M. (1989) Antidepressants for the relief of chronic pain: do they work?. Ann. Behav. Med., 11: 75–80.

Haas, L.F. (1977) Postherpetic neuralgia. Trans. Ophthalmol. Soc. N., 29: 133–136.

Hatangdi, V.S., Bond, R.A. and Richards, E.G. (1976) Postherpetic neuralgia: management with anti-epileptic tricyclic drugs. In: J.J. Bonica and D. Albe-Fessard (Eds.), Advances in Pain Research and Therapy, Vol. 1. Raven Press, New York, pp. 583–587.

Keczkes, K. and Basheer, A.M. (1980) Do corticosteroids prevent postherpetic neuralgia?. Br. J. Dermatol., 102: 551–555.

Kernbaum, S. and Hauchecorne, J. (1981) Administration of levodopa for relief of herpes zoster pain. J. Am. Med. Assoc., 246: 132–134.

Killian, J.M. and Fromm, G.H. (1968) Carbamazepine in the treatment of neuralgia. Arch. Neurol., 19: 129–136.

Kishore-Kumar, R., Schafer, S.C., Lawlor, B.A., Murphy, D.I. and Max, M.B. (1989) Single doses of the serotonin agonists buspirone and m-chlorophenylpiperazine do not relieve neuropathic pain. Pain, 37: 223–227.

Kishore-Kumar, R., Max, M.B. and Schafer, S.C. et al. (1990) Desipramine relieves postherpetic neuralgia. Clin. Pharmacol. Ther., 47: 305–312.

Kotani, N., Kushikata, T. and Hashimoto, H. et al. (2000) Intrathecal methylprednisolone for intractable postherpetic neuralgia. N. Engl. J. Med., 343: 1514–1519.

Laupacis, A., Sackett, D.L. and Robarts, R.S. (1988) An assessment of clinically useful measures of the consequences of treatment. New Engl. J. Med., 318: 1728–1733.

Lewith, G.T., Field, F. and Machin, D. (1983) Acupuncture versus placebo in postherpetic pain. Pain, 17: 361–368.

Max, M.B., Schafer, S.C., Culnane, M., Dubner, R. and Gracely, R.H. (1988a) Association of pain relief with drug side effects in postherpetic neuralgia: a single-dose study of clonidine, codeine, ibuprofen and placebo. Clin. Pharmacol. Ther., 43: 363–371.

Max, M.B., Schafer, S.C., Culnane, M., Smoller, B., Dubner, R. and Gracely, R.H. (1988b) Amitriptyline but not lorazepam relieves postherpetic neuralgia. Neurology, 38: 1427–1432.

McQuay, H.J., Trainer, M. and Nye, B.A. et al. (1996) A systematic review of antidepressants in neuropathic pain. Pain, 68: 217–222.

Merigan, T.C., Rand, K.H. and Pollard, R.B. et al. (1978) Human leukocyte-interferon for the treatment of herpes zoster in patients with cancer. New Engl. J. Med., 298: 981–987.

Nathan, P.W. (1978) Chlorprothixene (Taractan) in postherpetic neuralgia and other severe chronic pains. Pain, 5: 367–371.

Nathan, P.W. and Wall, P.D. (1974) Treatment of postherpetic neuralgia by prolonged electrical stimulation. Br. Med. J., 3: 645–647.

Perkins, H.M. and Hanlon, P.R. (1978) Epidural injection of local anesthetic and steroids for relief of pain secondary to herpes zoster. Arch. Surg., 113: 253–254.

Peterslund, N.A., Seyer-Hansen, K. and Ipsen, J. et al. (1981) Acyclovir in herpes zoster. Lancet, 2: 827–831.

Portenoy, R.K. (1990) Chronic opioid therapy in nonmalignant pain. J. Pain Symptom Manage., 5: 46–62.

Raftery, H. (1979) The management of postherpetic pain using sodium valproate and amitriptyline. Irish Med. J., 32: 399–401.

Riopelle, J.M., Naraghi, M. and Grush, K.P. (1984) Chronic neuralgia incident following local anesthetic therapy for herpes zoster. Arch. Dermatol., 129: 747–750.

Rowbotham, M.C., Reisner-Keller, I.A. and Fields, H. (1991) Both intravenous lidocaine and morphine relieve the pain of postherpetic neuralgia. Neurology, 41: 1024–1028.

Rowbotham, M., Harden, N., Stacey, B., et al. (1998) Gabapentin for the treatment of postherpetic neuralgia: a randomized controlled trial. J. Am. Med. Assoc., 280: 1837–1842.

Russell, W.R., Espire, M.L.E. and Morganstern, F.S. (1957) Treatment of postherpetic neuralgia. Lancet, i: 242–245.

Shepp, D.H., Dandliker, P.S. and Meyers, J.D. (1986) Treatment of varicella zoster virus infection in severely immunocompromised patients: a randomized comparison of acyclovir and vidarabine. New Engl. J. Med., 314: 208–212.

Sherlock, C.H. and Corey, L. (1985) Adenosine monophosphate for the treatment of varicella zoster infections, a large dose of caution. J. Am. Med. Assoc., 253: 1444–1445.

Sindrup, S.H. and Jensen, T.S. (1999) Efficacy of pharmacological treatments of neuropathic pain: an update and effect related to mechanism of drug action. Pain, 83: 389–400.

Sklar, S.H., Blue, W.T. and Alexander, E.J. et al. (1985) Herpes zoster, the treatment and prevention of neuralgia by adenosine monophosphate. J. Am. Med. Assoc., 253: 1427–1430.

Taub, A. (1973) Relief of postherpetic neuralgia with psychotropic drugs. J. Neurosurg., 39: 235–239.

Taub, A. and Collins, W.F. (1974) Observations on the treatment of denervation dysesthesia with psychotropic drugs. Adv. Neurol., 4: 309–315.

Taub, A. (1982) Opioid analgesics in the treatment of chronic intractable pain of non-neoplastic origin. In: L.M. Kitzhata and D. Collins (Eds.), Narcotic Analgesics in Anaesthesiology. Williams and Wilkins: Baltimore, MD, pp. 199–208.

Taverner, D. (1950) Alleviation of postherpetic neuralgia. Lancet, 2: 671–673.

Tennant, F.S. and Uelmen, G.F. (1983) Narcotic maintenance for chronic pain: medical and legal guidelines. J. Postgrad. Med., 73: 81–94.

Todd, E.M., Crae Jr., B.L. and Vergadano, M. (1965) Conservative treatment of postherptic neuralgia. Bull. LA Neurol. Soc., 30: 148–152.

Tyring, S., Barabash, R.A. and Nahlek, J.E. et al. (1995) Famciclovir for the treatment of acute disease and postherpetic neuralgia. Ann. Intern. Med., 123: 89–96.

Urban, B.J., France, R.D., Steinberger, D.L., Scott, D.J. and Maltbie, A.A. (1986) Long-term use of narcotic/antidepressant medication in the management of phantom limb pain. Pain, 24: 191–197.

Wan Lu, C., Urban, B., France, R.D. (1988) Long-term narcotic therapy in chronic pain. Presented at the Canadian Pain Society and American Pain Society Joint Meeting. Toronto, Canada, pp. 10–13.

Watson, C.P.N. and Babul, N. (1998) Oxycodone relieves neuropathic pain: a randomized trial in postherpetic neuralgia. Neurology, 50: 1837–1841.

Watson, C.P.N. and Evans, R.J. (1985) A comparative trial of amitriptyline and zimelidine in postherpetic neuralgia. Pain, 23: 387–394.

Watson, C.P.N., Evans, R.J., Reed, K., Merskey, H., Goldsmith, L. and Warsh, J. (1982) Amitriptyline versus placebo in postherpetic neuralgia. Neurology, 32: 671–673.

Watson, C.P.N., Evans, R.J., Watt, V.R. and Birkett, N. (1988) Postherpetic neuralgia: 208 cases. Pain, 35: 289–298.

Watson, C.P.N., Watt, V.R., Chipman, M., Birkett, N. and Evans, R.J. (1991) The prognosis with postherpetic neuralgia. Pain, 46: 195–199.

Watson, C.P.N., Chipman, M., Reed, K., Evans, R.J. and Birkett, N. (1992) Amitriptyline versus maprotiline in postherpetic neuralgia: a randomized double-blind crossover trial. Pain, 48: 29–36.

Watson, C.P.N., Vernich, L., Chipman, M. and Reed, K. (1998) Amitriptyline versus nortriptyline in postherpetic neuralgia. Neurology, 51: 1166–1171.

Whitley, R.J, Soong, S.J., Dolin, R., et al. (1982) Early vidarabine therapy to control the complications of herpes zoster in immunosuppressed patients. N. Engl. J. Med., 307: 971–975.

Whitley, R.J., Weiss, H., Gnann, J.W. et al. (1996) Acyclovir with and without prednisone for the treatment of herpes zoster, a randomized placebo-controlled trial. Ann. Int. Med., 125: 376–383.

Wood, M.J., Johnson, R.W. and McKendrick, M.W. (1994) A randomized trial of acyclovir for 7 days or 21 days with and without prednisolone for treatment of acute herpes zoster. N. Engl. J. Med., 330: 896–890.

Woodforde, J.M., Dwyer, B., McEwen, B.W., et al. (1965) The treatment of postherpetic neuralgia. Med. J. Aust., 2: 869–872.

Yanagida, H., Suwa, K. and Corssen, G. (1987) No prophylactic effect of early sympathetic blockade of postherpetic neuralgia. Anaesthesiology, 66: 73–79.

Zenz, M., Strumpf, M. and Tryba, M. (1992) Long-term oral opioid therapy in patients with non-malignant pain. J Pain Symptom Manage., 7: 69–77.

Herpes Zoster and Postherpetic Neuralgia, 2nd Revised and Enlarged Edition
Pain Research and Clinical Management, Vol. 11
Edited by C.P.N. Watson and A.A. Gershon

CHAPTER 23

Surgery for postherpetic neuralgia

John D. Loeser [*]

Departments of Neurological Surgery and Anesthesiology, University of Washington, Box 356470, Seattle, WA 98195, USA

1. Overview

There are no prospective, randomized, controlled studies of surgical procedures for the management of the pain of postherpetic neuralgia. It is, unfortunately, exceedingly unlikely that any will be undertaken. Indeed, only a very small fraction of the patients who have undergone surgery of any type have been reported in the literature; hence the true utility of any operation remains largely unknown. Even when reports of series of patients have been made, patient selection strategies often were unreported, the duration of follow-up was not stated or was obviously too short, the criteria for categorizing outcomes were not stated and the percentage of patients operated upon who were included in the follow-up was unknown (Sugar and Bucy, 1951; see also Tables I and II). Most of the articles about surgery for postherpetic neuralgia are case reports of a small number of patients who have failed the medical management offered to them and sought out additional pain relief. In general, experts in surgical management of pain have cautioned against ablative surgical procedures for postherpetic neuralgia (Falconer and Harris, 1968; Tasker, 1985, 1989).

Subsequent reports have rarely been as enthusiastic as the original descriptions of any operation utilized for postherpetic neuralgia. We have no data on the role of the surgeon's skills in leading to pain relief or surgical complications. Predicting the outcome for any operation is very hazardous, as there are no data that correlate the response to a medication or a nerve block with the surgical outcome. Nor has anyone looked at psychometric predictors of surgical outcome for this type of chronic pain. Since it is known that a significant fraction of the patients who develop postherpetic neuralgia undergo a spontaneous remission in their pain complaints, it is imperative that outcome studies control for the natural history of this disorder. The likelihood of remission is related to duration of pain complaint and age of the patient. None of the reports of surgical efficacy have considered these issues.

For the above reasons, this is a descriptive chapter that lacks statistical analysis. Along with the published data, I have included some of my own experiences in the surgical management of postherpetic neuralgia. As is true for so many aspects of the management of chronic pain, outcome studies of significant power are completely lacking. Moreover, recent texts rarely provide new information about treatment outcomes for PHN.

2. Undermining skin

Undermining the skin or elevating a skin flap in the painful region has been adequately reviewed by

---

[*] Correspondence to: Dr. J.D. Loeser, Department of Neurological Surgery, University of Washington, Box 356470, Seattle, WA 98195, USA. Phone: +1 (206) 543-3570; Fax: +1 (206) 543-8315; E-mail: jdloeser@u.washington.edu

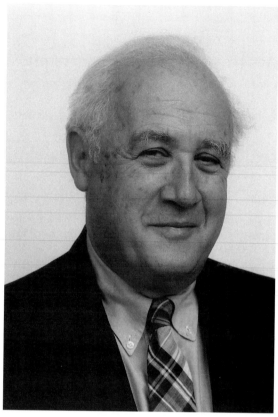

Dr. John D. Loeser

TABLE I

Operations used for postherpetic neuralgia

Undermining skin	Trigeminal tractotomy
Excising skin	Trigeminal nucleotomy
Peripheral neurectomy	Thalamotomy
Dorsal rhizotomy	Hypothalamotomy
Sympathectomy	Cingulumotomy
Dorsal root entry zone lesions	Corticectomy
Myelotomy	Transcutaneous stimulation
Cordotomy	Spinal cord stimulation
Medullary tractotomy	Deep brain stimulation
Mesencephalic tractotomy	Motor cortex stimulation

TABLE II

Survey of American neurosurgeons in 1946 treatment results for postherpetic neuralgia

Operation	Relief			
	None	Some	Good	Total
Retrogasserian neurotomy	29	2	2	33
Supraorbital n. avulsion	6	7	3	16
Alcohol inj. supraorbital n.	6	3	0	9
Trigeminal tractotomy	4	3	0	7
Cervical sympathectomy	3	2	1	6
Stellate block(s)	3	3	0	6
Radiation Gasserian ganglion	1	0	1	2
Alcohol inj. Gasserian ganglion	0	0	1	1

From Sugar and Bucy (1951).

White and Sweet (1969). Abbott and Martin (1951) undermined the skin of three patients with thoracic postherpetic neuralgia and reported that after at least 1 year, two had good results and one was only fair.

Subsequent information on an additional nine patients provided to White and Sweet (1969) suggested that only one had partial relief and the remaining eight were failures; therefore only two of 12 had good results. Farbman (1962) described a patient who had over 9 years of pain relief from such an operation. Verbiest and Calliauw (1963) described four failures to relieve pain by this technique; White and Sweet (1969) added three failures from experience at the Massachusetts General Hospital (MGH). Tindall et al. (1962) reported 11 patients, of whom three had good results, one was lost to follow-up and seven were failures.

This operation is probably not worthy of further study. Less than 20% of the 31 reported patients have had good long-term results. Permanent denervation of the skin is not usually obtained, and this was the reason for considering such a surgical approach. The lesions of postherpetic neuralgia involve central as well as peripheral structures and make the logic of such an operation questionable. The stimulation-driven component of postherpetic neuralgia might temporarily be alleviated, but this rarely suffices to solve the patient's pain problem.

3. Excision of skin

Removal of the painful skin region has been discussed for many years. Anecdotal success stories are common, but published results are not good. Verbiest and Calliauw (1963) had one of three patients with good long-term relief of pain. Tindall et al. (1962) described four patients who had skin excision: one had relief for at least 8 years, two were failures, and one had inadequate follow-up at the time of their report. Browder and De Veer (1949) reported five of 10 patients with good relief; in the ensuing discussion Kredel (1949) and Ray (1949) added four failures. White and Sweet (1969) add one success in three patients operated upon by Van Blaricom and Horrax. Weidmann (1976) reviewed the results of 10 of 16 patients: three cured, three improved and four failures. It is important to note that his successes included patients with short symptom duration whose natural history could have been quite favorable. Since many of the other reports do not mention duration of pain prior to surgery, this may be a factor in most of the good outcomes. On the other hand, when the patient describes immediate pain relief, it is hard to deny the role of the surgical procedure.

This operation does not appear to be of significant value, for reasons similar to those discussed above. Less than one-third of the 33 reported patients obtained adequate pain relief. It does not appear warranted to conduct further studies of its use.

Suzuki et al. (1980) described 10 of 14 patients with postherpetic neuralgia who had good or excellent pain relief from cryocautery of the painful regions. This led to a deep dermal burn and the loss of cutaneous hypersensitivity. All patients had experienced pain relief with local anesthetic infiltration in the painful areas prior to cryocautery. No subsequent reports of this technique can be found.

4. Peripheral neurectomy

There are very few case reports of patients who have had either trigeminal or spinal peripheral neurectomy for postherpetic neuralgia. Cushing (1920) reported one patient who had relief for 2.5 years and then 1 year from two peripheral trigeminal nerve avulsions. Barnard et al. (1981) reported that cryoablation of peripheral trigeminal branches gave pain relief for over 6 weeks in 42% of 26 patients, greater than 6 months in 3% and greater than 1 year in none. White and Sweet (1969) comment on the inadequacy of trigeminal procedures for postherpetic neuralgia.

In the absence of data, it is hard to evaluate peripheral neurectomy as a treatment for postherpetic neuralgia. As discussed above, the central nervous system pathology of herpes zoster makes it unlikely that a peripheral procedure will adequately address the generator(s) of postherpetic neuralgia. Furthermore, the trigeminal nerve has a tremendous propensity to regenerate, and peripheral avulsions are well known to yield only temporary sensory loss. In the spinal segments, there is significant overlap of the sensory fields of peripheral nerves, and regeneration is known to occur from sprouting and new central connectivity. Although there are no clinical trials, it seems unlikely that peripheral neurectomy will be a wise surgical choice for the patient with postherpetic neuralgia.

5. Sympathectomy

There are very few reports of sympathectomy as a treatment for postherpetic neuralgia. White and Sweet (1955) reviewed the experiences of Reichert, Hyndman and themselves and were dubious that cervical sympathectomy was useful for cranial postherpetic neuralgia. An occasional patient appeared to get temporary relief. Sugar and Bucy's (1951) survey found one patient out of three who had pain relief after cervical sympathectomy. Verbiest and Calliauw (1963) stated that sympathectomy was never successful. A judgment cannot be made on such limited published experience.

6. Dorsal rhizotomy

An occasional patient may get good long-term relief from spinal dorsal rhizotomy, but most do not. Individual case reports are infrequent; White and Sweet (1969) describe one good result in three patients.

Loeser (1972) reported two patients who did not obtain even temporary relief. Onofrio and Campa (1972) described one patient out of five who had long-term benefit from rhizotomy. Smith (1970) had two patients who received dorsal rhizotomy and spinal ganglionectomy who were relieved of their postherpetic neuralgia for an unknown period. Lazorthes et al. (1976) utilized a percutaneous thermocoagulation technique for rhizotomy and had one patient with good relief and one with none.

Meaningful data on cranial rhizotomy for postherpetic neuralgia are totally absent. Frazier and Russell (1924) and Peet (1929) reported a total of four unsuccessful trigeminal rhizotomies. Olivecrona (1947) reported four failures after trigeminal rhizotomy. Two of 33 patients obtained good relief in Sugar and Bucy's (1951) survey.

Gybels and Sweet (1989) state, without providing any supporting data, that percutaneous trigeminal rhizotomy may be successful in patients with postherpetic neuralgia and other atypical pains.

7. Dorsal root entry zone (DREZ) lesions

First described by Nashold and Ostdahl in 1979 (Nashold and Ostdahl, 1979), this operation has been utilized in large numbers of chronic pain patients in the past 14 years. Nashold's experience is the largest; his group has reported on 32 patients with postherpetic neuralgia (Friedman and Bullitt, 1988). Ninety percent of the patients had good early relief, but the pain recurred in 50% by 6 months. Only three patients have had some pain relief at 2 years or more of follow-up. Many of the patients report their pain recurrence as a new type of aching pain; the hyperpathia that is common in postherpetic neuralgia does not seem to be part of the pain recurrence. Most of these patients were elderly and had had pain for years; hence, the spontaneous remission rate would be expected to be low.

Young (1990) reported 16 patients with postherpetic neuralgia whom he had treated with DREZ lesions. Only mean follow-up was reported (about 4 years) and 50% of the patients were said to have experienced pain relief. This method of reporting outcome can obscure long-term failures.

Sindou and Daher (1988) described four patients with postherpetic neuralgia whom they had treated with Sindou's method of selective posterior rhizotomy in the dorsal root entry zone. All four had long-term relief of their spontaneous pain and their hyperalgesia. Thomas and Jones (1984) reported one unsuccessful DREZ lesion in a patient with postherpetic neuralgia.

The complication rate from DREZ lesions has been significant. There clearly is a learning curve for each surgeon, as described by both Nashold and Young. The technique of making the lesion has been debated in the neurosurgical literature: Nashold and many others use a series of radiofrequency lesions placed in the dorsal horn, others have used a laser or direct incisions into this region. Nor is the necessary extent of the lesion known: most advocate extending the lesions at least one-half neural segment above and below the painful dermatomes. In the best circumstances, a patient having a spinal DREZ lesion has at least a 10% risk of a significant neurologic complication.

Lesions can be made in the trigeminal nucleus so as to be functionally analogous with DREZ lesions in the spinal cord. Nashold's group has reported that nine patients with trigeminal postherpetic neuralgia have been treated with trigeminal nucleotomy and six have had excellent relief for 39 months (Bernard et al., 1988). Ishijima et al. (1988) also claimed that two patients with trigeminal postherpetic neuralgia were completely relieved of their pain for over 2 years by this operation. Siqueira (1985) and Plangger et al. (1987) each reported one patient with postherpetic neuralgia who obtained good long-term relief. Rath et al. (1996) reported that only two of 12 patients with postherpetic neuralgia got long-term relief. A series of radiofrequency current lesions are made with a 0.25-mm electrode 2 mm deep in the dorsolateral sulcus at 1-mm intervals from the most rostral C2 dorsal root to just above the obex. Exactly how this operation differs from trigeminal tractotomy is not clear, as the regions of the brainstem that are destroyed probably include the trigeminal tract, which is the target of trigeminal tractotomy as described below.

8. Cordotomy

Cordotomy is one of the oldest operations for chronic pain; there are many reports of long-term results. Kahn and Peet (1948) describe six patients, none of whom had a good long-term result. White and Sweet (1969) discussed the varying results in small numbers of patients reported by several neurosurgeons. J.C. White (1968) reviewed his experience, 374 cordotomies over a 30-year career, and identified seven patients with the diagnosis of postherpetic neuralgia, six of whom had a good early result and four of whom were classified as long-term successes. An additional two patients are included in White and Sweet's (1955) text, one of whom was a success and the other a failure. Mullan (1971) suggests that cordotomy is not likely to relieve the deep constricting pain of postherpetic neuralgia and that the hyperpathia is likely to recur in 2–3 years. He did not itemize his cases, however.

Percutaneous cordotomy has, in many institutions, replaced open cordotomy. The results for this procedure do not appear to differ significantly from the open operation. Lipton (1984) opined that cordotomy "... should not be used for such conditions as post-herpetic neuralgia ... "; Rosomoff (1982) reported on a personal series of over 1000 percutaneous cordotomies that included four patients with postherpetic neuralgia. Although the outcome for these four patients was not described, he stated that percutaneous cordotomy was "... not good for distressing dysesthesias."

9. Trigeminal tractotomy

Introduced by Sjöqvist (1938), this operation had significant complications in its early years. Sjöqvist (1948) reported two failures in patients with postherpetic neuralgia. Falconer (1949) reported four patients with postherpetic neuralgia whom he treated;

one died in the postoperative period and the other three were not benefitted. Sugar and Bucy (1951) found none of four patients in their survey got good long-term relief.

Stereotaxic trigeminal tractotomy was devised by Hitchcock (1970) and subsequently reported upon by Hitchcock and Schvarcz (1972) and by Schvarcz (1979, 1985, 1989) as well as by Fox (1973). About 3/4 of the patients with postherpetic neuralgia who have been treated with this procedure ($n = 21$) by Hitchcock and Schvarcz were reported to have good long-term relief of both the hyperpathia and the constant pain. Their lesion site was in the oral pole of nucleus caudalis. Fox (1973) did not achieve pain relief in his two patients with postherpetic neuralgia.

10. Midline myelotomy

Midline myelotomy has been utilized almost exclusively for bilateral pain associated with malignant diseases. It is usually performed via a laminectomy in the thoracolumbar region so as to expose the distal cord and conus. Hitchcock (1970) described a percutaneous high cervical approach, and his pupil Schvarcz (1978) mentioned its use in four patients with postherpetic neuralgia in a group of 14 with pain of non-malignant origin. Overall, this group had a 64% good result with follow-up of 6 months to 4 years. The results for those with postherpetic neuralgia were not specified. Papo and Luongo (1976) found that pain relief in a group of cancer pain patients was often of only weeks or months duration and suggested that this would not be a good procedure for patients with pain who did not have short life expectancy. Hence, it would appear not to be a wise choice in the patient with postherpetic neuralgia.

11. Mesencephalotomy

Originally utilized by Wycis and Spiegel in 1947, mesencephalotomy has been useful in a small number of patients with postherpetic neuralgia; its most common application has, however, been for pain due to head and neck cancer. By 1962, Wycis and Spiegel (1962) could report on seven patients, three of whom had significant long-term pain relief. Zapletal (1968) reviewed the published experience at that time and found 13 patients, three of whom were improved after mesencephalotomy. The review by Nashold (1982) suggested that about 50% of the patients with deafferentation pain who had had this operation obtained good pain relief for 3 years but many then relapsed; Tasker (1984) believed that 25% was a better estimate. For the neurosurgeon who frequently uses stereotaxic procedures, this operation may be helpful in patients with postherpetic neuralgia.

12. Thalamotomy and hypothalamotomy

Spiegel and Wycis (1953) reported one good long-term result with stereotaxic thalamotomy (VPM–VPL) for postherpetic neuralgia. Zapletal (1968) was able to find five reported patients, four of whom benefitted significantly from medial thalamotomy. White and Sweet (1969) added two more patients, one of whom had good long-term relief and the other is not further described. Medial thalamic targets such as centre median have been utilized with some success in a small number of patients (Tasker, 1984). Tasker (1989) thought that only about 25% of patients would get long-term benefit from this operation.

Sano (1977) described two patients with postherpetic neuralgia who had 'partial' relief from hypothalamotomy, but were followed for only 1 and 3 months. Siegfried (1977) reported that one patient in a group of four who had pulvinotomy was pain free more than 3 years later. However, hypothalamotomy and pulvinotomy were not thought to be effective for deafferentation pain in Tasker's (1984) review. I presume that postherpetic neuralgia would behave like other pains associated with nerve injury; medial thalamus is probably the target of choice and offers less than a 33% chance of long-term success. Like mesencephalic tractotomy, this operation may be useful in patients with postherpetic neuralgia.

13. Cingulumotomy

Cingulumotomy, which was derived from the no longer acceptable frontal leukotomy, has been extensively studied. It does not produce clinically significant cognitive deficits, but does seem to reduce suffering without altering the perception of a noxious stimulus. The relief of suffering is long-lasting and the risk of surgical morbidity is very low. Very few of the approximately 1000 patients who have been reported in the literature have had postherpetic neuralgia, but a significant number have had neuropathic pains. It seems reasonable to expect that cingulumotomy will be effective in reducing the patient's suffering in about three-fourths of the patients (Bouckoms, 1989). The furor about psychosurgery and subsequent administrative constraints have greatly reduced the willingness of neurosurgeons in North America to offer this operation to their patients.

14. Cortical excision

Excision of the parietal cortex has been repeatedly tried as an operation for pain relief after nerve, spinal cord or brain lesions (Le Beau, 1950). Although some good results have been reported, the consensus remains that this operation is unlikely to provide long-term relief. In the patient with intact neurological function, as in postherpetic neuralgia, the loss of parietal sensory function is too high a price to pay for a low chance of pain relief.

15. Neurostimulation

15.1. Transcutaneous

The earliest paper on the use of transcutaneous stimulation (TNS) in the treatment of postherpetic neuralgia was published by Nathan and Wall (1974). Eleven of 30 patients with long-standing postherpetic neuralgia were thought to have achieved good results. Two of them were thought to have been 'cured' and eight experienced "... an improvement in the course of the neuralgia." The natural history of postherpetic neuralgia could have been a significant factor in this apparent response to electrical stimulation.

Several of the early series of patients treated with TNS contain a few patients with postherpetic neuralgia. Loeser et al. (1975) reported that one of five patients obtained long-term benefit. Cauthen and Renner (1975) found that one patient did not benefit; Kirsch et al. (1975) reported that one of two patients was a success.

Long (1976) reported that four patients of a group of 197 had postherpetic neuralgia; three had short-term benefit and one did not. Of those with short-term benefit, two were still using their skin stimulator 1 year later; the other patient did not obtain long-term benefit. In an earlier review article, Long and Hagfors (1975) reported 12 of 16 patients to have long-term benefit. It is my belief that about 25% of patients with postherpetic neuralgia will obtain long-term and significant benefit from TNS. However, an equal number will report that their pain is aggravated by electrical stimulation of the skin.

15.2. Peripheral nerve

There are no reported cases of postherpetic neuralgia treated by peripheral nerve stimulation (PNS); nor do I have any such cases.

15.3. Spinal cord

Spinal cord stimulation has been clinically useful for over 30 years. Only a small fraction of the patients who have had stimulators implanted have been reported in the literature; very few patients with postherpetic neuralgia have been reported. Nashold and Friedman (1972) reported one patient with postherpetic neuralgia of 4 months duration who got an excellent result with a spinal cord stimulator. Clark (1975) had one patient who failed to get relief with spinal cord stimulation. Pineda (1975) also had one failure in a patient with postherpetic neuralgia. Nielsen et al. (1975) reported two failures. Meglio et al. (1989) reported on a series of 109 patients who re-

ceived spinal cord stimulators from 1978 until 1986, ten of whom had postherpetic neuralgia. Six of these ten patients reported good relief during stimulation trials and had implanted stimulators. The long-term results for these individual six patients cannot be determined, although the group experienced a 75% pain relief.

Sanchez-Ledesma et al. (1989) described a group of 49 patients (six of whom had postherpetic neuralgia), who were treated with spinal cord stimulation. Of this group, four had initial good results and were implanted with the stimulator. Of these four, only one had an excellent long-term result. Krainick and Thoden (1989) had one patient with postherpetic neuralgia in a group of 126 who were implanted with a spinal cord stimulator; this patient did not get significant pain relief.

Spinal cord stimulation has a small chance of alleviating the pain of postherpetic neuralgia. However, trial stimulation with percutaneously inserted electrodes and an external stimulator can be undertaken to identify those patients who might achieve long-term benefit and eliminate the 25–50% who do not even get immediate benefit. This procedure may have some utility in the patient with trunk or lower extremity postherpetic neuralgia who has failed medical management.

15.4. Deep brain

Electrodes have been stereotaxically placed most commonly in the lateral thalamus (VPL–VPM) and in the medial reticular formation, i.e. periventricular and periaqueductal gray matter (PVG–PAG). Most authorities believe that the lateral thalamic sites are more effective for neurogenic pain and the PVG–PAG better for somatic pain, such as that due to cancer. Some neurosurgeons implant patients with electrodes in both sites and then determine efficacy for the individual patient. Success rates for neurogenic pain in general and postherpetic neuralgia in specific have ranged widely from 25 to 80%.

Mazars (1975) reported five patients with postherpetic neuralgia in a group of 27; three of these appear to have had good long-term results of VPL stimulation. He then reported (Mazars, 1976) 9 successes out of 11 postherpetic patients. Richardson and Akil (1977) reported that one patient with postherpetic neuralgia got 'minor' pain relief from periventricular stimulation. Hosobuchi (1984) reviewed his experience in the prior decade; three patients with postherpetic neuralgia were subjected to lateral thalamic stimulation. Only one had a good initial response and was permanently implanted; this patient had pain relief for more than 6 months.

Siegfried (1982) studied 10 patients with postherpetic neuralgia of at least 1.5 years duration. Minimum follow-up was 7 months: five patients were rated as excellent results, three as good and two as poor. Patients used their stimulators for only a small fraction of the day (4–60 min) at frequencies of 33–195 Hz.

Dieckmann and Witzmann (1982) found that results did not seem to be dependent upon the site of stimulation for patients with deafferentation pain. In their group of 46 patients, there were three with postherpetic neuralgia: one had moderate and two marked response to stimulation; after implantation one had moderate, and one marked long-term response. The third patient's status was not stated. Young reviewed deep brain stimulation in 1989 and concluded that a total of 916 patients treated with brain stimulation could be found in the literature. He concluded that about 50% of the patients with deafferentation pain get pain relief but did not specify the results for patients with postherpetic neuralgia (Young, 1989). The complication rate for this operation is about 15% and the mortality rate about 2%. Most complications did not have long-term significance.

In summary, the number of patients with postherpetic neuralgia treated with deep brain stimulation reported in the literature is too small for meaningful analysis of efficacy. However, the impression from reviewing all neurosurgical procedures for pain relief in patients with postherpetic neuralgia is that this operation is probably more likely than any other to offer long-term benefit.

15.5. Motor cortex

This novel approach to neuropathic pain has been utilized for a little over a decade. Very few patients with postherpetic neuralgia have been included in the published series. The operation involves placing a stimulating electrode directly over the motor cortex in the epidural space. Good results have been reported for pain due to stroke and denervation of the face (Tsubokawa, 1995; Bendok and Levy, 1998). It could be a useful operation in some patients with postherpetic neuralgia, but further case series are required before a definitive statement can be made.

References

Abbott, K.R. and Martin, B.C. (1951) Surgical treatment of postherpetic neuralgia by subdermal denervation. Neurology, 1: 275–282.

Barnard, D., Lloyd, J. and Evans, J. (1981) Cryoanalgesia in the management of chronic facial pain. J. Maxillofac. Surg., 9: 101–102.

Bendok, B., Levy, R.M. (1998) Brain stimulation for persistent pain management. In: P.L. Gildenberg and R.R. Tasker (Eds.), Textbook of Stereotactic and Functional Neurosurgery. McGraw-Hill, New York, pp. 1539–1546.

Bernard, E.J. Jr., Mashold, B.S. Jr. and F. Caputi (1988) Clinical review of nucleus caudalis dorsal root entry zone lesions for facial pain. Appl. Neurophysiol., 51: 218–224.

Bouckoms, A.J. (1989) Psychosurgery for pain. In: R. Melzack and P.D. Wall (Eds.), Textbook of Pain. Churchill Livingstone, Edinburgh, pp. 868–881.

Browder, J. and De Veer, J.A. (1949) Herpes zoster: a surgical procedure for the treatment of postherpetic neuralgia. Ann. Surg., 130: 622–636.

Cauthen, J.C. and Renner, E.J. (1975) Transcutaneous and peripheral nerve stimulation for chronic pain states. Surg. Neurol., 4: 102–104.

Clark, K. (1975) Electrical stimulation of the nervous system for control of pain: University of Texas Southwestern Medical School experience. Surg. Neurol., 4: 16–166.

Cushing, H. (1920) The major trigeminal neuralgias and their surgical treatment based on experiences with 332 Gasserian operations. Am. J. Med. Sci., 160: 157–184.

Dieckmann, G. and Witzmann, A. (1982) Initial and long-term results of deep brain stimulation for chronic intractable pain. Appl. Neurophysiol., 45: 167–172.

Falconer, M.A. (1949) Intramedullary trigeminal tractotomy and its place in the treatment of facial pain. J. Neurol. Neurosurg. Psychiatry, 12: 297–311.

Falconer, M.A. and Harris, L. (1968) Surgical treatment of the cranial neuralgias. In: P.J. Vinken and G.W. Bruyn (Eds.), Handbook of Clinical Neurology, Vol. 5. North-Holland, Amsterdam, pp. 386–404.

Farbman, A.A. (1962) Surgical treatment of postherpetic neuralgia by subdermal denervation. J. Mich. Med. Soc., 61: 60–62.

Fox, J.L. (1973) Percutaneous trigeminal tractotomy for facial pain. Acta Neurochir. (Wien), 29: 83–88.

Frazier, C.H. and Russell, E.C. (1924) Neuralgia of the face: an analysis of 754 cases with relation to pain and other sensory phenomena before and after operation. Arch. Neurol. Psychiatry, 11: 557–563.

Friedman, A.H. and Bullitt, E. (1988) Dorsal root entry zone lesions in the treatment of pain following brachial plexus avulsion, spinal cord injury and herpes zoster. Appl. Neurophysiol., 51: 164–169.

Gybels, J. and Sweet, W.H. (Eds.) (1989) Neurosurgical Treatment of Persistent Pain. Pain and Headache, Vol. 11. Basle, Karger, pp. 1–444.

Hitchcock, E.R. (1970) Stereotactic cervical myelotomy. J. Neurol. Neurosurg. Psychiatry, 33: 224–330.

Hitchcock, E.R. and Schvarcz, J.R. (1972) Stereotaxic trigeminal tractotomy for post-herpetic facial pain. J. Neurosurg., 37: 412–417.

Hosobuchi, Y. (1984) Subcortical electrical stimulation for control of intractable pain in humans. J. Neurosurg., 64: 543–553.

Ishijima, B., Shimoji, K., Shimizu, H., Takahashi, H. and Suzuki, I. (1988) Lesions of spinal and trigeminal dorsal root entry zone for deafferentation pain. Appl. Neurophysiol., 51: 175–187.

Kahn, E.A. and Peet, M.M. (1948) The technique of anterolateral cordotomy. J. Neurosurg., 5: 276–283.

Kirsch, W.M., Lewis, J.A. and Simon, R.H. (1975) Experiences with electrical stimulation devices for the control of chronic pain. Med. Instrum. (Baltimore), 9: 217–220.

Krainick, J.-U. and Thoden, U. (1989) Spinal cord stimulation. In: P.D. Wall and R. Melzack (Eds.), Textbook of Pain, 2nd Edn. Churchill Livingstone, Edinburgh, pp. 920–924.

Kredel, F.E. (1949) Discussion. Ann. Surg., 130: 635–636.

Lazorthes, Y., Verdie, J.C. and Lagarrigue, J. (1976) Thermocoagulation percutanée des nerfs rachidiens à visée analgésique. Neuro-Chirurgie, 22: 445–453.

Le Beau, J. (1950) Experience with topectomy for the relief of intractable pain. J. Neurosurg., 7: 79–91.

Lipton, S. (1984) Percutaneous cordotomy. In: P.D. Wall and R. Melzack (Eds.), Textbook of Pain, 1st Edn. Churchill Livingstone, Edinburgh, pp. 632–638.

Loeser, J.D. (1972) Dorsal rhizotomy for the relief of chronic pain. J. Neurosurg., 36: 745–750.

Loeser, J.D., Black, R.G. and Christman, A. (1975) Relief of pain by transcutaneous stimulation. J. Neurosurg., 42: 308–314.

Long, D.M. (1976) Cutaneous afferent stimulation for the relief of pain. Prog. Neurol. Surg., 7: 35–51.

Long, D.M. and Hagfors, N. (1975) Electrical stimulation in the nervous system: the current status of electrical stimulation of the nervous system for relief of pain. Pain, 1: 109–123.

Mazars, G.J. (1975) Intermittent stimulation of nucleus ventralis posterolateralis for intractable pain. Surg. Neurol., 4: 93–95.

Mazars, G.J. (1976) Etat actuel de la chirurgie de la douleur. Neuro-Chirurgie, 22: Suppl. 1.

Meglio, M., Cioni, B. and Rossi, G.F. (1989) Spinal cord stimulation in management of chronic pain. J. Neurosurg., 70: 519–524.

Mullan, S. (1971) The surgical relief of pain. Clin. Neurosurg., 18: 208–224.

Nashold, B.S. (1982) Brainstem stereotaxic procedures. In: G. Schaltenbrand and A.E. Walker (Eds.), Stereotaxy of the Human Brain, 2nd edn. Thieme, Stuttgart, pp. 475–494.

Nashold, B.S. and Friedman, H. (1972) Dorsal column stimulation for control of pain. Preliminary report on 30 patients. J. Neurosurg., 36: 590–597.

Nashold, B.S. and Ostdahl, R.H. (1979) Dorsal root entry zone lesions for pain relief. J. Neurosurg., 51: 59–69.

Nathan, P.W. and Wall, P.D. (1974) Treatment of post-herpetic neuralgia by prolonged electrical stimulation. Br. Med. J., 1: 645–647.

Nielsen, K.D., Adams, J.E. and Hosobuchi, Y. (1975) Experience with dorsal column stimulation for relief of chronic intractable pain: 1969–1973. Surg. Neurol., 4: 148–152.

Olivecrona, H. (1947) The surgery of pain. Acta Psychiatr. Neurol. (Stockh.), Suppl. 46: 268–280.

Onofrio, B.M. and Campa, H.K. (1972) Evaluation of rhizotomy. Review of 12 years' experience. J. Neurosurg., 36: 751–755.

Papo, I. and Luongo, A. (1976) High cervical commissural myelotomy in the treatment of pain. J. Neurol. Neurosurg. Psychiatry, 39: 705–710.

Peet, M.M. (1929) Post-herpetic neuralgia: persistence of pain after section of sensory root of gasserian ganglion. J. Am. Med. Assoc., 92: 1503–1505.

Pineda, A. (1975) Dorsal column stimulation and its prospects. Surg. Neurol., 4: 157–163.

Plangger, C.A., Fischer, J., Grunert, V. and Mohsenipour, I. (1987) Tractotomy and partial vertical nucleotomy for treatment of special forms of trigeminal neuralgia and cancer pain of face and neck. Acta Neurochir. (Wien), Suppl. 39: 147–150.

Rath, S.A., Braun, V., Soliman, N., Antoniadis, G. and Richter, H.P. (1996) Results of DREZ coagulations for pain related to plexus lesions, cord injuries and postherpetic neuralgia. Acta Neurochir. (Wien), 138: 364–369.

Ray, B.S. (1949) Discussion. Ann. Surg., 130: 635.

Richardson, D.E. and Akil, H. (1977) Long-term results of periventricular gray self-stimulation. Neurosurgery, 1: 199–202.

Rosomoff, H.L. (1982) Stereotaxic cordotomy. In: J.R. Youmans

(Ed.), Neurological Surgery. Saunders, Philadelphia, PA, pp. 3672–3685.

Sanchez-Ledesma, M.J., Garcia-March, G., Diaz-Cascajo, P., Gomez-Moreta, J. and Broseta, J. (1989) Spinal cord stimulation in deafferentation pain. Stereotact. Funct. Neurosurg., 53: 40–45.

Sano, K. (1977) Intralaminar thalamotomy (thalamolaminotomy) and postero-medial hypothalamotomy in the treatment of intractable pain. Prog. Neurol. Surg., 8: 50–103.

Schvarcz, J.R. (1978) Spinal cord stereotactic techniques re trigeminal nucleotomy and extralemniscal myelotomy. Appl. Neurophysiol., 41: 99–112.

Schvarcz, J.R. (1979) Stereotactic spinal trigeminal nucleotomy for dysesthetic facial pain. In: J.J. Bonica et al. (Eds.), Advances in Pain Research and Therapy, Vol. 3. Raven Press, New York, pp. 331–336.

Schvarcz, J.R. (1985) Trigeminal glosso-vagal and high cervical post-herpetic neuralgia treated by stereotactic spinal trigeminal nucleotomy. Presented at 8th Int. Congr. on Neurological Surgery, Toronto.

Schvarcz, J.R. (1989) Craniofacial postherpetic neuralgia managed by spinal trigeminal tractotomy. Acta Neurochir. (Wien), 46: 62–64.

Siegfried, J. (1977) Stereotactic pulvinotomy in the treatment of intractable pain. Prog. Neurol. Surg., 8: 104–113.

Siegfried, J. (1982) Monopolar electrical stimulation of nucleus ventroposteromedialis thalami for postherpetic facial pain. Appl. Neurophysiol., 45: 179–184.

Sindou, M. and Daher, A. (1988) Spinal cord ablation procedures for pain. In: R. Dubner, G.F. Gebhart and M.R. Bond (Eds.), Proc. Vth World Congress on Pain. Elsevier, Amsterdam, pp. 477–495.

Siqueira, J.M. (1985) A method for bulbospinal trigeminal nucleotomy in the treatment of facial deafferentation pain. Appl. Neurophysiol., 48: 277–280.

Sjöqvist, O. (1938) Studies on pain conduction in the trigeminal nerve. A contribution to the surgical treatment of facial pain. Acta Psychiatr. Scand., Suppl. 17: 1–139.

Sjöqvist, O. (1948) Ten years' experience with trigeminal tractotomy. Brasil. Med. Cirurg., 10: 259–274.

Smith, F.P. (1970) Trans-spinal ganglionectomy for relief of intercostal pain. J. Neurosurg., 32: 574–577.

Spiegel, E.A. and Wycis, H.T. (1953) Mesencephalotomy in treatment of 'intractable' facial pain. Arch. Neurol. Psychiatry, 69: 1–13.

Sugar, O. and Bucy, P.C. (1951) Postherpetic trigeminal neuralgia. Arch. Neurol. Psychiatry, 65: 131–145.

Suzuki, H. et al. (1980) Cryocautery of sensitized skin areas for the relief of pain due to postherpetic neuralgia. Pain, 9: 355–362.

Tasker, R.R. (1984) Deafferentation. In: P.D. Wall and R. Melzack (Eds.), Textbook of Pain, 1st Edn. Churchill Livingstone, Edinburgh, pp. 119–132.

Tasker, R.R. (1985) Surgical approaches to the primary afferent and the spinal cord. In: H.L. Fields (Ed.), Advances in Pain Research and Therapy, Vol. 9. Raven Press, New York, pp. 799–824.

Tasker, R.R. (1989) Stereotaxic surgery. In: P.D. Wall and R. Melzack (Eds.), Textbook of Pain, 2nd Edn. Churchill Livingstone, Edinburgh, pp. 840–855.

Thomas, D.G.T. and Jones, S.J. (1984) Dorsal root entry zone lesions (Nashold's procedure) for pain due to brachial plexus avulsion. Neurosurgery, 15: 966–968.

Tindall, G.T., Odom, G.L. and Vieth, R.G. (1962) Surgical treatment of postherpetic neuralgia. Results of skin undermining and excision in 14 patients. Arch. Neurol., 7: 423–426.

Tsubokawa, T. (1995) Motor cortex stimulation for deafferentation pain relief in various clinical syndromes and its possible mechanism. In: J.M. Besson, G. Guilbaud, H. Ollat (Eds.), Forebrain Areas Involved in Pain Processing. John Libbey Eurotext, Paris, pp. 261–276.

Verbiest, H. and Calliauw, L. (1963) La chirurgie dans le traitement de la névralgie postherpétique du tronc. Psychiatr. Neurol. Neurochir., 66: 446–453.

Weidmann, M.J. (1976) Surgical relief of post-herpetic pain by excision of scarred skin. Med. J. Aust., 1: 472–473.

White, J.C. (1968) Operations for the relief of pain in the torso and extremities: evaluation of their effectiveness over long periods. In: A. Soulairac, J. Cahn and J. Charpentier (Eds.), Pain. Academic Press, London, pp. 503–519.

White, J.C. and Sweet, W.H. (1955) Pain. Thomas, Springfield, IL, pp. 522–526, 565–569.

White, J.C. and Sweet, W.H. (1969) Pain and the Neurosurgeon. Thomas, Springfield, IL, pp. 382–384, 474–477.

Wycis, H.T. and Spiegel, E.A. (1962) Long-range results in the treatment of intractable pain by stereotactic midbrain surgery. J. Neurosurg., 19: 101–107.

Young, R.F. (1989) Brain stimulation. In: P.D. Wall and R. Melzack (Eds.), Textbook of Pain. Churchill Livingstone, Edinburgh, pp. 925–929.

Young, R.F. (1990) Clinical experience with radiofrequency and laser DREZ lesions. J. Neurosurg., 72: 715–720.

Zapletal, B. (1968) Mesencephalotomy. Acta Neurochir. (Wien), Suppl. 16: 1–118.

Herpes Zoster and Postherpetic Neuralgia, 2nd Revised and Enlarged Edition
Pain Research and Clinical Management, Vol. 11
Edited by C.P.N. Watson and A.A. Gershon
© *2001 Elsevier Science B.V. All rights reserved*

CHAPTER 24

Suggestions for research and unanswered questions regarding postherpetic neuralgia

C. Peter N. Watson [1,*] and Mary Chipman [2]

[1] *Department of Medicine and* [2] *Department of Public Health Sciences, University of Toronto,*
Toronto, ON M9A 1T8, Canada

1. Introduction

Now, this is not the end. It is not even the beginning of the end. But it is, perhaps the end of the beginning.

Winston Spencer Churchill, 1942

Since the previous addition of this book, well-designed clinical trials in postherpetic neuralgia (PHN) have shown efficacy for oxycodone (Watson and Babul, 1998), gabapentin (Rowbotham et al., 1998), and a topical lidocaine patch (Rowbotham et al., 1996; Galer et al., 1999). These trials have successfully used the crossover method of several previous trials, a parallel design (Rowbotham et al., 1996) and an innovative, enriched enrolment process (Galer et al., 1999). The prospective investigator in PHN would be wise to consult data bases of clinical research reports, such as the Cochrane Database of Systematic Reviews, to avoid devoting energy to a question already settled or in progress and to be aware of the CONSORT guidelines regarding the reporting of clinical trials in the literature (Begg et al., 1996). Recent research has suggested different pathophysiological explanations for the pain experienced by PHN patients. A mechanistic approach has been suggested (Woolf and Decosterd, 1999). for tailoring treatment to disease mechanisms in the study of neuropathic pain. Examples of important issues addressed in this chapter are approaches to evaluating for the clinician how effective an agent is by utilizing such outcomes as the number of patients needed to be treated (NNT) to gain a moderate improvement and the value and pitfalls of testing for the blinding of a trial.

Despite the magnitude of the problem of neuropathic pain, we continue to need to find drugs which result in better pain relief with fewer side effects. All current approaches have a modest effect, often at the cost of significant side effects which are frequently not tolerated. The sole exception to this remains trigeminal neuralgia which appears to be a unique disorder in its clinical phenomenology and its highly successful responses to medical and surgical treatment. The chief clinical models for the investigation and treatment of other neuropathic pain remain painful diabetic neuropathy (PDN) and PHN. The latter continues to be an attractive model for neuropathic pain research because of its stereotyped

---

* Correspondence to: Dr. C.P.N. Watson, Department of Medicine, University of Toronto, Toronto, Ontario, Canada.
E-mail: peter.watson@utoronto.ca

nature and because adequate numbers of patients can be acquired even in a single centre if proper methods are used to recruit them. This chapter is not a comprehensive guide to clinical trials and for that the reader is directed elsewhere (Pocock, 1983; Max et al., 1991; Friedman et al., 1998). Much of what follows is based on one author's (CPNW) experience with the clinical investigation of the treatment of PHN in a single centre with limited resources in terms of personnel and funding. This chapter will not deal in any detail with clinical trials at the stage of herpes zoster which have their own problems, chiefly because of the large number of patients spontaneously improving over the course of the first month after the onset of the rash.

A recent review of the extensive literature on acute zoster pain and PHN shows that, in the past, there have been many putative remedies and illustrates the difficulties encountered in carrying out clinical trials in PHN. One of the main reasons for misleading, but favourable, results in uncontrolled trials is the inability to appreciate the natural history of improvement that occurs early on with postherpetic pain. When 90% of patients are pain-free at 4 weeks after the onset of the rash, any uncontrolled approach appears salutary.

2. Study design, sample size, and funding

In the clinical investigation of PHN, it is possible, in the authors' view, to keep the study simple and to confine the trial to a single centre since, as mentioned, adequate numbers of patient should be obtainable. If necessary, multicentre studies can be done, but these have their own problems (McKhann, 1989). After formulation of the research question, it is usually prudent to consult closely with a statistician. In working together, clinical and statistical researchers should (ideally) be able to blend theory and logistics to develop a workable project. The statistician can help at the planning stage by outlining the advantages and disadvantages of different possible designs to facilitate choice. The clinician can identify aspects of the clinical environment that

make some designs more feasible and logistically reasonable. Ultimately, the clinician has to decide, not only which is 'best', but which is manageable. The statistician can advise on many aspects of what is manageable as well; e.g. methods of data collection, storage to facilitate later analysis, and the resources for random and blind allocation of subjects to treatment.

One aspect in any design is the sample size required to obtain results which can answer the research question adequately. It has been remarked that "size is everything" (Moore, 2000) and that hundreds of patients may be required rather than the 20–50 found in many randomized, controlled trials in PHN. The authors certainly appreciate the logic in this and multicentre trials and meta-analyses are possible ways of obtaining larger numbers. However, it should be emphasized that nearly all our current information comes from the smaller trials and that larger numbers are difficult to accrue, particularly in PHN. Meta-analyses are strong primarily when the smaller studies that contribute have been carefully considered. Size, if overall quality is reduced, can merely compound problems of interpretation.

An 'enriched enrollment design' has been utilized in the study of the lidoderm patch in PHN (Galer et al., 1999). This utilizes patients previously determined to respond to the intervention (the patch) to study the efficacy of the patch alone versus the lidocaine-containing patch. This obviously reduces the number of patients required, but, of course, may give a falsely high estimate of the efficacy of the treatment as applied to the more general range of patients.

Pharmaceutical companies may request clinical investigation of an agent and can be important sources of funding and supply when other research funds are increasingly unavailable. An important issue is the development of guidelines for performing trials backed by the industry. This is especially true in light of a recent Canadian case which has gained international attention (Nathan and Weatherall, 1999). The pharmaceutical industry has an obvious interest in establishing the safety and effectiveness of their products and will benefit greatly from a commercial viewpoint when this occurs. It is important that clinicians and their industrial backers agree, in writing, beforehand on: (a) study design; (b) negotiating level of funding at the outset regardless of outcome; (c) agreeing on an independent industry funded analysis of the data; (d) agree that the results be published regardless of the outcome; and (e) agree regarding measures for protection of the investigator from legal action should that individual perceive any untoward events occurring and be at loggerheads with the company (see Intellectual Property Guidelines of the University of Toronto).

3. Choice of patients: pain duration and severity, recruitment

The proper choice of patients is one of the most critical factors determining the success of a clinical trial in PHN. Because postherpetic pain improves with time, especially in the first 4 weeks after the rash but slowly thereafter, it is necessary to choose patients with pain of at least 3 months' duration. Although this minimizes the problem, it will still be present in interpreting the results in non-blinded, uncontrolled trials. Random assignment of patients to each arm of a parallel or crossover trial will ensure that natural amelioration is likely to affect both arms equally. Fewer patients will be necessary to show a drug effect if the pain is reasonably stable over at least the few weeks of the trial. Stability can be actively assessed in a crossover trial. A comparison of first treatment (A or B) with second treatment (B or A) might reveal a change indicating a departure from the assumptions of a stable disease during the period of study or period effect. A comparison of AB versus BA might indicate a carryover effect for A, if patients in group AB appear to respond differently. Equal numbers in each treatment group will not protect from either effect, but will prevent confounding between the effects of order, period and treatment.

The choice of how severe the pain should be in patients eligible for the trial is a compromise between practicality and ethics. It will be much harder to demonstrate efficacy in patients whose pain is never more than mildly inconvenient, and this problem may be compounded by problems of compliance (lack of motivation to continue) and periods of absent pain in these subjects. Patients with moderate (disagreeable, uncomfortable) severity for at least half of the 12 waking hours are most suitable, especially for placebo-controlled trials.

Patients with PHN may have heterogeneous pain mechanisms as witnessed by different qualities of pain within and between patients. Woolf and Decosterd (1999) have suggested that we consider classifying pain on the basis of pain mechanisms rather than on the basis of disease. To this end they have suggested a qualitative pain assessment profile for clinical use based on an analysis of pain defined by mechanisms. This would supplement the standard history and physical examination including sensory testing. They have suggested an interview-based qualitative assessment of pain designed to establish if the patient has normal, hypo- or hyperbasal pain sensitivity and the extent to which the pain is spontaneous or evoked. For example, they state that "In a patient with PHN the aim would be to determine, by questioning, whether the patient has ongoing pain and, if so, if it is continuous or intermittent, if there is pain on transient contact with clothes, if sustained pressure, such as if a brassiere strap causes pain, and if cold relieves or exacerbates the pain." They state that intensity could be rated in a number of ways using standard rating scales and the quality of the pain determined by the sensory component of the McGill Pain Questionnaire, and then one could compare the patient's report of their pain with the results of simple sensory tests used in the physical examination using tests aimed to measure the presence and extent of any abnormal evoked pain sensitivity, such as allodynia.

Adequate numbers of patients may be generated by a single centre or from a reasonable population area if active recruitment is undertaken, otherwise accrual of patients may take considerable time. We have found that the memories of specialist colleagues and family physicians have been short in this regard and have had the most success from regular, repeated, paid newspaper advertisements or from solicited columns from journalists in the lay and medical press. The latter publicity has been gratis, but advertising costs may be incorporated with grant funding applications. Larger numbers of patients may be required, for example to study the effects of corticosteroids in preventing PHN when given at the stage of herpes zoster and multiple centres may be required. This type of trial has its own problems (Meinert, 1986; McKhann, 1989).

4. Outcome measures

In this section, we discuss a number of possible outcome measures that may be used in evaluating the results of a study: pain scales (for pain, pain relief, pain quality); sensory effects; depression; disability/side effects; and effectiveness.

4.1. Pain severity, pain relief, pain quality

Of the various outcome measures to be discussed, we have found that pain scales have been practical and effective when administered at weekly intervals and we also commonly use a diary for daily ratings. A number of scales are available for use in studies of chronic pain. The most commonly used of these for pain intensity are category scales, visual analogue scales (VAS), and the McGill Pain Questionnaire (Melzack, 1975). There is no good evidence for the superiority of any one of these (Bradley and Lindblom, 1989).

The four-point category scale of no pain, mild, moderate and severe is the oldest and most commonly used. This can be expanded with a 'very severe' category to give more choice, and we have found it useful to add in brackets qualifications such as mild (present, but not bothersome), moderate (uncomfortable), severe (unbearable and disabling), and to ask what percentage of 24 h is estimated as being spent in that situation; e.g. a response may be 'moderate for one-half of the day (12 h) with severe pain for 2 h'. A visual analogue scale (VAS) for pain severity marked 'least possible pain' at one end of the 10 cm line with the other extreme, 'worst possible pain', at the other is simple and easily un-

derstood and marked. We have found it useful to use both scales for pain severity. The category scale using everyday language is a useful check on the VAS in case of an error in marking the latter. The McGill Pain Questionnaire (Melzack, 1975) has been widely used in pain studies and is well-validated. Because it takes time to understand and complete, we have not found it useful in the PHN population when elderly people predominate and in the normal flow of office practice.

Category and VAS scales may also be used to assess pain relief. Although in acute pain these relief scales may be more sensitive than the category and VAS intensity scales (Sriwatanakul et al., 1983; Littman et al., 1985), they may not be so for chronic studies because they require a memory of baseline status, which is more remote in the chronic situation.

The pain of PHN often has three different aspects, a steady often burning component, brief jabs, and pain on tactile skin contact (allodynia). We have used the VAS and category scales for pain intensity to evaluate each of these (Watson et al., 1992). The frequency of application of these outcome measures for pain may vary from daily ratings with a mean calculated weekly to before- and end-of-treatment assessments. We have found it most practical and useful to see patients weekly for the collection of these measures.

4.2. Sensation

Although at our centre we have not been successful in devising a method to measure rapidly and reliably areas of sensory loss, heightened sensitivity (allodynia, hyperesthesia, dysesthesia) and sympathetic function, these are important characteristics of pain; e.g. with a potentially neurotoxic agent, such as capsaicin there is concern about increasing sensory loss. A centre with this expertise might consider incorporating this type of evaluation into a study.

4.3. Depression

Chronic pain and depression frequently co-exist. Antidepressant drugs have been shown to relieve PHN by an action independent of an antidepressant effect (Watson et al., 1982; Max et al., 1988b). Future studies will likely involve similar agents and the measurement and monitoring of depression may be important. Standard tools, such as the Beck, Zung and Hamilton rating scales have been designed for use in psychiatric patients and because of this questions are present which relate to sleep, fatigue, weight, and sexual activity. These are items likely to be affected directly by chronic pain as well as indirectly via depression, and thus a high score may lead to a factitious diagnosis of depression or falsely high value for the severity of the depression. Relief of pain may lead to a lower score because of these questions although there may be no real change in mood. The Hamilton rating scale may be modified to 20 questions if those items related to somatic symptoms are removed, but it takes about 30 min to administer. A VAS or 0–10 scale for depression is simple, quickly administered, reliable and valid. The Hospital Anxiety and Depression Scale (Zigmond and Snaith, 1983) is also a reliable, easily used and scored self-report for the detection and severity of depressed mood that is free of these somatically oriented questions.

4.4. Disability, side effects

A number of disability measures have been validated for use in chronic pain patients (Bradley, 1988). These include the Sickness Impact Profile, Functional Status Index, Health Assessment Questionnaire, Index of Functional Impairment, and SF-36 (Jette, 1980; Bergner et al., 1981; Fries et al., 1982; Ware et al., 1993). These may not, however, convey specific disability, such as not being able to tolerate a brassiere or other clothing and consideration could be given to designing disease-specific questions regarding PHN.

An open-ended assessment (volunteered) of side effects may lead to under-reporting and a pre-specified side-effect check list may lead to over-reporting. We have chosen to inquire about the commonest side effects listing them as tolerable or intolerable and then use an open-ended question for any others.

4.5. Effectiveness

An important issue for the clinician is effectiveness, that is, how many patients had acceptable pain relief without intolerable side effects. Simply asking the responders if they were satisfied with these aspects at each visit helps to clarify this. One can, for example, then define a good result as pain never worse than mild, no intolerable side effects, no significant disability, and an expression of satisfaction with the overall improvement achieved. Any of the above measures are more secure if the patients fill out the rating scale with the examiner present to review the result and verify that the scale is complete and done correctly.

The measure 'number needed to treat' (NNT) has been suggested to convey both statistical and meaningful clinical significance (Laupacis et al., 1988; Cook and Sackett, 1995). This evaluation is a description of an arbitrary therapeutic effort for a desired outcome (50% improvement or more) in one patient. It describes the difference between an intervention, such as a drug and a control treatment. It is expressed as the number of patients required to be treated for one desired favourable response (moderate or more than 50% improvement). This assessment and its use in systematic reviews has been discussed in acute and chronic pain studies (McQuay and Moore, 1997; Moore, 2000). A similar evaluation can be applied to adverse events and expressed as 'number needed to harm' (NNH). These measures still do not tell the clinician how many patients are satisfied with the pain relief and tolerability of side effects and may not be applicable to trials comparing a new drug with a standard therapy since there is no placebo in this type of trial.

5. Placebo control, standard of therapy

The first randomized, controlled trial of amitriptyline in PHN (Watson et al., 1982) was done with an inert, but carefully matched lactose placebo. The difficulty with drugs such as amitriptyline is that they produce side effects that threaten the blinding of the trial even though some patients on placebo complain of similar side effects. A clever innovation is to use an 'active' placebo (Max et al., 1991, p. 209) that produces effects similar to the common ones caused by the agent to be tested. For example, benztropine, an anticholinergic agent, and diazepam can be used (Max et al., 1991, p. 209) to produce dry mouth and drowsiness to mimic antidepressant side effects. Adverse effects may be less threatening to the validity of crossover trials than to parallel group trials if patients are blinded both to the order of administration and to the point of crossover.

Now that several trials have shown the efficacy of amitriptyline in PHN it is reasonable to consider this a standard of therapy and to compare any new drug to it. The argument that the new agent would require a large sample size or have to be very effective to show a difference is not really valid because amitriptyline only shows its effect in about 50–60% of those treated and rarely results in complete relief. If no difference occurs, the argument that both may be placebos should not be valid since one should be able to reproduce the results, at least with amitriptyline, of other trials (Watson et al., 1982; Max et al., 1988b) by similar methodology which demonstrate that 50–60% respond, a figure greater than the usual responsiveness to placebo.

Patients may also have previously used the standard therapy before the trial and be reluctant to use it again. An explanation to the subject as to our observation that the drug has often been used in too high a dose for too short a period will nearly always suffice to encourage entry into the trial. We agree with the argument that when a standard therapy exists for a severe pain problem, it is not ethical to use a placebo control (Pocock, 1983; Friedman et al., 1998).

The double-placebo or double-dummy technique is useful when two active agents cannot be matched completely, in which case two different placebos can be produced, one for each intervention. Patients are then randomized to take drug A and placebo B or drug B and placebo A. Blinding can then be preserved, although at the cost of more 'pill-taking', which might affect compliance. This method is also useful when two different routes or administration are compared, for example a topical agent versus a tablet, such as topical capsaicin versus amitriptyline.

6. Crossover design

The crossover design has been used repeatedly and successfully in PHN, a condition where if vigorous recruitment is undertaken, reasonable, but not large numbers of subjects are available at a single centre. This type of trial, in which treatments are compared over time within each patient, is statistically more efficient than a parallel groups design since random error is limited to variability within patients, not variability between patients. Important criteria for this type of design in chronic pain problems are: (1) that the patient's condition should be fairly stable over the course of the treatment period; (2) that the effect of each treatment is short-lived; (3) that side effects of either treatment are mild; and (4) that there be no interaction between treatments and their order of administration.

Patients with unstable pain will inflate the random variation of responses, and may not complete the study if their pain is resolved before both therapies have been tried. Persistent effects of either treatment may be managed with a washout period and the length of this period will depend on the duration of treatment effects. We have found with amitriptyline and related agents that a washout period of 2 weeks is enough to deal with any lingering effects from the first treatment period in most patients. Other studies have successfully not used a washout and have compared end of treatment values for each period.

If the occurrence of significant side effects is high, patients will either drop out or be withdrawn from the study in significant numbers. Since patients must complete both treatments for the analysis in a crossover design, such losses cause problems that would not arise in a study of parallel groups.

Finally, if order of administration appears to affect patients' responses to treatment, the results of a crossover design may be difficult to interpret. Order effects may be due either to a carryover effect from period 1 to period 2 or the difference between the two treatments actually changing as the study progresses (i.e. a time by treatment interaction). Ideally, order effects should be ruled out on a priori biological or pharmacological grounds; statistical tests should, of course, look for carryover effects, but they have been criticized as being less sensitive than treatment comparisons because they rely on between-patient comparisons (Brown, 1980; Pocock, 1983). When the ordering of treatments is discovered to have an effect, a method of statistical analysis has been suggested by Grizzle (1965). With this, period 2 data are discarded and analysis is based on period 1 data alone; i.e. use treatment comparisons between rather than within patients. Although this approach is inefficient, it is a method of salvaging at least some information on treatment effect.

It has been suggested that "ultimately the crossover design is vulnerable to psychological carryover and alternate designs should be considered when the measurement of treatment differences relies on subjective reports" (Woods et al., 1989). It would seem reasonable that this effect can be minimized or negated in blinded trials when the duration of washout and the timing of the crossover is not known to the patient or observer. When clinical research or experience suggests that the assumptions upon which the crossover design depends are not valid, expanded designs have been suggested (Max et al., 1991, p. 212). If several other treatment sequences or a third treatment period are added, unbiased estimates of treatment effects are possible even if an ordering effect is present (Laska et al., 1983). We have not encountered problems with order or period effects in the simple two-period crossover design either due to natural history effects or pharmacological carryover when a 2-week washout is interposed. Dropouts have not been a problem despite the potential for side effects when careful titration of antidepressants is observed. We believe this 2×2 crossover design is usually practical and that the complexities of the modified crossover designs with the increased risk of patient dropout deters their use in practice.

7. Parallel design

When the assumptions of a crossover design are in doubt (major concerns about carryover, changing natural history of the pain) the simpler parallel-groups design is preferred. Although it requires more patients the problem of subject withdrawal is less. In our experience with PHN, it is probable that a multicentre trial will be necessary with this type of design in order to generate the increased number of patients required. A baseline consisting of several observations on no treatment increases the power of treatment comparisons and helps to reduce variability (Lavori et al., 1983; Kaiser, 1989).

8. Case series

The medical literature has a long history of reports of series of cases (longitudinal observation studies) that may be prospective as well as retrospective. Having studied a number of chronic pain problems in this regard, one being PHN (Watson et al., 1988b), we can attest to the labour and difficulty of this approach for the sparseness of useful data acquired and would question whether anything much new can be gleaned unless the trial is a careful, prospective one, with very focused aims in terms of new information desired.

Historical control studies are, of course, no substitute for a randomized controlled clinical trial. Patient characteristics as well as methods of treatment administration change in subtle ways over time and have the potential to introduce bias. Any bias in the open, uncontrolled observations of new therapy (compared to the memories and records of reported pain among past patients) is likely to favour the new treatment, and such studies may indeed be used to justify the 'promise' of a new drug. If this enthusiasm also promotes a properly controlled clinical study, well and good. But otherwise, uncontrolled or historically controlled studies have little to recommend them — particularly for such subjective data as reported pain.

The attractions of case series are speed, low cost

and an efficient means of gaining field experience to plan a randomized controlled trial when preliminary results suggest it may be warranted. The ethical issues in such a study shift from treating some patients with a known placebo to treating all patients with an agent of unknown efficacy.

Since only one treatment is involved, double-blinded assessment is not possible and the opportunities for biased response are much greater for both the subject and the observer. It is important to treat a population with stable, chronic pain of some duration to guard against the natural history of improvement that occurs. It would be reasonable that a beneficial treatment effect be inferred if significant pain relief occurs in a population with chronic stable pain of more than 6 months' duration over the short period of such a trial. Caution should be taken as well not to treat only patients who fail other treatments so that a misleading negative result is obtained in a selected intractable group. As with randomized controlled trials, it is important to prepare a protocol beforehand, carefully defining the disorder and population to be studied (age, pain duration, exclusion criteria), choosing reliable and valid outcome measures and optimally limiting the study to one or two knowledgeable investigators in a single centre with careful monitoring to discourage dropouts.

9. Dose, dose increments, dose ranging

It is clear from our experience with clinical trials of antidepressants in PHN that dose overestimation for the best response is quite common, even if one escalates by small increments (10–25 mg) every 3–5 days. This is not unexpected given the delay in onset of effect in many patients with this type of agent. This overestimation of dose and blood level associated with pain relief has been evident when after study completion we titrate the dose down in order to reduce side effects and determine the minimum effective analgesic dose and blood level. This relatively short period between dose increments has to be accepted in our view to keep the trial of reasonable length. Less frequent dosage increments,

however, pose a problem particularly with crossover trials because they, of course, may make the trial excessively long and cause problems with compliance and dropouts. The range of doses (10–250 mg) seen in pragmatic trials with patients from the general population with neuropathic pain poses a major problem for planned dose–response studies crossing over different doses in random order, in terms of overdosage and lack of compliance because of side effects. Dose titration in order to achieve maximal analgesia and minimal untoward side effects is a delicate business, particularly with antidepressants. One would at least have to stratify patients for age and give a lower range of doses to the older population. An alternative — ascending titration designs — is more attractive, with free titration to maximum response or side effects and then assignment of responders to several treatments randomly of 25–100% of the maximum dose. We have been puzzled and disturbed by the frequent failure to recapture initial good responses on retreatment with the same dose. The reason for this is uncertain, but it could be a result of the natural history (progression of disease), the placebo effect, tolerance, or some chronic change in receptors related to the drug.

10. Data analysis

Inevitably, the results of a clinical trial include considerable selection bias in screening patients for entry. This can, of course, result in both selecting out patients who might respond less favourably (the aged or those with other medical problems) and those who may respond (patients obtaining some benefit with opioids who cannot endure opioid withdrawal prior to entering an opioid trial). Much selection is not preventible, however, patients may drop out after entry because of side effects or lack of relief. Recent trials have had an intent-to-treat (ITT) data analysis as a primary evaluation (Cook and Sackett, 1995). This includes all patients exposed to treatment regardless of whether they dropped out for any reason, such as adverse events and perceived lack of benefit. Thus, it more closely duplicates clinical practice. An efficacy analysis limited to all those completing the trial may also be reported. Increasingly, NNT and number needed to harm (NNH) figures are being utilized in reporting clinical trial results (Laupacis et al., 1988; Cook and Sackett, 1995). Although this does not convey to the clinician the number of patients actually satisfied with pain relief and adverse event tolerability, it does give a measure of treatment effect for the clinician which can be compared with other approaches. Thus, in designing the trial, it is useful to be able to determine the arbitrary response of those obtaining 50% or greater benefit as this is used in this measure.

The blinding of patients and assessors may be threatened in trials where agents with significant side effects are involved, such as topical capsaicin (for which no active placebo can be found) or with an inert placebo. The integrity of the blinding can then be tested by asking the subject and investigator to guess in which phase the active agent was used. If this is done, it is important to also ask whether the guess was made because of side effects or pain relief.

11. Unanswered questions

Although we have made significant gains since the previous volume, particularly regarding putative mechanisms and treatments of PHN, much remains to be achieved. The direction of this work appears clearer now from what has been done.

We still require an answer as to why some HZ patients develop intractable PHN (especially older patients) and the majority do not. We still have not answered Henry Head's question (Head and Campbell, 1900) about predilection for involvement of certain ganglia (the ophthalmic division of the trigeminal and thoracic) and why the dorsal part of the ganglion is affected.

Further studies are necessary to fully explain the areas of sensory loss and allodynia far exceeding a single dermatome with practical measures to determine if changes occur with treatment. The clarification of mechanism-based sub-groups may help to tailor therapy. There may be a sub-group with

sympathetically maintained pain, but, to date, this has not been clarified. The significance of the recent findings of bilateral involvement with clinically unilateral disease remains to be elucidated (Watson et al., 1991; Baron et al., 1997; Oaklander, 1998; Watson et al., 2000).

Because of the intractability of PHN, as evidenced by the fact that 40–60% of patients respond poorly or not at all to our best treatments, we need to look closely at preventive measures (Watson, 1998, Chapter 19). Although the incidence of zoster appears lower after varicella vaccination, we do not know as yet whether this approach or vaccinating the elderly will reduce the incidence of PHN. A trial is currently in progress regarding the latter. There is evidence that antiviral agents have a modest preventive effect. Other preventive approaches are the early use of antidepressants, opioids, and nerve blocks to relieve acute pain. These approaches appear to be reasonable and safe. It is obvious that we need to explore newer therapeutic approaches for established PHN as all the treatments currently available have, at best, a moderate effect. Newer anticonvulsants can be considered based on the experience with gabapentin. Antidepressants, particularly those that potentiate norepinephrine and serotonin, need to be explored. Further trials of opioids or drugs acting on opioid receptors, such as tramadol, seem appropriate. Agents that more effectively and safely block sodium channels or NMDA receptors should be evaluated. Further research might also profitably focus on blockers of channels characteristic of hyperexcitable neurones, selective blockers of damaged axons, and on neurotrophins which may ameliorate afferent nerve damage. These approaches are described in more detail by Dr. Wall in Chapter 17. Topical agents, such as lidocaine and capsaicin, may be made more effective by improving transdermal delivery or finding ways to deal with the burning sensation induced by capsaicin. Since all current drugs seem to act in different ways, it may be that combinations of agents are useful for some patients and each may be better tolerated at lower doses in combination therapy. Comparative trials have not been of great interest to the pharmaceutical industry for obvious reasons. However, the ethics of using a placebo when a standard of treatment is available in a clinical trial has to be raised and from a scientific point of view it is useful to know about the relative efficacy of these drugs. We believe that any new approach which seems reasonable and safe should be studied in these intractable and often desperate patients. Both the empirical approach of the clinician and the study of new therapeutic agents from the laboratory seem to be reasonable in the search for new treatments.

12. Summary

This chapter suggests that PHN continues to be a good model for the study of neuropathic pain and makes suggestions for research based on the authors' experience and on the literature on the subject. Aspects discussed here are study design, sample size, funding, patient choice, outcome measures, and controls. The chapter concludes with an outline of some of the important questions yet to be answered by research into this difficult neuropathic pain problem.

References

Baron, R., Haendler, G. and Schulte, H. (1997) Afferent large fiber neuropathy predicts the development of postherpetic neuralgia. Pain, 73: 231–238.

Begg, C., Cho, M. and Eastwood, S. et al. (1996) Improving the quality of reporting of randomized controlled trials. Consort Stat., 276: 637–663.

Bergner, M., Bobbitt, R.A., Carter, W.B. and Gibson, B.S. (1981) The sickness impact profile: development and final revision of a health status measure. Med. Care, 19: 787–805.

Bradley, L.A. (1988) Assessing the psychological profile of the chronic pain patient. In: R. Dubner, G.F. Beghard and M.R. Bond (Eds.), Proc Vth World Congress on Pain. Elsevier, Amsterdam, pp. 251–262.

Bradley L.A. and Lindblom U. (1989) Do different types of chronic pain require different measurement technologies? In: C.R. Chapman and J.D. Loeser (Eds.), Issues in Pain Measurement. Raven Press, New York, pp. 445–454.

Brown, B.W. (1980) Statistical controversies in the design of clinical trials — some personal views. Control. Clin. Trials, 1: 13–27.

Cook, R.J. and Sackett, D.L. (1995) The number needed to treat: a clinically useful measure of treatment effect. Br. Med. J., 310: 452–454.

Friedman, L.M., Furberg, C.D., DeMets, and D.L. (1998) Fundamentals of Clinical Trials, 3rd edn. Springer, New York.

Fries, J.F., Spitz, P., Kraines, R.G. and Holman, H.R. (1982) Measurement of patient outcome in arthritis. Arthritis Rheum., 25: 1048–1053.

Galer, B.S., Rowbotham, M.C., Perander, J. and Friedman, E. (1999) Topical lidocaine patch relieves postherpetic neuralgia more effectively than a vehicle topical patch: results of an enriched enrollment study. Pain, 80: 533–538.

Grizzle, J.E. (1965) The two-period change-over design and its use in clinical trials. Biometrics, 21: 167–180.

Head, H. and Campbell, A.W. (1900) The pathology of herpes zoster and its bearing on sensory localization. Brain, 23: 353–523.

Intellectual Property Guidelines for Graduate Students and Supervisors at the University of Toronto School of Graduate Studies, 63/65 St. George Street, Toronto, ON, Canada M5S 2Z9.

Jette, A.M. (1980) Functional status instrument: reliability of a chronic disease evaluation instrument. Arch. Phys. Med. Rehabil., 61: 395–401.

Kaiser, I. (1989) Adjusting for baseline: change or percentage change?. Stat. Med., 8: 1183–1190.

Laska, E., Meisner, M. and Kushner, H.B. (1983) Optimal crossover designs in the presence of carryover effects. Biometrics, 39: 1087–1091.

Laupacis, A., Sackett, D.L. and Robarts, R.S. (1988) An assessment of clinically useful measures of the consequences of treatment. New Engl. J. Med., 318: 1728–1733.

Lavori, P.W., Louis, T.A., Bailar, J.D. and Polansky, M. (1983) Designs for experiments — parallel comparisons of treatment. New Engl. J. Med., 309: 1291–1298.

Littman, G.S., Walker, B.R. and Schneider, B.E. (1985) Reassessment of the verbal and visual analogue ratings in analgesic studies. Clin. Pharmacol. Ther., 38: 16–23.

Max, M.B., Schafer, S.C., Culnane, M., Dubner, R. and Gracely, R.H. (1988a) Association of pain relief with drug side effects in postherpetic neuralgia: a single-dose study of clonidine, codeine, ibuprofen and placebo. Clin. Pharmacol. Ther., 43: 363–371.

Max, M.B., Schafer, S.C. and Culnane, M. et al. (1988b) Amitriptyline, but not lorazepam, relieves postherpetic neuralgia. Neurology, 38: 1427–1432.

Max, M.B., Portenoy, R.K. and Laska, E.M. (Eds.) (1991) The design of analgesic clinical trials. In: Advances in Pain Research and Therapy, Vol. 18. Raven Press, New York.

McKhann, G.M. (1989) The trials of clinical trials. Arch. Neurol., 46: 611–614.

McQuay, H.J. and Moore, R.A. (1997) Using numerical results from systematic reviews in clinical practice. Ann. Int. Med., 126: 712–720.

Meinert, C.L. (1986) Clinical Trials: Design, Conduct and Analysis. New York: Oxford University Press.

Melzack, R. (1975) The McGill Pain Questionnaire: Major properties and scoring methods. Pain, 1: 277–299.

Moore, R.A. (2000) Understanding clinical trials: What have we learned from systematic reviews. In: M. Devor, M.C. Rowbotham and Z. Wiesenfeld-Hallin (Eds.), Proc. 9th World Congress on Pain. Elsevier, Amsterdam.

Nathan, D.G. and Weatherall, D.J. (1999) Academia and industry: lessons from the unfortunate events in Toronto. Lancet, 353: 771–772.

Oaklander, A.L., Romans, K. and Horasek, S. et al. (1998) Unilateral postherpetic neuralgia is associated with bilateral sensory damage. Ann. Neurol., 44: 789–795.

Pocock, S.J. (1983) Clinical Trials, A Practical Approach. Wiley, Chichester.

Rowbotham, M.C., Davies, P.S., Verkempinck, C. and Galer, B.S. (1996) Lidocaine patch double-blind controlled study of a new treatment method for postherpetic neuralgia. Pain, 65: 39–44.

Rowbotham, M.C., Harden, N. and Stacey, B. et al. (1998) Gabapentin for the treatment of postherpetic neuralgia: A randomized controlled trial. J. Am. Med. Assoc., 280: 1837–1842.

Sriwatanakul, K., Kelvie, W., Lasagna, L., Weis, O.F. and Mehta, G. (1983) Studies with different types of visual analogue scales for measurement of pain. Clin. Pharmacol. Ther., 34: 234–239.

Ware, J., Snow, K.K., Kosinaki, M., Gavdek, B. (1993) Health Survey: Manual and Interpretation Guide. Boston, MA. The Health Institute, New England Medical Center.

Watson, C.P.N. (1998) Postherpetic neuralgia: the importance of treating this end-stage intractable disorder. J. Infect. Dis., 178(Suppl. 1): S91–S94.

Watson, C.P.N. and Babul, N. (1998) Oxycodone relieves neuropathic pain: a randomized trial in postherpetic neuralgia. Neurology, 50: 1837–1841.

Watson, C.P.N., Evans, R.J., Reed, K., Merskey, H., Goldsmith, L. and Warsh, J. (1982) Amitriptyline versus placebo in postherpetic neuralgia. Neurology, 32: 671–673.

Watson, C.P.N., Evans, R.J. and Watt, V.R. (1988a) Postherpetic neuralgia and topical capsaicin. Pain, 33: 333–340.

Watson, C.P.N., Evans, R.J., Watt, V.R. and Birkett, N. (1988b) Postherpetic neuralgia: 208 cases. Pain, 34: 289–298.

Watson, C.P.N., Deck, J.H., Morshead, C., Van Der Kooy, D. and Evans, R.J. (1991) Postherpetic neuralgia: further postmortem studies of cases with and without pain. Pain, 44: 105–117.

Watson, C.P.N., Chipman, M., Reed, K., Evans, R.J. and Birkett, N. (1992) Amitriptyline versus maprotiline in postherpetic neuralgia: a randomized, double-blind, crossover trial. Pain, 48: 29–36.

Watson, C.P.N., Midha, R., Devor, M. et al. (2000) Trigeminal postherpetic neuralgia postmortem: clinically unilateral, pathologically bilateral. In: M. Devor, M.C. Rowbotham and Z. Wiesenfeld-Hallin (Eds.), Proc. 9th World Congress on Pain, Vienna.

Woods, J.R., Williams, J.G. and Tavel, M. (1989) The two period crossover design in medical research. Ann. Intern. Med., 110: 560–566.

Woolf, C.J. and Decosterd, I. (1999) Implications of recent advances in the understanding of pain pathophysiology for the assessment of pain in patients. Pain, Suppl. 6: 141–147.

Zigmond, A.S. and Snaith, R.P. (1983) The hospital anxiety and depression scale. Acta Psychiatr. Scand., 67: 361–370.

Herpes Zoster and Postherpetic Neuralgia, 2nd Revised and Enlarged Edition
Pain Research and Clinical Management, Vol. 11
Edited by C.P.N. Watson and A.A. Gershon
© *2001 Elsevier Science B.V. All rights reserved*

Subject Index